T0180240

Clinical Insights and Examination Techniques in Ophthalmology

Thomas Kuriakose

Clinical Insights and Examination Techniques in Ophthalmology

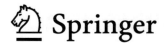 Springer

Thomas Kuriakose
Professor of Ophthalmology
Eye Department
Christian Medical College Vellore
Schell Campus
Vellore
India

ISBN 978-981-15-2892-7   ISBN 978-981-15-2890-3   (eBook)
https://doi.org/10.1007/978-981-15-2890-3

© Springer Nature Singapore Pte Ltd. 2020
This work is subject to copyright. All rights are reserved by the Publisher, whether the whole or part of the material is concerned, specifically the rights of translation, reprinting, reuse of illustrations, recitation, broadcasting, reproduction on microfilms or in any other physical way, and transmission or information storage and retrieval, electronic adaptation, computer software, or by similar or dissimilar methodology now known or hereafter developed.
The use of general descriptive names, registered names, trademarks, service marks, etc. in this publication does not imply, even in the absence of a specific statement, that such names are exempt from the relevant protective laws and regulations and therefore free for general use.
The publisher, the authors, and the editors are safe to assume that the advice and information in this book are believed to be true and accurate at the date of publication. Neither the publisher nor the authors or the editors give a warranty, expressed or implied, with respect to the material contained herein or for any errors or omissions that may have been made. The publisher remains neutral with regard to jurisdictional claims in published maps and institutional affiliations.

This Springer imprint is published by the registered company Springer Nature Singapore Pte Ltd. The registered company address is: 152 Beach Road, #21-01/04 Gateway East, Singapore 189721, Singapore

Dedicated to my Father Dr. E. T. Kuriakose, the Ophthalmologist before me and my first teacher and to my other teachers and students all of who have taught me more ophthalmology than they think they may have.

Preface

During ward rounds (yes, we still have them for training our postgraduates) one day, I was upset that a particular case was not diagnosed in a certain way. After the rounds one of my bright colleagues came and told me that there is no point getting upset as not everybody can think the way I do. The assumption here I think was that clinical thinking is genetically endowed, a position I was not willing to accept. To prove clinical thinking and diagnostic skills in Ophthalmology can be inculcated; I looked for a resource I could direct my students to so that they can learn from it. I could not find any single source to direct them to, yet, all what I practice and know were sourced from the writings of other authors in various books or articles.

It is very unlikely that the ideas in this book are my own; it is more likely that these are reflections of the 'Ha ha' moments I have had when reading other authors or listening to people speak. This book is a compilation of practices I have gathered over years and is an effort to try and prove that anybody who can finish medical school can become a good clinician, especially a good clinical Ophthalmologist.

To be a good clinician, it was clear to me that the basic skill one requires for the practice of good Ophthalmology was clinical skill. 'Hutchison's Clinical Methods' [1] and 'Das' Clinical Surgery' [2] were the two books that gave me my first glimpse of clinical medicine. As an ophthalmologist, I felt a book of similar nature would go a long way in honing the clinical skills of the Ophthalmologist who are training or trained. It is my hope that this book will do that and more for the ophthalmic community. Most clinical books in Ophthalmology discuss the subject, disease wise. That is, the illness is discussed first and then the signs and symptoms related to it. In real life, patient comes with symptoms and signs from which one has to deduce the disease. I am hoping that this book through its discussion on symptoms and signs will enable the doctor to come up with a sensible list of disease probabilities and look at other dedicated books to study each disease entity in more detail.

Two books that changed the way I thought as a doctor was Clinical Epidemiology—A Basic Science for Clinical Medicine by Sackett et al. [3] and George Eisner's Eye Surgery—An Introduction to Operative Techniques [4]. These books gave a lot of answers as to why we did things the way we did and provided the foundation on which this book was written. Knowing the 'why' of the various clinical tests we perform makes the understanding of the test and its interpretation more exciting.

In this day of readymade information made available on the internet, I was not sure if there will be enough people who would have the patience to read a book. Information does not translate to knowledge unless people understood the thought process behind the information generated and internalise it. It is my hope that with practice of what is written in this book, it will give knowledge rather than information. As a corollary to that, this book is not an easy to access information book written in point form so that it can be read and memorised in the shortest possible time; reproduced in an exam and finally forgotten in an equally short time!

In some countries 'competitive exams' have become a curse of their education system. These exams in order to discriminate (to select the 'best' memory storage disc) ask for the most irrelevant details in the exams. So much so the student memorises both the relevant and irrelevant (even more) details. Six months after the exams, both are forgotten and the application of what they have learnt becomes difficult. What I have included in this book is only information I have needed on a day-to-day basis in the hope the student understands and retain what is needed in the clinics, rather than all the information one may need to be successful in a competitive exam.

This book is meant for the 'students' of Ophthalmology (whatever their stage in life) so that they can appreciate clinical Ophthalmology and the principles underlying it as they pursue Ophthalmology and put into practice what they have learnt.

It is never late to pick up insights and so this book could be a good resource for people who did not have access to such a resource and was looking for a single source compilation of clinical methods in Ophthalmology. I believe that this book will also be a good resource for teachers who need some scientific backing for practices they have adopted consciously or unconsciously.

A book on cooking and recipes is of no use unless you put them into practice. So is the case with this book. Repeated clinical examination of both the sick and healthy is needed to hone one's clinical skill and thinking.

'Assessment dictates learning' is an oft-repeated quote in training programmes on education. While this may be true till the undergraduate level of education, that should no longer be the criterion for postgraduate training. Adult learning is self-driven. Medical postgraduates should be doing the course because they love the subject and want to treat the patients they come across. Being able to have a comfortable life as a by-product is not something anybody is going to complain about! Passing or failing an examination at the postgraduate level or the marks obtained in it is unlikely to decide how good a doctor one will be. The only advantage of passing in the first attempt is that you can stop doing all the dirty work you have to do as an apprentice trainee! So enjoy this book for Ophthalmology and clinical medicine's sake rather than with the objective of passing an exam.

'There is always a better way', said Thomas Edison. This book can be better. Your disagreements with ideas in this book and suggestions for improvements will be greatly appreciated. Many reading this book will find it difficult to accept some of the concepts given in the book because of years of training otherwise. Not all seeds strewn on the ground germinate. Only the ones that fall on fertile soil will. This book is in search of that soil.

My 'Gurus', students and my colleagues who interacted with me over the years are my biggest teachers. Knowingly or unknowingly they have given me insights through their statements or questions. To them I owe much of what is written here.

Further Reading

Glynn M, Drake WM, Hutchison R. Hutchison's clinical methods: an integrated approach to clinical practice. Elsevier Health Sciences; 2012.

Das S. A manual on Clinical Surgery (S. Das 2015).

David L Sackett, R Brian Haynes, Gordon H Guyatt, Peter Tugwell; Clinical Epidemiology: A basic science for clinical medicine. 2nd ed; Little Brown & Co; 1991.

Eisner G, Telger TC, Schneider P. Eye surgery: an introduction to operative technique. Berlin: Springer; 2013.

Vellore, India   Thomas Kuriakose

Acknowledgements

There are only a limited number of institutions that give time off to write a book. I would like to thank Christian Medical College Vellore for grooming me to be the Ophthalmologist I am today and for not only giving me the time to write this book but also providing me access to the library and the clinical material to help produce this book.

Dr. Swetha Sara Philip, who I co-authored with to write the chapter on Examination of the Child, was so prompt with her submission that it inspired me to move faster. A big thanks to her for helping with this difficult chapter.

This book would not have been possible if not for the generous help and support of many colleagues and friends of mine. Thank you to my friends and colleagues who modelled for me to demonstrate the various clinical tests done on patients. My thanks are also due to Dr. Senthil V Maharajan, Dr. Sanita M Korah, Dr. Lekha Abraham, Dr. Jayanthi Peter, Dr. Jeyanth Rose and Dr. Nancy Magdalene Rajasekaran who reviewed some of the chapters and gave me critical inputs. My gratitude to Mr. M. Dinesh Kumar and Mr. Nirmal Raj Mohan for helping with recording and getting together the clinical photos required for the book. Thanks to Ms. Jagjeet Kaur Saini and Ms. Saanthi Shankhararaman from Springer publications for all the guidance to write this book and for patiently waiting for my submissions. Thanks to them also for directing the layout and production of this book.

This book would not have been possible if I did not have my family's support to take time off work to do this book. To my wife Jenny, son Naveen and daughter Nimmy a big thank you for what you mean to me.

Contents

About the Author

Thomas Kuriakose, MBBS, DNB, FRCSEd completed his graduate and postgraduate studies at the Christian Medical College (CMC) in Vellore, India followed by 3 years of ophthalmology training in Edinburgh, UK. His initial sub-speciality exposure was in the cornea, and gradually shifted to an interest in the posterior segment. In addition, he has maintained his interest in general ophthalmology, which was essential for teaching CMC's undergraduate and post-graduate students. He joined the faculty of CMC Vellore in 1992 and went on to become a professor of ophthalmology there. He has been an examiner for the Royal College of Surgeons Edinburgh, University of Malaysia and several Indian universities including the National Board of Examinations. He has over 30 publications in peer-reviewed journals and his work has been referred to in ophthalmology textbooks.

e-mail: kuriakoset@gmail.com

Introduction

1.1 Clinical Ophthalmology an Exciting Detective Work

It was the clinical skill of an Ophthalmologist that inspired Sir Arthur Conan Doyle to write his famous Sherlock Holmes detective series. What can be more exciting than becoming Sherlock Holmes every day of our lives when we try to solve the diagnostic riddles of the patients who walk into our clinic? Holmes did not inherit this skill, we see him keeping himself well informed about all that is to be known in his field and also practise his skills.

This book tries to help in the how and why of collecting the clues or clinical evidence needed to solve the mystery diagnosis. Without practice, however, one cannot perfect the art of collecting evidence and is something one will have to learn on real patients, volunteers or even clinical simulators. This book will only deal with collecting the clues to make the diagnosis.

Power of observation, range of knowledge and power of deduction makes a physician good in making clinical diagnosis. The eye does not see what the mind does not know, so depth and range of knowledge is needed to know what to look for. In the same vein, once you know what to look for unless you look for it, one may not see it. It is very easy to miss a faint corneal scar on the cornea unless you are consciously looking for it. One can easily miss vitreous cells if you are not looking for it. Just because you have looked through the vitreous to see the retina does not mean there were no cells. There is, however, a downside to this too. The mind sometimes sees what it wants to see even if it is not there!

Before we discuss further the art and science of making a diagnosis, there are a few terms that will have to be made clear so that all of us are thinking of the same thing when the term is used.

1.2 Definitions

- *Test*: The Webster dictionary defines test as—a critical examination, observation or evaluation. In the clinical setting, it is an evaluation done to rule in or rule out a diagnosis. A test is also done to quantify the function/abnormality we are looking for.
- *Clinical test and clinical investigation*: In this book, a **clinical test** (classically known as clinical examination) is an activity done by the physician or an authorised person and makes use of their own sensory skills to make observations. The reason why the term clinical test has been used for clinical examination (history and physical examination) is to look at this also as a test which it really is. Any test requiring sophisticated equipment and not needing the physicians skill we will call it **Clinical Investigation**. The distinction between a test and investigation is not clear-cut and one could debate the categorisation.

© Springer Nature Singapore Pte Ltd. 2020
T. Kuriakose, *Clinical Insights and Examination Techniques in Ophthalmology*,
https://doi.org/10.1007/978-981-15-2890-3_1

Clinical trials are sometimes called clinical test but for this book it is not the same.

- *He:* Means a person and is meant for all genders. He is used instead of she as it has one letter less!

1.3   Diagnosis Making Process

Disease is the diagnosis to make or mystery to crack. In trying to figure out the clinical problem or making a diagnosis, it is important not to lose sight of the patient who has the problem. The patient's social support systems, psychological make-up, economic background, the disability due to the clinical problem, all should be kept in mind when diagnosing and managing the patient. For example, if an apprehensive patient comes for reading glasses and you find an early harmless pterygium the patient has not noticed, it may be best not to direct the patient's attention to it.

The history (symptoms) and signs are the first clues to help make a diagnosis. Clinical investigation (beyond the scope of this book) is the next clue one looks for and if this too is not helpful, then as a physician one tries a therapeutic trial to make a diagnosis. If the patient responds to the treatment for a particular disease, there is a possibility that the person had the disease. It is also possible that it was a placebo effect or time the great healer with the help of the body's own defence systems cured itself. Physicians should

therefore be careful when taking credit for their therapeutic trial.

In their book on clinical epidemiology by Sackett et al., the authors mention four ways by which we make a diagnosis. **(1)** The strategy of exhaustion used by the novice involves taking a history according to the classical textbooks, i.e. presenting complaints, history of presenting complaints, past history, medical history, personal history, family history and social history and noting them all. Examination involves looking at all the systems of the body noting down all abnormalities. Once all this is noted down the information is scanned to look for a pattern that fits a diagnosis. This strategy may be alright in the early years of training as a medical student but should be abandoned as soon as possible without feeling guilty about it. The reasons for this will be mentioned in the chapter on history taking. **(2)** Called multiple branching strategy by the authors, this method is more like an algorithm that is followed when a patient is seen. Figure 1.1 shows such an algorithm followed for the diagnosis of a patient with a red eye. This strategy is used when the diagnosis making responsibility is delegated, for example to nurses or junior doctors in an emergency room. Though a useful tool if developed keeping all clinical evidence in mind, creating an algorithm can be very difficult. In fact, all non-AI (artificial intelligence) computer-based diagnostic programmes are based on such algorithms. **(3)** Pattern recognition is a method that is used by more experienced clinicians in selected cases. When looking at the

Fig. 1.1 Flow chart to make a diagnosis of conjunctivitis

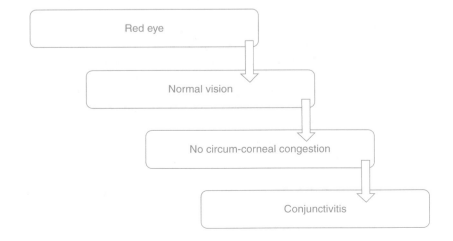

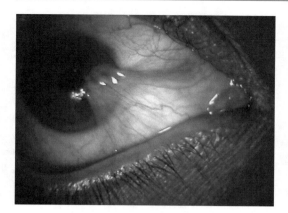

Fig. 1.2 Triangular mass of tissue on the medial aspect of the cornea of the right eye suggestive of a pterygium

use normal vision to rule out the other conditions rather than rule in conjunctivitis. Authors have opined that we normally work with three or four hypothesis at a time. Even if we managed to bring down the possibilities to one, it would only be a fool who is 100% sure of the diagnosis. In my early years of dealing with corneal ulcers, I was quite sure what the aetiology of the ulcer was when I saw one. As I saw more cases, I became less sure of the probable aetiology! The more we know we realise how little we know! Thus, the possibility of something we have not thought about or an unusual presentation should be kept in mind when making a diagnosis.

1.3.1 Dealing with Uncertainty

Human beings find uncertainty very difficult to deal with. We prefer a definite explanation for everything, and if one is not forthcoming we invent one and stick with it as though it is absolute truth. A classic example seen even today in some remote parts is people attributing the 'common cold' they have to the food they have had the previous day. 'Medicine is a science of uncertainty and an art of probability. Absolute diagnoses are unsafe and are made at the expense of the conscience' wrote William Osler. Besides being unsure of the diagnosis what is often not appreciated is that any test including those we do to elicit clinical signs is fallible and may be elicitable in some patients but not in others with the same clinical diagnosis. This uncertainty is not restricted to medicine or biology, with the advent of quantum physics, even physics which we once thought was exact science is all about probabilities. A chapter on epidemiology and statistics has been added in the hope that it will help the student deal with this uncertainty and also understand the epidemiologic basis of clinical medicine.

eye of the patient in Fig. 1.2, clinicians who have seen such cases before can immediately say it is a pterygium. The problem with pattern recognition is that one may jump into a conclusion without considering all possibilities and as has been written before it is more 'reflexive than reflective'. In addition, all diseases are not amenable to pattern recognition. Besides visual, pattern recognition can be through sound (a bruit), touch (palpation characteristics), smell (classical odour in atrophic rhinitis) and even taste (not used in the present day). **(4)** The most common method used by all clinicians for making a diagnosis is however the hypothetico-deductive strategy. Here depending on the patient's circumstances, story or findings, the clinician thinks of the possibilities for a diagnosis and then takes action (ask more questions or do more clinical tests) to remove or add to this list till the list can be reduced to one or two. Unlike in scientific experiments where we disprove hypothesis (which may be a better strategy), the human brain naturally looks for more evidence to support our thinking rather than looking for evidence to rule out the other possibilities on the list. For example, when one sees a patient with red eye one would normally think of conjunctivitis, uveitis, corneal ulcer or angle closure glaucoma (the list of hypothesis). Now you check the vision and if it is normal you would deduce that you are more likely to be dealing with conjunctivitis rather the other three conditions. It is suggested (will be explained in the chapter on epidemiology) that it is better to

1.3.2 Emperor's New Clothes

As children we are taught to believe everything that is written in print in our textbooks and not to question it. This mindset continues all our life and very few are encouraged to question things written in books. In the fable story of 'Emperor's new clothes' while everybody in the court was admiring the emperor's new clothes, only an innocent unconditioned child's mind could point out that the emperor had no clothes on. Literature has clinical tests which have not been questioned by new authors who have reproduced them in their books. Every student of medicine should question what is written in print and be bold enough to point out the rubbish if it does not make sense, rather than feeling guilty or inadequate because the test does not make sense to you. Before discarding the test, however, one should examine the possible reasons for the disagreement and rule them out. There are many reasons why a test does not make sense.

1.4   When Clinical Tests Do Not Make Sense

Racial variations in clinical findings—a red rash on the face will be obvious in a lightly pigmented patient and will not be noticeable in a darkly pigmented individual. When I first read that one could make out the cornea through the lids in the condition called levator dissertation, it did not make sense in the heavily pigmented lids of the patients I normally see. It was only when I finally saw the cornea through the lid in a lightly pigmented patient did it make sense. Thus, one has to match the diagnostic environment of the test originally described.

Use of inappropriate aids in the diagnosis: A poor light source in a slit lamp will not show the cells in the anterior chamber. Use of pin on the skin may not pick up subtle loss of sensation.

Faulty sensory organs of the clinician, e.g. colour-blind person may not pick up changes in the colour of the conjunctiva and sclera. If in doubt, best ask a clinician colleague to check your findings.

Incorrect method of doing the test and interpreting it: When looking for a relative afferent pupillary defect, if the torch is quickly moved from one eye to the other, the results can be misleading.

The main aim of this book is to bring together in one book all **relevant** clinical tests we do in Ophthalmology, describe them and give reason

for doing the test in the way described. An effort will also be made to review literature (failed most of the time) to see how good the tests are in clinical practice.

In this book, clinical tests that have not been found useful (tests with poor sensitivity and specificity or those that do not give any added information) in the clinic have not been mentioned. To list all the clinical tests ever described is not the intention of this book. By keeping these tests out, it is hoped that the clinician does not lose sight of the useful tests.

1.5   Natural History of Disease and Clinical Presentation

1.5.1   Knowing Natural History

The way a disease progresses from the earliest stage of its onset to its termination in cure, recovery, disability or death is called the Natural History of Disease. The signs and symptoms of the disease can vary depending on the stages of the disease. Similarly, the culmination of the disease in recovery, disability or death varies depending on the severity of the insult, patient's genetic make-up and how the body responds to them. It may be humbling to know that many diseases recover by themselves due to the bodies own ability to fight disease and heal itself. Clinical presentation therefore varies depending on the stages of the disease and one should be wary of criticising a colleague who may have missed a diagnosis because he would have seen the patient very early in the course of the disease. Likewise, when treating a disease be wary of taking credit for the cure. For all you know, the resolution may have been part of the natural history of the disease and not due to one's treatment!

1.6   Medical Etiquette

When a patient walks into your room, there is an implied consent that he is willing to be examined and treated by you. This, however, does not give us the freedom to do whatever we please with the patient. In Ophthalmology, ensure privacy for the patient especially when they are telling us their history or story. Lack of privacy will prevent the patient from giving history that may be relevant for diagnosis, for instance, an assault by the spouse or a visit to a sex worker may not be forthcoming unless the patient trusts you and feels there is privacy. One of the ways to create trust is to give dedicated time to your patients without being distracted by various electronic devices like phone in your room. Distraction while examining the patient is also not good for the thinking process of the physician. For the doctor it may be the 1000th case of a simple viral conjunctivitis walking through the door but for the patient who has no idea about eye diseases; the apprehension is, what if he loses his eye due to this horrible condition! So instead of considering the patient as a fussy person it is important for us as doctors to put the patient at ease and answer their questions that may appear silly to us. Empathy is a trait worth developing to become a successful doctor. Respect your patients because they are your real teachers. Reading a book like this without practising it on patients will never make one a good doctor. It is a good practice to tell the patient what you are going to do and immediately after the test give the result as the patient will be eagerly waiting for it. For example, before you measure the intraocular pressure (IOP) tell the patient what you are going to do and after measurement inform if the IOP is normal or abnormal. If there are trainees or other people in the room during the examination tell the patient who they are and get a consent for them to be around. After the examination, give your working diagnosis and why you think so and what next. It is alright to tell the patient that you do not have a working diagnosis and more tests or consultation with a colleague or senior is needed. A doctor should be honest and honesty inspires confidence in the patients. Keeping the patient's information confidential is a must by law.

1.7 Recording and Interpreting Your Findings

Note the findings accurately and not our interpretation of the same as the latter can be wrong, e.g. describe a corneal lesion with margins having tentacle-like extension as such instead of calling it a viral ulcer. Alan Mortiz stated—'If evidence is properly gathered and recorded, then mistakes in its interpretation can be corrected if needed'.

1.8 Normal

In a clinical examination, one is looking for abnormalities that will give us a clue to the diagnosis. This brings us to the issue of what is normal? Is anybody normal? Is black, white, yellow or brown skin colour normal? The whole issue of what is normal is made even more complex with moral and philosophical implications added and is beyond the scope of this book. Doctors should, however, be aware of the complexities of defining normal in the context of biology and at what point is a test result abnormal. More on this will be looked at in the chapter on statistics and epidemiology. One thing, however, should be clear at this stage. Normal in biology is not a single number; it is a range. Normal vision cannot be 6/6; normal temperature cannot be 37 °C. The absurdity of a single number 'normal' becomes obvious if one made a statement that normal weight is 60 kg when even having a meal can change one's weight! A good clinician should be aware of all the variations of normal before identifying abnormal findings.

Clinical medicine is complex and an inexact science by itself. If to this we add physicians' ignorance the consequences are for anyone to guess. There is so much at stake and an approaching examination cannot be the only reason for a physician to gain clinical competence! Finally, in closing this chapter which already looks like a sermon in places, one cannot but remember Alvan Feinstein's advice '**To advance art and science in clinical examination the equipment a clinician most needs to improve is himself**'.

Further Reading

David L Sackett, R Brian Haynes, Gordon H Guyatt, Peter Tugwell; Clinical epidemiology: a basic science for clinical medicine; 2nd ed. Little Brown & Co; 1991.

Overview of Statistics and Epidemiology for Clinical Diagnosis: Connecting the Dots

Introduction-The Connection

A chapter on statistics and epidemiology in a specialty book on clinical methods is most unusual. A world renowned epidemiologist once said that it was 'amoral to combine epidemiology with clinical practice'. The reason for this one presumes is: epidemiology deals with the population and clinical practice deals with managing the individual patient that comes to your clinic.

There was this patient who went to a doctor with a serious surgical condition. After examining the patient, the doctor said that he needs a very complicated surgery but would survive. The patient asked how the doctor was so sure and the doctor replied, 'Statistical studies have shown that one out of 10 patients with this condition survive after surgery. Since his last 9 patients have died the concerned patient should survive!' This story highlights the thought that epidemiological studies are fine for the population but not for the patient in front of you. Today that thinking has changed. The discipline of clinical epidemiology integrates epidemiology with clinical practice and explains the science behind clinical medicine.

Today with the evolution of clinical epidemiology, one wonders how anyone can practise clinical medicine without the knowledge of clinical epidemiology. Concepts in clinical epidemiology and biostatistics, help us understand better what we as clinicians do and give it a more scientific backing. It gives us the science behind the art of medicine and demystifies it in a sense. It will also help the clinician to understand the strengths and limitations of the clinical diagnosis making process and evolve strategies to improve the effectiveness of clinical tests.

It is numerophobia that drives some people to become doctors! Being numerophobic and dyslexic myself, discussing statistics with numbers will be avoided as much as possible!

An assumption that is made here is that the reader in the past has been exposed to some statistics during the school days and some biostatistics during the medical school days. Normally, the various aspects of statistics are taught in separate silos. Even if the teacher did tell the connection between the chapters, it does not normally register in one's head! The attempt here will be to describe concepts of statistics and epidemiology in English and keep use of numbers to minimum possible. By putting together all the relevant topics in one chapter, it is hoped that the student can see the connection between the various concepts. With a broad understanding of the principles governing the use of statistics and epidemiology, it is possible to apply the principles of statistics and epidemiology where needed without going into the mathematical details or its derivations. This understanding should not only help the reader understand literature containing statistical and epidemiological terms better but also see clinical medicine in a more scientific manner.

This chapter is not a substitute for a standard textbook on medical statistics and epidemiology.

© Springer Nature Singapore Pte Ltd. 2020
T. Kuriakose, *Clinical Insights and Examination Techniques in Ophthalmology*,
https://doi.org/10.1007/978-981-15-2890-3_2

Students should refer to specialised books in this field for more detailed understanding. Books listed in the additional reading list will be a good starting point. This chapter has insights which dawned on me later in life and which was not obvious during the earlier stages of study of books on the subject.

The border between statistics and epidemiology is blurred for me and one seems to merge into the other. **Statistics** is the branch of science that deals with the collection, analysis and interpretation of data. **Data** (the starting point in statistics) is discrete observations of attributes that carry little meaning when considered by itself. **Statistics compiles and analyses this data and converts it into information.** It is a disservice to say that statistics is math. Statistics is logic explained in terms of numbers. The central concept of 'null hypothesis' comes from logic and not math. Logic says one can never prove a hypothesis. It is, however, possible to disprove a hypothesis which then becomes a proof for the opposite. So if the **null hypothesis** states that there is no difference between *A* and *B*; disproving it means there is a difference.

Epidemiology has many definitions. At first, it was supposed to be 'a study of distribution and determinants of disease in a population and application of this study to control health problems'. From this it has grown in many directions and **clinical epidemiology** tries to marry epidemiology and clinical medicine. **One could say that the information generated by statistics is interpreted intelligently through epidemiology to make decisions**. Now if one were to put together statistics and epidemiology in the context of clinical diagnosis, then the signs and symptoms are the data (each standing alone does not mean much) which are put together (converted to information) to figure out the organ at fault. This information is then interpreted based on probabilities to make a diagnosis. The connection of statistics and epidemiology to clinical medicine thus becomes clear and one would even suggest it is 'amoral' not to see them together!

Given below are some basic concepts in statistics and epidemiology so that the reader gets a bird's eye view of the various concepts and tests done in statistics and epidemiology.

2.1 Population and Sample

With statistics and epidemiology, the idea is to study a **population** (any collection of objects), say a population of diabetics. However, it is not practical to study the population as a whole due to the limited resources available. The alternative therefore is to study a **sample** from the population of interest and then generalise the sample results to the population. Intuitively, one can say that every sample we study will give a different result, which in turn will be different from the real population result. This is due to **sampling variation** with its consequent errors. The problem with studying only a sample from the population is the sampling error. This occurs because the sample studied will not be exactly the same as that of the population if it were to be studied as a whole. Minimising sampling errors and predicting the confidence with which one can apply the results of the sample studied to the population is what we often do in statistics. What aspect of the population one needs to study will dictate the type of study, the sampling techniques, the type of data collected and the method of analysis.

2.1.1 Selecting the Sample

If the objective is to study the population from which the sample is taken, then the sample should be representative of the population. To get an unbiased and representative sample, one needs to use strategies like simple random sampling, systematic sampling, stratified sampling, age match sampling, multistage sampling, random allocation, blinding, etc. Along with the type of sample the number of samples collected is also important. Very few samples may not be representative of the information needed. Too many samples will waste resources and put more patients at risk of the bad outcomes of the study. In clinical medicine, too many investigations will likewise put patients at unnecessary risk and be a financial burden. The number needed for the sample will depend on the type of study, the prevalence/incidence of the data being studied, the standard deviation, the amount of difference we expect to see between groups and the confidence with which we need to state the findings. Formulas using the preceding parameters exist, based on which the sample size is calculated. Some of the information needed like standard deviation is got from previous studies in the area or from pilot studies.

Bias is a systematic deviation from the truth. **Information bias** is when there is an error in collection of data like when using a faulty apparatus (giving high/low values). **Selection bias** is when the sample you select is not representative of the population you want to study. For example, selecting your friends to be volunteers in a study to assess the normative data of the population.

2.2   Data

From the sample selected we get the data. The world around us is made up of 'things' and not numbers. What we are interested in are these things and not numbers. For analysis, however, we need to convert these 'things' into numbers. To begin to understand statistics, one needs to understand the data being studied. The type of data we are studying and the way it is distributed in the population defines the strategies to study them.

2.2.1   Data Types

Data can be **qualitative** (categorical or discrete), e.g. place of residence, number of males and females. **Discrete or qualitative data** move in a stepwise fashion and is in whole numbers. For example, 40 males or 41 males, it cannot be 40.5 males. Data can also be **quantitative data** (numerical or interval). **Continuous data** has a graded continuous progression, e.g. weight, which can be 40 or 40.1 kg. In Ophthalmology vision in Snellen notation, type of corneal ulcer, cause of uveitis, etc. are all examples of discrete data. Vision in LogMAR values, intraocular pressures, etc. will be continuous data.

2.2.2   Data Distribution

Like the type of data, an idea of its distribution in the population is also needed for analysis. **Normal distribution** of data (**parametric data**) is when the data is distributed in a symmetrical pattern in what is called a bell-shaped curve. With data that is normally distributed, majority of data points have one value and the remaining lie on either side of this value in a symmetrical fashion (Fig. 2.1). Data that is not distributed

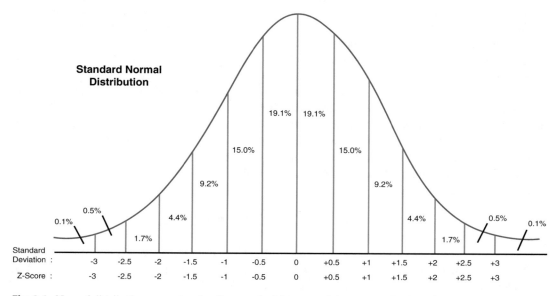

Fig. 2.1 Normal distribution curve showing the spread of data around the centre point (mean)

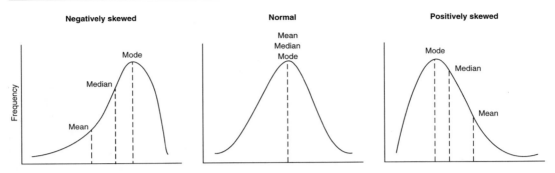

Fig. 2.2 Data distribution in normal (parametric) and skewed (non-parametric) distribution

symmetrically is called **non-parametric data**. The data may be skewed. When the maximum number of data points lies to one side of the distribution curve and is not symmetrical, it is positively or negatively skewed. Depending on the location of mean, median and mode (measure of central tendency) in this distribution curve, one can figure out the type of distribution of the data (Fig. 2.2). There exists other non-parametric distribution of data like bimodal, J shaped, etc., but will not go into it here. As we will see later, the test one uses to analyse data will depend on the type and distribution of the data.

One should also be aware that the formulas derived in statistics assume random selection of subjects. An understanding of the strategies to ensure random selection of data is as important as the knowledge that, for the formulas to be valid, random selection is important. Matching the type of data to the appropriate statistical test also depend on what is being studied. The flow chart in Fig. 2.3 gives the broad division of the types of data and some examples the appropriate tests used for each. In medicine, normally data collected is used to look at averages; difference between averages, correlation between data sets, any association between factors affecting the data, rate of occurrence, survival analysis, etc.

2.3   Central Tendency or Average

Multiple individual data points are difficult to remember and make sense if it is just listed in a document. To summarise the data and make sense

out of it, we use statistics. One of the commonest exercises done to summarise data is to find the central tendency or average of the data. **Mean** is the mathematical average where all the values are added and divided by the total number of data points. If the data is arranged in ascending or descending order, the data point in the middle is the **median**. If the data set is even, then the average of the middle two values is taken. **Mode** is the data value that occurs maximum number of times in the data set. If the data set is normally distributed (parametric data), then the mean, median and mode will be the same value as shown in the central graph in Fig. 2.2. The pattern of distribution of mean, median and mode in skewed data (non-parametric data) is also shown in Fig. 2.2.

Mean is the preferred measure of the central tendency especially for continuous variables because it is amenable to mathematical and statistical manipulation. Median is used when there are extremely high or low values in the data set as this shifts the mean so much that it is not representative of the data set. Mode is used rarely and is especially useful when you have non-linear data which cannot be added and divided like continuous variables. Vision of patients in the Snellen notation is a typical measurement where mode is useful.

2.3.1   Precision

By itself the central tendency may not make sense if the spread of the data is not known. For example, a data set of 5, 5, 95, 95 will have an average of 50 which is not really representative of the data set. Measuring the spread of data in its simplest form is done by mentioning the lowest and highest value of the data set and is called the **range**. The range, however, does not give us any idea of the data in between. To get a better picture of the entire data set, the mean of the data set is calculated first, and the distance of each data point from this mean is then calculated. The mean of the square of this distance gives the **standard deviation** (spread). From the sample mean, when one wants to extrapolate to the population mean, using the spread of only one data set to estimate it would not be appropriate. Instead one would prefer to get the spread of means if multiple samples were taken from the population. The spread of these means is given by what is called **standard error (SE) of the sample mean**. The sample mean of the study plus or minus the product of standard error and Z value (Fig. 2.1) gives the confidence interval within which the population mean is likely to be. Normally, the 95% confidence interval is given. In a study if it is mentioned that the mean is 6.4 ± 1.2 and a Z value of 1.96 is used, it implies that the population mean will lie between 5.2 and 7.6, 95% of the time. When the mean of a set of data is given with the confidence interval, it means that the real mean can lie anywhere within this range with equal chance and does not mean it is more likely to be closer to the mean of 6.4.

When the distribution of the population to be studied follows a normal distribution curve, then the percentage of population under the curve follows a pattern. Figure 2.2 shows the percentage of population under the curve for each standard deviation (SD) from the mean value. What one needs to note is that 95.5% of population lies within 2 standard deviations from the mean. 99.9% of population lies 3 SDs from the mean. One of the ways normal is defined is, as those lying within 2 SD of the mean. When clinical labs give the range for normal values of a test, what they give is the values 2 SD from the mean on either side. This does not mean that the values outside this are necessarily pathological. It just means that this value is not, what is seen in 95% of the normal population.

2.3.2   Confidence Intervals

When one is dealing with the mean value of the sample studied and wants to apply it to the larger population from which the sample was taken, then one gives a confidence interval between which the population mean lies. If one wants a 95% confidence level, the interval is between 2 SEs below the mean and 2 SEs above the mean. For example, it will be written as '95% confidence limit is $X \pm Y$ where X is the mean of the sample and Y is $2 \times$ SE. For categorical data, proportions are used and the confidence interval for a single proportion is calculated using binomial distribution (the sampling distribution seen with proportions) or normal distribution. There are tests of significance available comparing two proportions and giving confidence interval (Fig. 2.3).

2.4   Hypothesis Testing

When statistical tests are done on results of sample studied and data sets are compared to see if they are different or if the data sets are related to each other, there is a possibility that the differences or associations have occurred by chance. As mentioned previously, with logic one cannot prove that two data sets are different but can disprove that they are the same (null hypothesis)! Null hypothesis testing gives the 'p value' which is the chance that the null hypothesis is true. A p value of less than 0.05 means that there is less than 5% chance that the null hypothesis is true and so we reject the null hypothesis and accept the reverse.

2.5   Comparing Means

If one wants to compare two means, e.g. intraocular pressure before and after treatment, to see if they are different, there is a possibility that the difference in the two means we got is due to sampling variation of the two samples. It could also mean that the difference between the two means (however small they are) is actually different and

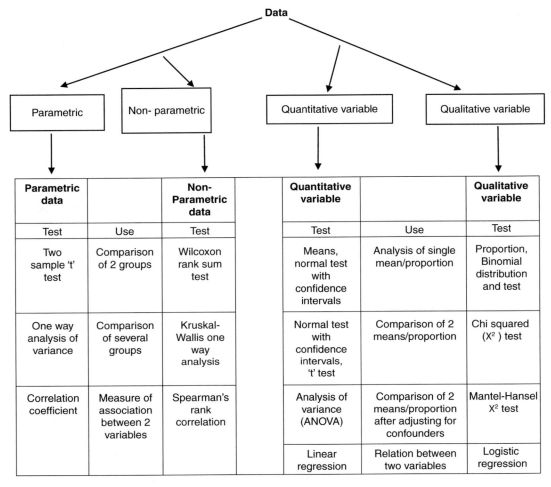

Fig. 2.3 Chart showing the broad types of data and some of the more common statistical tests that are done to evaluate them

is beyond the normal sampling variation possible. We use a *'t'* **test** to compare means for continuous variables. If the sample size is less than 15, we use the **student** *'t'* **test** to compare means. If the two sample sets are related, e.g. vision before and after surgery in an eye, then we use a **paired** *t* **test**. It is also possible to know what is the amount of difference and the confidence interval of the difference. Some people think this is more useful than *p* values.

If more than two means need to be compared, then an **analysis of variance** (ANOVA) is used. (Fig. 2.3)

2.6 Correlation and Survival Analysis

To see if there is a relation between two types of data from a sample, e.g. operating time and anterior chamber reaction as measured by intensity of the flare measured, a **test of correlation** is done. This association is measured by 'correlation coefficient' *r*. The value of the correlation is between −1 to 0 to +1. Zero means no correlation. −1 means perfect negative correlation, that is if one value goes down the other goes up. +1 is the opposite and means perfect positive correlation. The measure of the correlation is done by doing a regression analysis. **Linear regression** measures how one continuous variable is related to the other. **It is important to understand that the presence of a correlation or association does not mean that one causes the other**. To prove causality (i.e. one event causes the other), one needs to fulfil the cox postulates. If we are interested in the dependency of one variable to several variables, then a **multiple regression** is done.

If we are comparing two categorical data, they can be put into a 2/2 contingency table and then a **Chi-squared test** or something similar is done to look for differences and associations. If sample size is less than 40 between the four cells or if one cell has less than 5 values, then a **Fischer's exact *t* test** is used. The equivalent of paired t test here is **matched pair design**. **Mantel–Haenszel chi-squared test** is used to compare multiple 2×2 tables. **Logistic regression** is the equivalent for multiple regression for continuous variables.

Time event data is the time followed up before the event occurs. One can get median time to death from this type of data. To study survival (not necessarily related to living or dead), one does what is called **survival analysis** like **Kaplan–Meier plot**. For example, to study how long a trabeculectomy bleb functions one does a survival analysis.

2.7 Epidemiological Concepts for Clinical Medicine

2.7.1 Probability

Probability is the chance of something occurring. Our brain is constantly taking decisions based on probabilities either consciously or unconsciously. We decide to cross a road in spite of seeing a car coming from a distance; it is because our brain has calculated that the probability of the car hitting us while crossing is minimal. Probability (*x/y*) is the number of times an outcome will be *x* if the experiment is done *y* times. So probability of something happening is between 0 and 1. It can also be represented in percentage from 0% to 100%. For example, there is 65% chance that history alone will give us the clinical diagnosis. In life, for daily activities our brain is consciously or unconsciously calculating probabilities before we take a decision. In clinical medicine, we come to the conclusion as to the most likely diagnosis the patient has by weighing the probability of each of the differential diagnosis and then choosing the most likely one out the list. **Pre-test probability** is the probability of a hypothesis/diagnosis before a test is done. **Post-test probability** is the probability of the same hypothesis/diagnosis after the test is done. The Bayesian approach to statistics tries to quantify the change in probability based on the test result. Though methods exist to calculate exactly the post-test probability for every test done, it is difficult to put this in practice in the clinic for every patient that comes. The human brain, with experience works out this probability and it is this ability that is interpreted as the art of medicine. May be a day will come when the 'hospital electronic medical records (EMR)' will incorporate usefulness of test data (sensitivity and specificity) from the literature and the hospital disease prevalence data, to work out the probability of a particular disease in a patient in front of you!

The probability of two things occurring together is the product of each of the individual probabilities. The product of two fractions is always less than either of them. So much so since the value of probability is between 0 and 1 (a fraction) the chances of somebody having two diseases together is less than having only one of the diseases. So think of only one diagnosis rather than two when examining the patient. For example, if there are two differential diagnoses for a set of clinical tests, it is more likely the patient has one of this rather than have both at the same time. The probability of one or the other hypothesis being true is the addition of each of the probability.

2.7.2 Incidence and Prevalence

Incidence of a disease is the number of new cases occurring in the susceptible population (population at risk) over a specific period. Therefore, if we are studying the incidence of cataract the denominator should not include people who have already had cataract surgery as incidence of cataract in patients who have had cataract surgery makes no sense. Incidence is more useful to study acute short duration diseases.

Prevalence is the number of affected patients in the community at one point in time (**point prevalence**) or over a period of time (**period prevalence**). Prevalence depends on the incidence and also the duration of the illness. Prevalence of a disease in the community we are administering a test will dictate how predictive the test will be for that disease. This concept will be further clarified in the section on clinical testing.

2.8 Diagnostic Test and Diagnosis

Any tool to collect data to make a diagnosis is called diagnostic test. As will be explained, even history is a tool to collect data from the patient. When we make a diagnosis or give a set of differential diagnosis, we are essentially classifying the diagnostic data under question into the category of disease that has these test results as its feature. This classification is based on the data we collect from the patient and looking at the probabilities to see into which group the data collected fits best.

2.8.1 Validity and Reliability

To make a diagnosis, the quality of data you collect is important. The first thing to be sure is that the data you collect is **valid** for what you are looking for. Taking history from a relative instead of the mother or carer of a child will not be valid. Measurement of blood pressure is not a valid

measurement to assess intraocular pressure (IOP). Though this may seem an obvious fact (given to drive home the point), it may not be obvious in real life. A poorly trained doctor may be taking such a poor history that he never manages to get the real presenting complaints from the patient!

When collecting data, there should be **consistency** or it should be **reliable**. If a tonometer gives readings varying from 2 to 30 mm of Mercury on the same patient in a span of 5 min, it is not reliable. **Data collected therefore should be both valid and reliable**.

One of the problems with clinical examination is that it is very dependent on the examiner, his knowledge, training, mental state at that time of the day, etc. This variability in validity and reliability of clinical tests done by them coupled with commercial interest and a lack of self-confidence in one's clinical finding is what takes away from the powerful tool of clinical examination, its due.

No test, clinical or equipment assisted will be positive for all the patients with disease or be negative for all healthy patients. Familiarity with epidemiological terms associated with a test is useful to understand the significance and limitations of the test we do for our patients.

The term '**gold standard**' has its origins in the gold that was the standard on which money was based initially. McGraw-Hill Concise Dictionary of Modern Medicine defines gold standard as 'The best or most successful diagnostic or therapeutic modality for a condition, against which new tests or results and protocols are compared'. In other words 'gold standard' is that indicator/standard which is most suggestive of the definition of the disease of interest and any new innovation has to be compared to that. For example, culturing the organism from corneal scraping is the gold standard for diagnosis of bacterial corneal ulcer. It could also be a set of signs or symptoms that defines a disease. Acute onset of eye pain, high IOP, closed angles on gonioscopy and oval pupils could be the gold standard for acute angle closure glaucoma.

The ability of a test (symptom, sign or laboratory result) to classify individuals into a particu-

Table 2.1   The 2 × 2 table used for evaluating diagnostic test

Test	Disease		Total
	Positive	Negative	
Positive	a (22)	b (3)	$a + b$ (25)
Negative	c (20)	d (55)	$c + d$ (75)
Total	$a + c$ (42)	$b + d$ (58)	Total sample 'n' $a + b + c + d = 100$

Sensitivity = $a/a + c$; **Specificity** = $d/b + d$; **Positive predictive value** (PPV) = $a/a + b$ (88%); **Negative predictive value** (NPV) = $d/c + d$

lar disease or no disease category depends on the test itself, the magnitude of the test result and how common that condition is in the community. Two parameters of a test, namely **Sensitivity** and **Specificity** give us an idea as to how good the test is in '*ruling in*' or '*ruling out*' a disease. **Sensitivity** is the proportion of people with the disease that test positive with the test. **Specificity** is the proportion of healthy people that test negative with the test. Sensitivity and specificity of a test remains the same irrespective of the population you do the test on. Table 2.1 is a two by two contingency table for diagnostic tests. It shows the results of a test done on a sample of population with and without the disease. Horizontally across, the boxes are in rows and depict the number of people who tested positive and negative. Vertically, the boxes arranged in columns contain the number of people with and without the disease. The presence of disease is confirmed by applying the gold standard parameters. The total across the rows and columns are given in the margin. The total of all the boxes is given in the right bottom which is the total number of people on whom the test was done (**n**).

Prevalence of the disease in the sample tested is all disease positive divided by the total (*n*). **Sensitivity** is true positives divided by all positives. **Specificity** is the true negatives divided by all negatives. It is obvious from the table that some people with the disease did not test positive and all patients who tested positive did not have the disease. To decide the significance of a positive test in a patient, we need what is called the **positive predictive value (PPV)** of the test which is the true positives divided by all positives. The **negative predictive value (NPV)** is all patients testing negative among the non-diseased

people. These values (PPV & NPV) unlike sensitivity and specificity changes with the prevalence of the disease in the population we are testing. Table 2.2 shows the same test as in Table 2.1 done on a population with a higher prevalence of the disease. Here, one will note that the positive predictive value increases and the negative predictive value decreases when prevalence increases. The opposite happens when the prevalence decreases. One would be tempted to think that it is better to use PPV when prevalence increases and NPV when it decreases. In the clinic situation, however, when the prevalence of a disease increases to over 80% the clinician also gives a high pre-test probability after going through the symptoms and signs. The added value of another test, therefore, may be only 5% more probability. On the other hand, when the pre-test probability is around 40–60%, the change in post-test probability is much more. Figure 2.4 show the same idea in number terms.

Unlike tests which are just reported as positive or negative, in tests which can be quantified, e.g. IOP it may be possible to get different sensitivity and specificity for a disease depending on the level of IOP one keeps the cut off at. If one were to plot a graph using the sensitivity and '1 − Specificity' values at different value levels of the test, one gets what is called an **ROC curve** (receiver operator characteristic) Fig. 2.5 (green curve). The point at the top and left most of the graph will give the value of the result (e.g. IOP) at which the test is most useful. The area below and right of the curve is called the **area under the curve or AUC**. Closer the top left point on the curve is to the top left of the graph, larger is the area under the curve and the better the sensitivity and specificity of the test. The red straight

Table 2.2 The 2 × 2 table showing results for the same test as in Table 2.1 in a population with higher prevalence of the disease (42% vs. 60%)

| Test | Disease | | Total |
	Positive	Negative	
Positive	a (31)	b (2)	$a + b$ (33)
Negative	c (29)	d (38)	$c + d$ (67)
Total	$a + c$ (60)	$b + d$ (40)	Total sample 'n' $a + b + c + d = 100$

Positive predictive value (PPV) = $a/a + b$ (93%)

line in the graph represents a test that is of no value to make a diagnosis and is only as good as throwing up a coin to decide if the patient has a disease or not.

Understanding the concept of pre- and post-test probabilities, sensitivity and specificity of tests and how prevalence affects it will help us understand the science behind the clinical art. It is definitely not in one's mental make-up to think numbers as patient walks into the consulting room. When a patient walks into the clinic with a red eye, it is difficult to start thinking 'Right, this guy has a pre-test probability of corneal foreign body of x%, conjunctivitis y% and angle closure glaucoma of Z%. Now I will ask him a question with a% sensitivity and b% specificity with the knowledge of c% prevalence to come up with f% post-test probability'. What clinical experience does is to give the doctor a feel for these probabilities without actually articulating them. The junior doctors also go through these mental exercises, but the values of the probabilities need refining. If as a clinician one thinks this clinical exercise is not something that comes to mind naturally, it is possible to go through the process in a more conscious manner and think of the numbers as one proceeds through the clinical exercise. The main problem with such conscious working out is that data is not available for a large number of clinical conditions and one will have to make an extra effort to get the numbers locally. In the not too distant future, there will be computer programmes or electronic medical records with all these numbers fed in to give us the final probability of the diagnosis being considered! Will the art of clinical diagnosis then be taken over by machines? Who knows! Till the time machine take over we can continue enjoying clinical medicine just like

we enjoy driving without having to make conscious complex mathematical calculations before we decide to overtake a vehicle!

Any test (symptoms, signs or laboratory tests) has variations in their outcomes. Observation by themselves can vary between different observers (**inter-observer variation**). When the same test is done repeatedly by the same person, the results can vary. IOP measured by the same person repeatedly can be different (**intra-observer variation**). Agreement between the results done by different people and by the same person done at different times can be analysed by **kappa statistic**. Using Kappa statistics, one can quantify this variation to get the inter- and intra-observer agreement. In clinical medicine, one should be aware of the existence of this variation. Clinicians should also have a sense of the Kappa values of the tests done. If the inter-observer variation of a test is high, then you should not be surprised if your colleague's findings are different from yours. This should also make one humble about ones finding and willing to re-evaluate one's findings when there is a disagreement!

2.9 Regression to Mean

When a test is abnormal, it should be repeated to ensure that the abnormality is real. More often than not the repeat test result will be closer to the normal value. This regression to mean should be looked for before labelling a test/clinical observation as abnormal. Circadian variations, intra- and inter-observer variations and regression to mean are some of the reasons to take multiple measurements/observations before labelling someone abnormal.

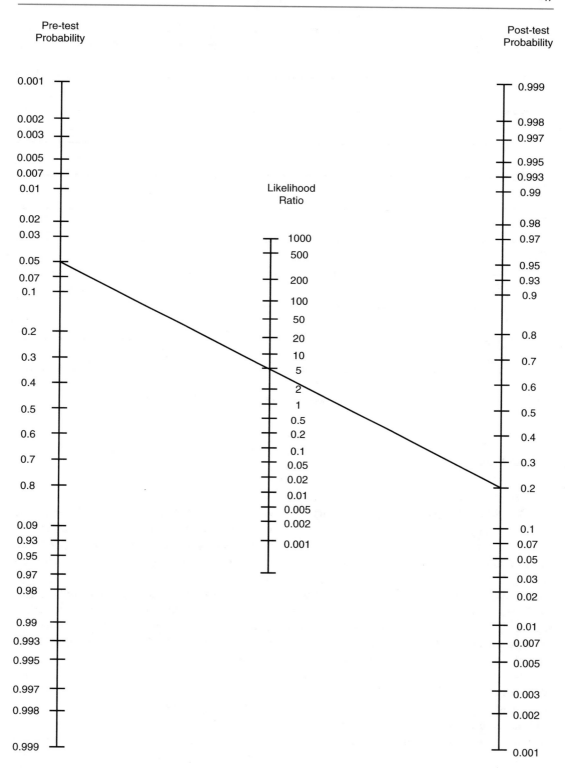

Fig. 2.4 Graph showing change in post-test predictive values depending on the likelihood ratio of the test being positive or negative

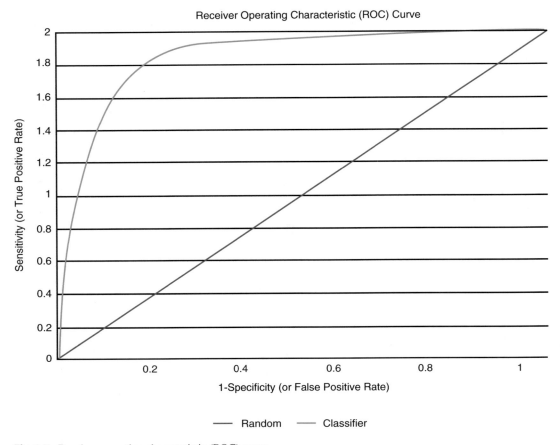

Fig. 2.5 Receiver operating characteristic (ROC) curve

2.10 Some Strategies for Making Diagnosis

Maximum probability of something happening is 100%. If we have three differential diagnosis (DD), all cannot have a pre-test probability of 50% or thereabout as it will add up to 150%! So compare the DDs, try and make forced choice as which is more unlikely and reduce its probability. This will reduce the DD to 2 and is easier to handle.

Our brains are normally wired to rule in a diagnosis. Statistically more effective is, to rule out a diagnosis. So look for clues to rule out some of the differential diagnosis so that what is remaining becomes the probable diagnosis by default.

What if we make a mistake in the assessment of pre-test probability? A wrong assessment of

the pre-test probability will affect the predictive value of the subsequent test we do and unless one attributes very high or very low pre-test probability, subsequent testing can correct the probabilities.

At what post-test probability should we stop testing further? The value of post-test probability at which one stops test depends on the seriousness of the disease and the consequence of misdiagnosis or late diagnosis.

2.10.1 Diagnostic Possibility

One will be relieved to know that this at least is not epidemiology! Before we even think of pre-test probability, the possibility of a diagnosis even being considered depends on familiarity with the condition. This familiarity comes with reading textbooks, looking at atlases especially for ophthalmic and dermatology doctors, exposure to such cases in the past and reading journals.

This chapter is meant to give a bird's eye view to the clinician the concepts so that they get the broader picture of the subject and see how this relates to day-to-day clinical work, research and teaching. *Statistics and epidemiology is all about chance and probabilities, one can never be 100% sure and that is a humbling and sobering thought.* As clinicians, except for the gifted few, getting a good understanding of statistics and epidemiol-ogy is difficult with one reading. Repeated reading and internalisation is required for majority of us to understand it enough to direct clinical medicine and research. It is best to get help from statisticians and epidemiologists to give the finer inputs when doing the actual research.

Further Reading

Kirkwood BR. Essentials of medical statistics. Malden, MA: Blackwell Scientific Publications; 1988.
David L Sackett, R Brian Haynes, Gordon H Guyatt, Peter Tugwell; Clinical epidemiology: a basic science for clinical medicine; 2nd ed; Little Brown & Co; 1991.

History Taking: The Most Important Clinical Test

History is his/her story and should be heard with the same delight one hears any story. History taking in medicine is probably as old as the practice of medicine itself. It was never considered a test and was therefore never looked at from that point of view. If we accept the definition of a clinical test (Chap. 1), it becomes clear that **history taking is a test** used to rule in or out a disease and one can even quantify disease by asking the patient if they are better or worse. **Studies have shown that it is the most important clinical test one can do to make a diagnosis.** In a medical clinic, it was observed that from history alone one could make a diagnosis in 56% of the cases that presented. As a patient walks into the physician's office, he could have any disease. He gives his presenting complaint and then you have a fair idea of the system involved. Further questioning will start giving the clues as to possible diseases one may be dealing with. From the pre-test probability of near zero as the patient walks into the room you have after history a post-test probability of your differential diagnosis at around 40–50% at least 6 out of 10 cases. What is also useful is that you will order test in such a way that the pre-test probability is high for the disease being tested, and this makes the positive predictive value of the test even more useful.

It is usually only books on general medicine that discusses history taking in any detail. The possible symptoms are so many in medicine that to cover them all, one would take a whole book in itself. The subtleties in history taking are therefore left to the clinician to figure out and then when it is figured out by serendipity it is called an art!

Traditional teaching has it that the history is taken first and then the examination. While this is true to an extent one should not hesitate to ask more questions depending on what you find in examination. So after a stage, **history taking and clinical examination are done together**.

History taking is an art and a science: History-taking skills is not inherited, the good news is that it can be learned. **There is a difference between history taking and what is called information collection**. Information collection from patients is in a way a passive exercise with no analytical thinking on part of the interviewer. Information like age, presenting complaints, history of diabetes or hypertension, allergies, list of drugs being used, past surgeries in the eye, etc. is collected one after the other and can be done by a clinical assistant or a novice doctor in training. This is collected according to a protocol, irrespective of what presenting complaint the patient has. Since it can be protocol driven, the person collecting this information **need not** be very knowledgeable about various diseases. It is almost like filling out a questionnaire. If one went back to Sherlock Holmes stories, the person who collects information is Dr. Watson and it takes Holmes himself to ask a few more directed questions (history) to increase the value of the information collected.

© Springer Nature Singapore Pte Ltd. 2020
T. Kuriakose, *Clinical Insights and Examination Techniques in Ophthalmology*,
https://doi.org/10.1007/978-981-15-2890-3_3

History taking is an active and involved exercise. It is **directed questioning** and need not be exhaustive. It requires a good insight into all the diseases and their pathophysiology. Every question of the doctor including age and presenting complaint is a test in a way. It 'rules in' a certain condition and 'rules out' others. A 5-year-old child is unlikely to have age-related macular degeneration and may be ruled out. The answer for each question gives a clue to the post-test probability of the conditions you are considering as diagnostic probability. The answer also gives an idea of the pre-test probability relevant to the next question you will ask. In fact, each question and its response guides us to the next question we need to ask the patient. For example, if the presenting complaint is disturbance in near vision in a 40-year-old man, it is not necessary to ask about a history of flashes and floaters. Instead one would explore the type of difficulty he has with near vision and other related symptoms like headache.

The interview process to take history is also a bond-building exercise where the patient–physician relationship is established. The time and attention we give sends them the message that we care about them. Intelligent-targeted questioning improves the patient's confidence in you. The patient will almost think you are a magician and have him wondering how you knew about the symptoms you are questioning him about!

The objective of a good history is to figure out the diagnosis, assess the severity of illness, decide what specific clinical examination and investigations are required, figure out how the patient and family is affected by the disease and finally to chart out the appropriate treatment modality.

Besides the primary objective, history taking gives the doctor a clue to the patient's perception of the disease, his expectation from the treatment and also the type of personality the patient is.

Ophthalmic history taking is similar to any other medical specialty. The broad headings under which history is taken are listed and explained. How one goes through the checklist will depend on the expertise of the person involved in the exercise. As a new trainee, one could go through the list to make sure all areas are covered. Sooner

Table 3.1 Components of 'history' taking

No.	Broad heading	Salient points
1	Introductions	Introduction of physician and others in the room
2	Demographic details	Name, age, occupation, race, etc.
3	Presenting complaints	List of problems that brought the patient to clinic
4	History of presenting complaints	Details of the problems
5	Past medical history	Previous medical/ ophthalmic problems patient has had
6	Personal history	Habits and lifestyle like use of alcohol, smoking, etc.
7	Review of systems	Associated medical problems like diabetes, arthritis, etc.
8	Treatment history	Medical/surgical treatment patient has had or is currently on
9	History of allergies	Known allergies especially medications
10	Family history	Similar illness in the family, consanguinity
11	Social history	Living conditions, earnings, insurance, etc. that is relevant

than later, one should evolve from an information collector to a history taker and the checklist should be **abandoned**. Table 3.1 gives the list of headings under which history is normally taken.

3.1 Demographic Details

Knowing the age of the patient is important, as the type of disease and its aetiology can be dependent on age. One would not think of a high pre-test probability of age-related macular degeneration in a 5-year-old child complaining of decreased vision. Likewise, if a 30-year-old patient comes with complaints of difficulty in reading one would think of hypermetropia having a higher post-test probability compared to presbyopia.

Eye diseases too like other medical conditions can have sex predilection. Thyroid eye disease is more likely to be seen in females.

Knowing the place of stay of patient can be important not only for making a diagnosis but also for advocacy or social intervention. In the days when trachoma was more prevalent, patients from certain localities had higher chances of being diagnosed with it due to the endemicity and lifestyles of people of that locality. Suppose it was noticed in the clinic that all the vitamin A deficiency cases were coming from one area it calls for the physicians to alert the authorities for social intervention.

It is becoming increasingly evident that there are racial differences in the incidence and severity of diseases. Angle closure glaucoma is more prevalent in the Asian population.

3.2 Presenting Complaint

Presenting complaint is the reason why patient comes to you. Most of the patients will tell you directly the reason or reasons for the visit. One would think that this would be a straightforward exercise and patient would straight away tell you this. Far from it, some patients will never tell you the real reason why they have come, and it takes the detective skill of the doctor to figure that out. Therefore, when recording PC it is best to keep some space blank so as to record it when patients open up or the physician has figured it out indirectly. There was a young educated gentleman who came complaining of decreased vision, and his vision was noted to be 6/6. Finally, it turned out that he wanted an eye check-up to rule out HIV infection! Disturbance of vision, redness of eye, ocular discomfort like irritation, watering of eye, injury to the eye, headache, eye swelling, referral by a physician, routine eye check-up, etc. are the common presenting complaints in an eye clinic. There are some patients who knowingly or unknowingly will not reveal the reason for their coming. It is almost like they are challenging the doctor to find out their presenting complaint! Like they say 'it takes all varieties to make the world go around'. It is worth reiterating that the presenting complaint may not be forthcoming easily in the beginning of the consultation even though that is your starting point or the first test

question. Sometimes, the patient will tell you his 'diagnosis' instead of his problems. He will say I have cataract (probably diagnosed by his neighbour or internet) instead of saying his vision is poor. At this stage, you will have to remind him gently to tell you his problems and you will make an effort to figure out the diagnosis! A 'know it all' patient should be dealt with tact rather than irritation.

3.3 History of Presenting Complaint

Once the type of problem the patient has is known, its duration would be the next concern. Is it acute, chronic or recurrent? If the exact time of start of the problem is not forthcoming, a good question to ask is 'when was the patient perfectly well'. Sometimes, especially in older patients it may be a good idea to ask the patient if he has had an eye check-up in the past and what was the reason for the same. One of the problems of onset of disease in Ophthalmology is that only one eye is required for most visual needs and we have two of them! Having a spare one is a great help for the patient and a greater help for the Ophthalmologist who has a spare one to work with! There is a difference between the onset of decreased vision being of 1-week duration and having **noticed** decreased vision in one eye only for a week. It is therefore useful to ask how the patient noticed that vision was less. It is not uncommon for patients to say that they noticed that problem eye had decreased vision when they closed the good eye when dust went in. Sometimes, the problem eye would have had an injury and patient would have closed the good eye to check if vision is normal in the injured eye. Noticing decreased vision in one eye accidently could mean the problem was longstanding. It is not necessary to have vision of 6/6 (20/20) to lead a normal life. Quite often children spend many years of their life without knowing they do not have the vision Ophthalmologist think they should have. It is only when their friends can read the board, and they cannot or parents notice that the child is going close to the TV or they had a school screening test, they realise they do not fit the world norms. At times due to social stigma of wearing glasses, patients do not reveal they have a problem with vision and come not too long after marriage with complaints starting only after marriage! In such a situation, it is in nobody's interest to convince the patient or the relative that the refractive error (condition requiring glasses to correct vision) has been there for a long time and is better to play along with the complaints as they are presented.

Duration of illness gives us an idea of the diagnosis and aetiology. A recent onset deviation of the eye in a young adult would suggest a paralytic squint with a more sinister aetiology that requires more investigations compared to a patient with history of deviation of eye from childhood. Long duration of illness will give the doctor an idea of the patient's coping skills. It should also raise the question as to why the patient decided to seek your opinion now. It could be an impending marriage for a cosmetic defect or an army recruitment for colour-blind patients. At times, it is difficult to come to a conclusion on the duration of illness. In some cases, when applicable one may have to look at old family photographs. In our department, we call it the FAT scan or family album tomography!

3.3.1   Details of the Symptom

When investigating the details of the symptoms, the first thing to ensure is that both the doctor and the patient are talking about the same thing, This is especially important in today's globalised world where there are people from so many different backgrounds visiting a single clinic. To make things more complicated, the internet throws up words with their own meanings. Even today, I am not sure what a 'dude' really means. Mild diplopia may be called blurring of vision by some patients. Funny sensation in the eye could be itching or irritation. Distinguishing photophobia from glare is important in making a diagnosis. It is the doctors' job to really make sure that he understands what the patient is saying. The 'diagnosis' of the right meaning again can come from probabilities of the diseases you are thinking of at that point in the history taking. If the patient and physician speak different language, then the services of an interpreter should be got.

Once you are sure both you and patient are talking about the same thing more details about the symptoms like the exact location of pain, change in character or frequency of symptom, rate of progression or any such details that may be relevant should be gone into. When assessing the location of pain, one has to keep in mind referred pain. A corneal foreign body can give the sensation that there is something under the lid. Orbital apical lesions can refer pain to the frontal region. Pain in the orbit can be due to a sinus infection. It is useful to get the patient's perception of their problem. This will help make better decisions on the treatment and communicate more effectively with the patient. The same size pterygium can affect two people very differently. A 30-year-old lady may be very upset due to its cosmetic disfigurement as opposed to a 60-year-old man who would not be bothered about it too much.

Severity of the symptoms, besides giving an idea of the aetiology will also give us an idea of the aggressiveness required for the treatment. A very painful corneal haze with some epithelial defect is more likely to be Acanthamoeba keratitis rather than the relatively painless viral ulcer. How quickly you start treatment including giving pain-relieving measures depends on the severity.

Constancy of symptoms is a useful clue to make a diagnosis in Ophthalmology. A constant foreign body sensation in one location of the eye is more likely to be due to an actual foreign body in the eye. As opposed to this, intermittent irritation is more likely to be due to dry eye. Frequency and persistence of headache can give an idea of the type of headache. One-sided headaches that last for a day or few hours may be migraine compared to cluster headaches which last much longer. Intermittent decrease in distant vision is more likely to be due to spasm of accommodation rather than myopia which is more constant. The time of onset of recurrent symptoms can also give a clue to the diagnosis. Ocular irritation and discomfort more in the evening can be due to dry eye. Headache early in the morning on being woken up suddenly can be migraine.

Factors that bring on a symptom or relieve it give hints to its aetiology and management. Ocular symptoms which are triggered when the patient is working in the garden are more likely due to allergic origin and lifestyle modifications may be needed in addition to the medications to manage the condition. A patient saying he has more trouble when watching TV or working on the computer monitor with symptoms being relieved with washing of the eye may be suffering from dry eye. Headaches triggered by the classical triggers like lack of sleep, hunger, anxiety, being suddenly woken up from sleep, etc. can be attributed to migraine.

3.3.2 Associated Symptoms

When a patient complains of a particular symptom, it does not mean he has no other associated symptoms. Sometimes, the associated problem is minor, and it slips his mind during the interview. Often the patient thinks his other symptoms are due to another disease and need not bother an eye specialist with it. History of joint pains could be significant in a patient with dry eye or uveitis; both of which could be associated with autoimmune disorders. A patient on long-term hydroxychloroquine for joint pains could come with complains of decreased vision and may not volunteer to tell us about it. Due to the stigma, patients may not volunteer to inform us about the tuberculosis or HIV infection he has.

3.3.3 Extent of Disability

6/6 vision is not a must for all to lead a comfortable life. Neither is it the only goal for all eye doctors. Knowing what the patient wants to do with his vision and what he cannot manage at present goes a long way in the management of the patient as a whole. A professional driver with posterior subcapsular cataract and a vision of 6/6 may require surgery if his night driving is affected. On the other hand, a farmer who comes for a pair of glasses may be quite happy with his best corrected vision of 6/18 and can wait for sur-

gery. When there is irreversible retinal damage; knowing patients' needs will help us define the goals for a low vision aid.

3.3.4 Rechecking History

After or during the examination, if the history is not consistent with the findings it is imperative to recheck the history. This is especially seen in cases of trauma. Medico-legal implications, traumatic stress and social circumstances surrounding the trauma could all be the reasons why the history may not be right. Getting the history from a witness to the injury may be helpful in such cases.

3.4 Past History

Past systemic or ocular problems could have a bearing on the reason why the patient has come to the eye specialist. Decreased vision in one eye may be related to the squint surgery the patient has had as a child. The squint may have been associated with amblyopia (decreased vision without an obvious ocular cause) and after surgery now only the decrease vision remains. The current divergent squint may be due to the correction of the convergent squint as a child. Past history of recurrent redness and blurring of vision is suggestive of recurrent viral keratitis or uveitis and may give a clue to the current corneal lesion the patient has. Any surgeries the patient may have had in the eye or elsewhere may be relevant. The current episode of central retinal artery occlusion may be related to the heart surgery the patient may have had in the past. Quite often questions on past medical history have to be directed, after having examined the patient.

Working in a tertiary care centre can pose a problem with patients showing you the details of the consultations they have had recently in other places. To see the previous records before one makes, an independent assessment can affect one's thinking process. It also robs one of the pleasure of doing one's own detective work and drawing conclusions! When patients hand you these reports before you ask them, politely tell them that you want to think fresh about their case and do not want to be biased. Patients appreciate that opportunity to be re-evaluated afresh. However, you will have to see all the reports at the end to see if there is a different line of thinking or if you have missed something that your colleague has picked up or there has been a change in findings over time. Humility is not a bad quality especially in medicine!

3.5 Personal History

A knowledge of the patient's profession helps in unravelling some of the patient's visual problems. Decreasing vision in one eye of a patient working in a metal workshop should raise the possibility of an intraocular metallic foreign body which the patient never even felt going into the eye. Patient's lifestyle may have a bearing on the clinical problem. There was a young bank employee who came with anterior subcapsular cataract. Questioning him on exposure to toxic vapours or hot furnaces did not reveal any contributory factors. Finally, it turned out he was using a tanning bed which exposed him to ultraviolet light, and he was not using the recommended eye protection in order to get a tan around the eye too! Dietary habits, history of smoking and dependence on alcohol are all other questions one may need to ask depending on the condition one is dealing with.

3.6 Medical History/Review of Systems

Eye is the window of the body they say, and it is true in more ways than one. There are many systemic diseases and their treatments that affect eye. Eye manifestations of diabetes could be the commonest problem one may encounter in the clinic. In addition, the medications you give may exacerbate or mask systemic illness. If the patient is undergoing an eye surgery, then systemic conditions may have to be kept in mind. It may be a useful practice to enquire about diabetes, autoimmune diseases, pulmonary airway disease, neurological and cardiovascular disorders in patients over 40 years of age. Knowledge about renal functions may be useful in a diabetic.

3.7 Treatment and Allergies

The list of medications the patient is on and the allergies they may have is useful to look for the drug effects on the eye. It will also give us an idea of the other diseases the patient has. Modifications or stopping of drugs like anticoagulants may be needed prior to an eye surgery if it is planned. When prescribing new drugs, drug interactions and allergies have to be kept in mind.

3.8 Family History

Most diseases except trauma probably have a genetic basis. History of similar disease in the family is helpful both for making a diagnosis and predicting the course of the disease. When younger patients with retinitis pigmentosa ask about the future course of the disease, a good guide could be the features of the disease in the previous generation if they have the disease. Progression of diabetic retinopathy could be similar in a family. A family history of glaucoma should make one more suspicious of the disease being present in the patient. Certain practices in the family may also have a bearing on the disease. Consanguineous marriages are more likely to bring out the recessive disease traits. Sun worship could be the reason for the macular scar seen on examination. Family history of a diagnosis of glaucoma is a routine question all patients above 40 years should be asked as a part of the targeted glaucoma screening. Senior members of the family are better at giving family history and if available should be questioned.

3.9 Social History

A doctor's responsibility is more than that of the organ or even the sub-organ they are treating. No man is an island. Every patient and his disease is a by-product of the society they live in. Besides the patient, the health of the society from which the patient comes from should also be a concern to a good doctor. The reason why a person waited and came to you after the cataract became mature in both eyes should be explored. Unhealthy nutritional practice leading to vitamin A deficiency should be explored and flagged to the authorities. An idea of patient's finances and social support system is needed to suggest appropriate treatment when they are not covered by the state or insurance policies. At the end of the interview, one should try to make an assessment of the type of patient you are dealing with and his background.

The amount of questioning one does depends on the presenting complaint. The questions are directed to rule in or rule out diseases and to achieve the other objectives of history taking mentioned previously.

3.10 Documentation and Confidentiality

Ensure, especially in a busy clinic with multiple patients having the same name that the right patient's details are being entered. Entries should be dated and timed. Details of the history can be entered under the various headings given so that it is more structured. If a targeted history (which is what all should eventually aim to take) is taken, only the relevant details need to be entered. As much as possible, use patient's language in the history. Putting it in a way all can understand is acceptable. Besides having space for free text entries in medical records, tick boxes will also help to facilitate entry and also be a reminder system. Documenting signs will be dealt with in chapters they are discussed. Remember that the medical record is also for another doctor who may see the patient in your absence. Confidentiality of the patient records is important.

3.11 History as a Test and Other Issues

As has been mentioned earlier, history is really a test. Unlike the normal tests that come to one's mind, this test is done using two very tempera-

mental and at times unreliable machines, namely the doctor and the patient. It is this unreliability and a false sense of reliability on machines created in the minds of public by clever marketing that has prevented giving history taking its rightful place in the medical management of patients. With no machines to sell, research into its usefulness is also limited! Be that as it may, history taking can be discussed like any other test. Every doctor in training would have experienced that the history we got was very different from what the consultant has elicited. One would have also noticed that patient gives a different history when we repeat the history taking in the ward. One way to minimise this inter- and intra-observer variation is to repeat this history taking. The differences in the story (history) may be due to the difference in interview techniques, patient's confidence, level of sensorium, mood of the patient, recall bias (patient may not recollect a history of trauma the first time it is asked but later he recalls the same), etc. In spite of all these limitations, history continues to be the most important clinical test.

It is often written that only open-ended questions should be asked. That may be a good idea if the patient was a physician himself and there was unlimited time. That is not the reality. Patients do not really know what is important for the physician to know. After the first one or two open-ended questions depending on the answers and the post-test probabilities, it is best to ask directed questions. This directed questioning also keeps the physicians mind focused rather than letting it drift while listening to the answers of the open-ended questions. The counter-argument for missing information that may have come out in response to open-ended question is that the physician would not register its significance any way if he was not aware of it, and if he was aware of the importance of such information it would have been part of the directed questioning!

The balance between documenting what is being said and maintaining a conversation is not easy. Warning the patient that you will be taking down notes will be reassuring.

The role of bystanders/relatives can be very cultural. In some cultures, an entire battalion of relatives and well-wishers will come with the patient. In others, it will only be the patient. After ascertaining their relation to the patient, one or maximum two bystanders may come into your room if the patient so wishes and there is space in your examination room! Getting information patients may not know, like snoring at night suggestive of sleep apnoea or nocturnal exposure of the eye can only be got from people close to the patient. Corroborating history from relatives can also be useful. It is unethical to use underage relative as an interpreter or source of information.

Distractions in the clinic, when with the patients should be minimised. Long conversation on the phone or with a colleague should be avoided and is disrespect to the patient and his time. Apologise for the interruption when you restart with the patient.

Association with a disease is different from causation of the disease. According to the patient's belief system, patients could attribute various reasons for their disease. It is for the physician to decide if factors in the history are the association or causation.

Though examination is discussed after history in all books, examination should start even before one takes a history. As the patient walks into the room, while greeting him, look to see how he is looking at you. Does he fix his eye on you? Does the person have a blank look with roving eye movements? Or does he seem to look somewhere else when he is looking at you (eccentric fixation or squint)? These pre-assessments can be very useful at times.

Over-reliance on investigations partly driven by the industry diminishes the importance of history taking. The rapport one creates with the patient during history taking gives the human touch patients crave for and reduces the chances of litigation.

3.12   Analysing the Interview Result

At the end of the interview, one should figure out the significant positive and negative findings. Some symptoms like red eye may be present in multiple diseases and acquires its significance in the presence of other significant findings like keratic precipitates on the endothelium of the cornea. Try to figure out which part of the eye may be at fault and then think of a few differential diagnoses before planning the examination strategy. In the early days of training, one will not know enough to give the differential diagnosis. Initially try to figure out which part of the eye is at fault and one can slowly build on that. As a rule, think of one diagnosis that fits in with all the symptoms. While in training, play it like a game and see how often you can get it right. Discuss with your teachers and argue with them about the possibilities and do not take 'It is so because I said so' for an answer. The luxury of counterchecking with a senior is something a trainee should use to the maximum.

3.13   Beyond History Taking

History taking and examination time also gives the physician the opportunity to connect with the patient. Making that connection with a fellow human being is also one of the satisfactions we get as clinicians. Making that connect is also necessary to be a successful clinician. The first step towards this is to focus on the patient and not be distracted by the computer or the mobile electronic devices with you. Patient details if any available should be looked at before the patient enters the room. Before starting to make notes look at the patient and ask the first few questions. During the interaction with the patient, try to assess the patient's response to the illness and suffering. 'Alternative medicine' practitioners depend heavily on talking to patients to achieve healing. So use communication in the form of reassurance and encouragement to foster healing. A pet coming towards us and touching us is very therapeutic. Depending on the cultural practices in the area where you work, appropriate touch or a pat can be very comforting to the patient. Humour and laughter in your interaction with the patients can put patients at ease and make the connect. Finally, as mentioned before showing empathy is different from being emotionally involved. Empathy makes the patient feel there is somebody who can understand them and feel their pain.

Clinical Testing

The following chapters will deal with the actual clinical examination or testing. Tell the patient what test you are going to do and why you are doing it. Then proceed to tell him what to expect and reassure him. After the test, tell him the results as they are quite anxious and worried that the test may show some abnormality. For example, before checking the intraocular pressure by applanation you should tell the patient that you are going to check the pressure to see if it is high or low. Then you tell them that the anaesthetic drop you are going to put may sting, and it is put to numb the eye so that when you touch the eye they will not feel it. After the measurement, tell them immediately if the pressure is normal as they will be eager to know.

Visual Function and Its Assessment

People often think that the eye is the organ that sees things in front of us. In reality, the brain is the seeing organ of the body. The eye is only a transducer which converts analogue signals (images of the outside world falling on the retina) to digital signals so that it can be processed by the nervous system to give us the sensation of vision and the ability to the rest of the body to interact with the world view of the brain. In other words, when we stretch out our hand to pick up an object in the outside world, our hand centres are feeding into the vision centres and making adjustments depending on how the brain perceives the world outside. Theoretically, therefore, any electronic transducer (digital camera) bypassing the eye and interfacing with the brain should enable us to see. Will Ophthalmologist then become redundant?

4.1 Visual Processing

The reflected light from object in the environment after refraction by the optical system of the eye falls on the light-sensitive rods and cones of the retina like an image on a screen. There are about 5 million cones (sub-serves colour vision) and 90 million rods that receive the light to be converted to digital form. After a series of interaction within the neuronal layers of the retina, only about 1 million nerves (axons of the ganglion cells) leave the eye as the optic nerve with signals to be processed by the brain. 50–53% of the optic nerve fibres cross over in the chiasm to form the optic tract along with the uncrossed fibres of the opposite eye. It is the nasal fibres sub-serving the temporal half of the visual field that crosses over. The optic tract relays information from the opposite half of the field (right optic tract has information from the left half of the field of the patient) to the neurons in the lateral geniculate body whose axons then form the optic radiation. Fibres of the optic radiation sweep through the temporal and parietal cortex to reach the occipital cortex (area 17) to relay in the neurons there. From the occipital cortex fibre radiate to the secondary visual cortex (areas 18.19) and other control centres of the brain. These connections and processing is complex and not fully understood as yet. Figure 4.1 shows the visual pathway and the field defects caused by lesions at various points in the pathway.

4.2 Attributes of Vision

Visual perception has many complex attributes and testing each of them is difficult. The value of measuring each of them is not known fully and only some of them are tested routinely. Minimum visible (ability to detect small differences in brightness), minimum perceptible (ability to make out the existence of the smallest object in a background), two point separation, vernier acuity (ability to make out a misalignment in two lines),

© Springer Nature Singapore Pte Ltd. 2020
T. Kuriakose, *Clinical Insights and Examination Techniques in Ophthalmology*,
https://doi.org/10.1007/978-981-15-2890-3_4

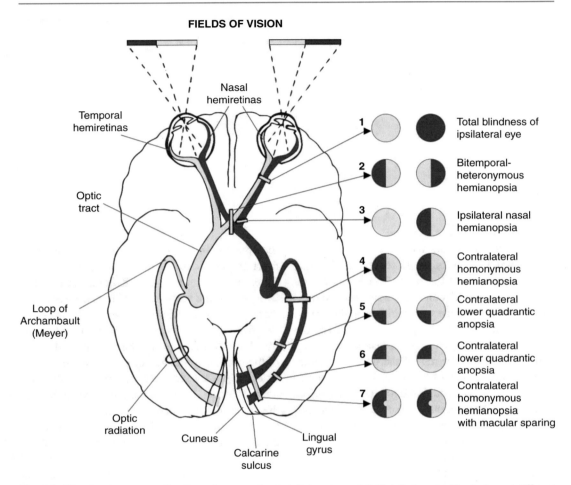

Fig. 4.1 Visual pathway extending from the eye to the occipital cortex and field defects caused by lesions at different locations in the pathway

minimum legible (spatial resolution or sense), colour vision and field (extent of surrounding areas seen at a time) are some of the better known attributes. Some of these attributes even overlap in their function. Except visual fields and colour vision other attributes in an indirect way is measured by the standard visual acuity testing. Visual acuity testing primarily tests the spatial sense or resolution. The three important aspects of vision tested routinely in the clinic are visual acuity, visual fields and colour vision. Binocular field and assessment of stereopsis are two other tests done for specific reasons.

Tests of visual function check patient's perception of the world around. The psyche of the patient therefore plays a role. **Psychophysical**

tests are those tests having a mental and physical component. Visual function testing is a psychophysical test. Since patient's mental status also plays a role, it is not strictly an objective test. One therefore needs to keep this in mind when interpreting these tests.

4.3   Visual Acuity Testing

The ability to make out form is tested by measuring the VA. This is tested using various vision testing charts available that have letters, numbers or figures of various sizes printed on it. The letters of these charts are designed in such a way that their images subtend specific angles at the eye. The popular Snellen chart which assumed normal vision as 6/6(20/20) was actually designed based on a wrong interpretation of Helmholtz study on the visual angles. In fact, according to Helmholtz study on visual grating one should have a vision of 6/3(20/10). Though this was pointed out by Tshering as early as 1898, 6/6(20/20) continues to be regarded as normal vision by many.

4.3.1 Normal Vision

As was alluded to, normal vision cannot be a single value of 1.0, 6/6 or 20/20 depending on the testing notation one follows. 6/6 vision is not even a population-based normal vision. It is interesting that in spite of studies showing that normal vision is better than 6/6, it remains the standard for normal vision one aims for. Calling somebody with very good vision of 6/4 or better abnormal would be counterintuitive. Likewise, it will be very difficult to prove that people with vision of 6/9 is at any great disadvantage compared to those with vision of 6/6. Therefore, anybody with a vision of 6/7.5 or above could be considered as having normal vision. The 6/6 letter just means that what normal people can read at 6 m the patient too can read at 6 m. The large 6/60 letter means normal people can read that letter at 60 m, but the patient can only read it at 6 m distance. The 6/6 letter on the chart was originally designed by Snellen so that the full letter would subtend 5 min of an arc at the eye and each stroke of the letter 1 min of an arc when the letter is kept at 6 m. Therefore, the overall size of a 6/6 letter would be 8.73 mm in size. 1 minute of the arc was chosen with the wrong assumption that it is the minimum resolvable angle by the eye. 6 metres was a compromise reading distance chosen instead of keeping the target at infinity. At 6 m from the source the divergence of rays is −0.16 D instead of the 0 vergence of light (parallel rays) from infinity. The probable reasons why we continue with 6/6 as normal vision is because it is the vision level at which all functions of daily living can be done. It is a level of vision that is easy to achieve after most eye surgeries making

both patients and doctors happy! It has also been noted that the normal vision in the older age group (60 years and above) is 6/6 due to degenerative changes. If the bar of normal vision is raised, there would be more patients who would be mentally unhappy. If the standard of normal vision level is raised, one would also have to investigate all patients with vision of 6/6 or less because they have subnormal vision and that would not yield any useful results. VA we measure is the vision when the retinal image is on the foveola which has only cone receptors that are packed closely. At the fovea, there is also a one-to-one connection to the ganglion cells. Outside the fovea, rods also start to be seen and multiple photoreceptors connect to one ganglion cell. Visual acuity thus rapidly starts dropping if the image falls outside the foveola and reaches 6/60 at the edge of the fovea. In conditions where the fovea is diseased, the vision drops significantly even if the rest of the macula is normal. The graph in Fig. 4.2 shows how visual potential drops as one goes further away from the foveola.

4.4 Vision Checking Charts and Measurement of Vision

Figure 4.3 shows a classical Snellen chart with English letters. Instead of a language letter, one could have Roman numerals or the letter 'E' placed in different directions and patient asked to identify the direction, or Lancelot 'C' where again the direction of the opening of the 'C' has to be identified. The recording of vision here follows a fraction notation where the numerator is the distance at which the letters are being read and denominator is the distance at which a normal person would read that line. America measures distance in feet and the UK in metres. Europe converts this fraction into decimals. Thus, 20/20, 6/6 and 1 all represent the same visual acuity

The problem with the Snellen chart is that the change in size of letters from one line to the next does not follow a linear progression. In addition, the number of letters in each line and the space in between letters is not constant. The absence of linear progression of letters and difference in the

Fig. 4.2 Posterior pole of the retina with the potential for vision possible in each area. Note how the potential for vision drops as one moves away from 0° (location of foveola)

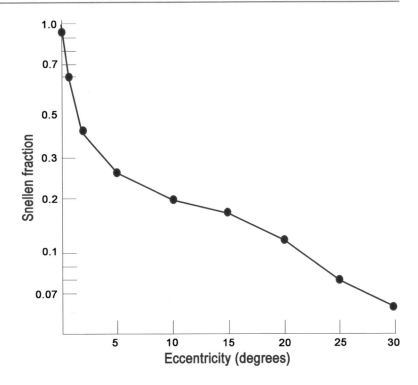

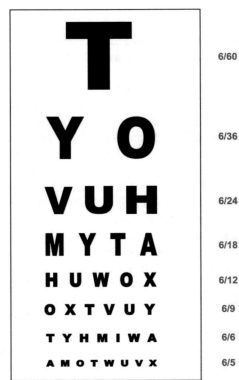

Fig. 4.3 The classic Snellen chart

number of letters in each line makes statistical studies difficult as vision measured with this would not be a continuous variable. Calculating statistical means and related parameters is therefore not possible. Varying the number of letters in each line varied the probability of getting the letters right by chance for each line. The space variation can affect the ability to read letters due to a phenomenon called **crowding**.

To overcome these problems, Bailey created a chart where there was a linear progression of letter sizes between lines and the number of letters in each line was the same. These charts used only letters with equal reading difficulty (H, N, V, R, U, E, D, F, P, Z; Arial bold font) to maintain consistency. The ETDRS (Early treatment of Diabetic retinopathy study) chart is a modification of this and is tested at 4 m so as to save clinic space. Here too the target can be alphabets, numbers, 'E's or 'C's. Picture though possible may not be amenable to the exact sizes in which the letters are drawn. Also in alphabets, there is a difficulty factor in making out the letters, and this is taken into consideration when deciding which letters are used. For example 'I' is a simple letter

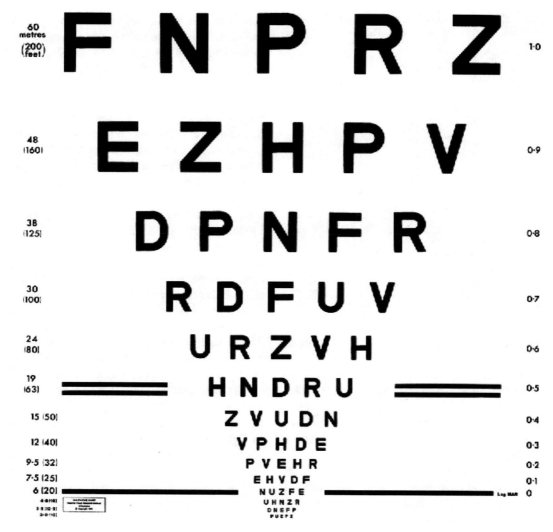

Fig. 4.4 LogMAR chart

to make out and 'B' is difficult. The ETDRS and Bailey charts are called LogMAR charts (Fig. 4.4) because the vision is recorded in log values of the minimum angle of resolution (MAR) and can be subjected to statistical calculations like any other continuous variable. The LogMAR equivalent to all letters read in the 6/6 line is 0. If a complete line is read, then the vision given on the side of the line is taken as the patients' vision. If two additional letters are read on the lower line, then weightage is given as follows. Each single letter read correctly is assigned a LogMAR value of −0.02 log unit and subtracted from the value of the line where every letter was read correctly. If the 6/6 line is read correctly, the vision in LogMAR is 0. Now, if in addition the patient reads 2 more letters in the line below, then $0.02 \times 2 = 0.04$ log units have to be subtracted from 0 and the final LogMAR vision will be −0.04. Table 4.1 from ICO (International Council of Ophthalmology) shows the vision comparison between the different systems.

Due to the variations in the results of vision testing, only a 5 letter or 'one line' difference (using LogMAR chart) in vision can be considered a change in vision when tested again.

Table 4.1 Comparison of visual acuity notations of the more commonly used assessing systems

Visual acuity notations					
Snellen (6/6)	US feet (20/20)	UK matric (6/6)	EU matric (5/5)	Decimal notation (1.0)	LogMAR (0)
6/3	20/10	6/3	5/2.5	2	−0.3
6/4	20/12.5	6/3.8	5/3.2	1.6	−0.2
6/5	20/16	6/4.8	5/4	1.25	−0.1
6/6	20/20	6/6	5/5	1.0	0
6/7.5	20/25	6/7.5	5/6.3	0.8	0.1
6/9	20/32	6/9.5	5/8	0.63	0.2
6/12	20/40	6/12	5/10	0.5	0.3
6/15	20/50	6/15	5/12.5	0.4	0.4
6/18	20/63	6/19	5/16	0.32	0.5
6/24	20/80	6/24	5/20	0.25	0.6
	20/100	6/30	5/25	0.2	0.7
6/36	20/125	6/38	5/32	0.16	0.8
6/48	20/160	6/48	5/40	0.125	0.9
6/60	20/200	6/60	5/50	0.1	1.0

Differences less than that could be just normal biological variations.

The fact that there are so many systems for recording vision suggests that none is perfect. Considering all factors, LogMAR chart is accepted to be the best method to record vision especially when one needs to do statistical analysis.

Besides the letter sizes and spacing the illumination of the chart is also important. LogMAR charts are created so that the space between letters and between lines are standardised. Charts are also available where the light is also calibrated.

Ideally, one should make the patient read from the biggest letter seen down to the smallest possible letter seen. In the clinic, practically patients are asked to read out from the line which has the smallest visible letters. When that is identified, make the patient read from one line above till the smallest possible letters he can see. Tell the patient not to guess. The vision is checked with one eye at a time. It is not correct to occlude the eye not being tested with the hand as one may be able to see between the fingers. It is best to use an opaque occluder. If the vision is so poor that even the biggest letter cannot be read, then ideally the patient should be brought closer to the chart till he can make out the big-

gest letter. Since that can be difficult in a busy clinic, often the examiner's hand is brought close to the patient till he can count the fingers and recorded as counting fingers at the distance finger counting was possible.

For patients who cannot even count fingers, one should look for perception of light, projection of light and hand movements close to face.

Examination of **light perception** (PL) to see if the eye perceives any light at all is important for clinical decision-making. As mentioned earlier, the brain is the seeing organ and it can imagine a lot of things including perceiving light when there is no light! The common phrase 'I saw stars' is not just a figure of speech. One can really see stars if you get knocked on your head. Patients who do not perceive light find it difficult to accept that they do not even see light in their eye and clutches on to every input to try and make out if there is light. Examination for PL should be done in a dark room. The eye not being tested should be closed by the palm and not by the approximated fingers of the examiner's hand so that no light goes between the fingers of the examiner. Patients hand should not be used. A closed eyelid alone is also not enough as light can be seen through closed lids. The brightest possible source of light (usually the indirect light) available in the clinic is used for testing. Patient should be asked to say when he perceives light and it is not a good idea to ask the patient if he sees light just after you have switched on the bright source of light. Your question and the noise of the switch being put on can be hint for the patient to respond affirmatively. It is also not right to bring the light close to the eye as the heat of the light may also be a hint that the light is present and patient may respond to that. The patient should be questioned multiple times with and without the presence of light. The number of right answers (more than 50% of the time) will give an idea if the patient is perceiving light or not. This test in not as simple as one would think it is. This result is recorded as PL +ve or PL −ve.

If one is sure that the patient is perceiving light, then one should check to see if he can say from where the light is coming. One tests the superior, inferior, nasal and temporal parts of the

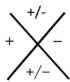

Fig. 4.5 Vision recording of a patient who has inaccurate projection of light in the nasal quadrant of the right eye. The projection is doubtful in the superior and inferior quadrants and accurate in the temporal quadrant

field. If he identifies all quadrants correctly, then it is recorded as 'PR (projection) accurate'. If inaccurate, one should mention which quadrant is inaccurate (Fig. 4.5). Projection accurate in the temporal half of the eye or projecting light to the temporal half irrespective of the position of the light is typically seen in end-stage glaucoma.

Perceiving hand movements need not be better vision than inaccurate projection of light. When checking for hand movements, the hand must not be between the patient and a light source. If that is the case, one is actually testing light perception as the patient will interpret the light being cut out intermittently with the hand as hand movements.

4.4.1 Near Vision Testing

In conditions where the normal human lens accommodative effort is not effective like in presbyopia, near vision needs to be assessed both to evaluate the functional disability and to give the necessary glasses. The near vision charts originally used were devised with the idea of assessing functional vision. To do this, printing blocks used by the printing industry were used to develop the near vision optotype. Progression of the decrease in letter size, the difficulty in reading the print style or the type of letters used were not considerations in deciding on the type of print used. Even the distance at which the patient kept the near vision chart was not fixed. Patients were told to keep the chart at their normal reading distance and read. Jaeger charts and N-notation charts are two popular non-logarithmic near vision charts. The largest letter in the Jaeger chart is denoted as J 11 and the smallest J 1. With the N-notation charts, it is N 48 to N 5. These charts are enough in the clinic setting where one is only

looking to give glasses to improve functional near vision. However, for standardisation and research this is inadequate.

To overcome the standardisation problem, LogMAR charts with logarithmic progression like those for distance vision have been developed for near acuity testing. Since reading is more than just recognising the optotype, it has been suggested that these charts be given a different name. **LogRAD** or **log reading acuity determination** charts will also convey the message that similar LogMAR and LogRAD values are not exactly the same. To standardise the reading distance, these charts come with a string attached to it so that the reading distance can be fixed at 40 cm. For low vision prescriptions, the charts may have to be brought closer. Colenbrander reading charts and RADNER reading charts are two of the standardised near reading charts available.

4.4.2 Vision Testing in Special Situations

The way vision testing is done depends on the objective of the test. The patient's age, mental capabilities and type of patient being tested are factors that decide the testing strategies. An illiterate person will not be able to read the letter or number chart however good his vision may be! An 'E' chart or similar will be required for evaluating a person who cannot read.

Examining vision in normal **children** and those with cerebral visual insufficiency need special skill and require special charts to evaluate their vision. This is discussed in the chapter on examination of the child.

In **low vision clinics,** the idea is not to see if the patient has normal vision or compare the patient's vision with normal people. Here the diagnosis is already known. The objective of vision testing here is to assess the **functional vision** with the objective of using that information to maximise visual function. In other words, the assessed vision decides the type of low vision assistance needed to maximise function. If the functional vision problem is 'not able to read the computer screen', then that is looked at and solutions like changing font colour/size, the brightness, etc. is looked for. The entire assessment is done with the knowledge of the patient's eye pathology, e.g. diabetic retinopathy or retinitis pigmentosa so that appropriate solutions can be found and counselling is given. When indicated special charts are used to assess low vision.

4.5   Pinhole Vision and Other Macular Function Assessments

4.5.1   Pinhole Vision

When vision of a patient tested is less than expected, the first thing to do is to see if the vision improves with pinhole. A pinhole size of around 0.75–1 mm diameter may be the best compromise between having an ideal pinhole and the problems of diffraction at the edge of the pinhole which blurs the image. In a person whose vision is normal without glasses, divergent light from every point on the object of regard is refracted by the eye's optical system and focused back to a point on the retinal image. There is thus a point-to-point representation of the object on the retina (Fig. 4.6). This point-to-point representation is absent when there is refractive error and the image is blurred. With pinhole theoretically only

one ray of light from each point on the object is let into the eye via the pinhole. Thus, irrespective of the refractive state of the eye only a single ray of light from a point on the object of regard hits the retina giving a point-to-point representation on the retina like one sees with appropriate correction. Theoretically, this should give a well-defined image. Practically, there are three problems with this. First, since the number of rays representing a point has been reduced, the contrast/brightness is significantly less. It is this loss of contrast that actually drops the vision with pinhole when patients have macular pathology. Second, diffraction at the edges of the pinhole blurs the image. Finally, even though theoretically only one ray is supposed to pass through, many more pass through even a 0.5 mm pinhole. In patients with higher refractive errors therefore, the defocusing of the small pencil of light that enters the PH is much more than in those with lower refractive errors. This is the reason that visual improvement with PH does not touch even the 6/9 or 20/40 level in high refractive errors. With the degradation due to diffraction, a vision recording of 6/7.5 is what majority of people read with pinhole. If vision improves with PH, it means there is a refractive error that can be corrected to improve vision. On the other hand, if vision drops with PH it means the patient is either not looking through the PH correctly or that the

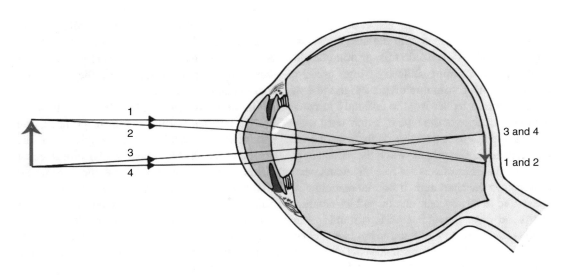

Fig. 4.6 Point-to-point representation of the object of regard on the retina

patient has a macular pathology that is causing the decrease in vision.

4.5.2 Macular Stress Test

At a time when equipment like optical coherence topography (OCT) was not available, photo-stress test was a useful test to see if the patient's complaint was due to a macular pathology. This is more useful if the fellow eye is normal as one would have a comparator. After recording the vision with and without pinhole, the light from a direct ophthalmoscope is shown into the eye and the patient is asked to look at the light for about 10 s. Soon afterwards, the patient is asked to look at the vision chart and asked to read again. The time taken for the patient to read the smallest line read before the light was shown is measured. The light causes bleaching of the retinal pigments and the decreased vision initially. Normally, one should recover within 50 s. If the recovery takes more than 90 s, then the photo-stress is positive and suggest a macular pathology. In conditions like diabetic macular oedema and macular degeneration, the time for recovery is prolonged.

4.5.3 Macular Function Test

Macular function tests were popular tests when cataract surgeries were done only after the cataract was advanced and there was no ultrasound to scan the posterior segment. The idea here is to check the macular function preoperatively to give the prognosis for surgery. When macular function testing is required to be done, besides a brisk pupillary reaction, an easy and practical test that can be done in the clinic is the Maddox rod test. Today with earlier operations and other sophisticated scans to evaluate the macula macular function tests are done rarely.

4.5.4 Maddox Rod Test

The Maddox rod is available as a red wavy lens in the trial set. It is like a set of glass rods stacked one on top of the other. When a bright spot light passes through this glass, a streak of light perpendicular to the stacked glass rods is seen. When kept in front of the eye, a patient with cataract should also be able to see this red line which is continuous without any breaks. In people who are colour blind, the colour may be confusing but the line would still be seen. Normal patients will report no break in the line and will give the direction of the line correctly.

Entopic phenomenon, Haidinger's brush, etc. are other tests described. These are tests not easy to make patients understand and do not add any value. A very useful test which will be described in the chapter on pupil is the checking for relative afferent pupillary defect (RAPD) in the eye with cataracts. If the suspect eye has no RAPD and the fellow eye is healthy, then the chances are that the macula is healthy.

4.6 Visual Fields Testing

Visual acuity predominantly assesses the vision sub-served by the macula or more specifically the fovea. WHO (World Health Organization) defines blindness not only using visual acuity but also the visual fields. The importance of seeing the surrounding areas at the same time as the central area for effective visual function is highlighted by the WHO definition.

When one is examining the fields, one should be aware of the types of field defects possible and the lesions that cause them. Familiarity with the anatomy of the visual pathway (Fig. 4.1) will help localise lesions depending on the type of field defect. From the anatomy it is clear that any pathology behind the chiasm will affect only one half of the field, namely right or the left half. If the field defect is due to a vascular lesion in the eye, it will affect the upper or lower half of the fields. In glaucoma, the fields obey the horizontal meridian because of the arrangement of the nerve fibres which enter the optic nerve from above or below the horizontal meridian. Bringing the testing target along the vertical or horizontal meridian of the eye should therefore be avoided when testing fields. Scotomas or field defects that do not follow these rules are due to pathology restricted to the retina or optic nerve like a chorioretinitis or optic neuritis. Thus from the type of field defect one should be able to tell the possible site of lesion.

In each eye, the normal visual field extends about 100° temporally, 50° superiorly and 60° nasally and inferiorly. Since the temporal field is a 100°, it means that one can even see slightly behind the level of the eye. Confrontation field testing is the classical bedside field testing that is taught. Unfortunately, the classical confrontation field testing has pitfalls and simpler methods of testing is enough to uncover the gross field defects that confrontation test is capable of unravelling compared to the more accurate automated perimeters. Classically, it has been taught that in confrontation method of field testing, one needs to bring the target from the non-seeing area to the seeing area while being seated about a metre away in front of the patient. Sitting a metre away from the patient, makes it impossible to achieve this temporally as one has to go behind the patient to reach the non-seeing area.

Scotoma is a non-seeing area in the field surrounded by seeing area. A field defect on the other hand is a non-seeing area contiguous with the peripheral sea of blindness (the non-seeing area beyond the normal extant of the field mentioned above).

If available, static automated perimetry (SAP) is the current gold standard for examination of the fields. Trying to quantify and delineate a scotoma exactly by clinical examination is a waste of time and effort because its reliability and repeatability is not comparable with SAP. Clinical examination of fields should only be used as a quick screen to detect obvious field defects. Trying to refine it by spending time as described in older textbooks should be avoided. Classical confrontation method of field examination requires the examiner to compare his field with that of the patients. Assuming that the clinician is normal can be dangerous! Screening of visual field in the clinic should not take more than 2 min per eye for a patient. One suggested way to achieve this is to seat the patient about 40 cm in front of you. Closing the patient's eye with the palm of your hand ask if he can see

your face fully or if any part is missing or appear distorted (assuming your face in not distorted to start with!). This is done to check for any central scotoma or metamorphopsia seen in patients with macular lesions. Next, bring the target you are going to use for peripheral field testing (your finger or better still a red bead on a steel pin) into the patient's seeing area so that he knows what to expect. Once the patient knows what to look for, move a bit closer and bring the target from behind the patient's head in the four quadrants (supero-nasally, supero-temporally, infero-nasally and infero-temporally) till the patient spots the target. In the superior and inferior nasal side, when the target is in line with facial bone the patient should be able to see the target. Temporally, if the eye is very prominent one may have to bring the target one finger width anterior to the zygomatic bone; otherwise, the patient will see the target when it is at the level of the Zygomatic bone. Except in cases were the facial bones are absent, this end point is standard and one needs no other reference point like the examiners own fields. The other advantage of testing fields with the target coming from behind the patient and using patient's facial bones as the boundaries of the visual fields is that it can be done at the bedside when patient is lying on the bed. Once the outer margins of the fields are delineated and the patient does not show any obvious field defect, then one should look for simultaneous perception. For this, the patient's own hand or that of the clinical assistant should be used to close one eye of the patient at a time. On either side of the vertical meridian, in the upper or lower half of the field of vision show asymmetrical number of fingers (say two fingers temporally and one nasally) simultaneously and ask the patient to say how many fingers he sees totally. If he sees three fingers, it means he is seeing in both fields. If either one or two is mentioned, then it means he is not appreciating the finger in the other field. Besides fingers one could also use two similar red coloured pins in the two halves of the field. Patient may report that the colour of the pin in one half of the field seem drained out. Simultaneous perception can bring out the more subtle hemianopia in patients.

Binocular field testing is not done for diagnostic purpose. This is done to look for suitability for activities of daily living like driving, etc. and is best to do a field analysis using an automated machine with both eyes open.

4.7 Colour Vision Testing

Colour is not a property of the electromagnetic radiation that causes it. It is a feature of visual perception by an observer. In fact, there are people who perceive colour when the sensory input is sound and not light (synaesthesia). Perception and experience of colour is a complex process thereby making its testing far from simple. There are people who go through a good part of their life not realising they have a problem with colour vision. Testing as part of recruitment for a job or screening for drug toxicity are some of the occasions people realise they have a colour vision problem. From the type, and amount of pigments in the retinal cone, to the neural processing occurring in the brain, all affect the perception of colour. Though there has been some success in classifying the type of colour defect, quantifying change has not had much success. In addition to the problem of the subjects tested, the other problem is colour itself. Anybody who has selected a dress and worn it for a few years would realise how the colour changes depending on the light being used and how over time colour fades. Coloured lights behave differently from coloured pigments. Therefore, difficulty in the standardisation of testing conditions (production of colour plates, deterioration of colour plates, lighting changes) make colour test a crude one.

The primary site for signalling colour differences is the cones of the eye. Normally, there are three types of cones L, M and S which respond maximally to wavelengths near red, green and blue colours, respectively. In congenital colour blindness, defects of the opsins (light-sensitive molecule) in the cones cause defects in colour perception. Absence of these opsins cause protanopia (red blindness), deuteranopia (green blindness) and tritanopia (blue blindness). If there is only small alteration in the opsins, then one gets an anomalous perception, e.g. protanomaly. Tritanopia and tritanomaly are extremely rare. Red and green deficiencies are due to genetic causes and are congenital. Acquired colour vision defects due to drugs and diseases like glaucoma occur in the blue spectrum and are called tritan defects. In optic nerve pathologies, the red colour looks washed out. Many tests are available to evaluate colour vision but the results can be very variable. This inconsistency in the results is the reason for the availability of different types of testing methods. Defining the gold standard is another problem when one wants to evaluate the various tests. Currently, the gold standard for evaluating colour vision is an 'anomaloscope' where subjects try to match the colour on one half of a screen with a combination of primary colours in the other half of the screen.

One can start colour vision testing by first seeing if the patient can name the standard colours by showing them red, green, blue and yellow objects.

Isochromatic Charts or confusion charts are based on the observation that patients with colour deficiencies confuse certain shades of colours. To take advantage of this, plates are made in a way that the target to be made out is in a background of coloured dots with which the patient can confuse the target pattern.

Ishihara's Isochromatic Charts are the most commonly used charts in clinic to test colour vision. This was developed primarily to detect congenital colour blindness. The test consists of making patients read numbers or trace pattern on plates which has coloured dots (Fig. 4.7). Patients with colour defects either cannot make out the number at all or see a different number or pattern according to the colour defect they have. The instruction booklet given along with the plates helps one interpret the colour defect depending on the response of the patient. When using isochromatic charts, it is important that the lighting mimics sunlight. With time these charts tend to fade and that should be kept in mind.

Farnsworth-Munsell 100 hue or Farnsworth Panel 15-D test was developed with the idea that it will better assess acquired colour vision disorders. The 100 hue test is time-consuming and

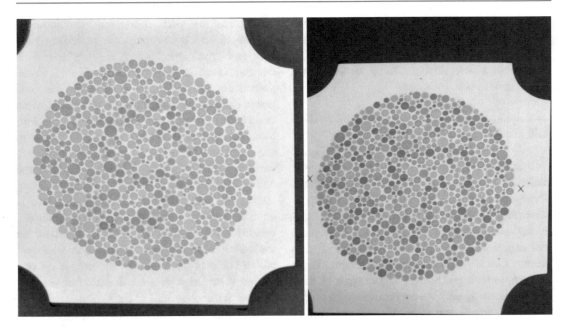

Fig. 4.7 Ishihara's colour testing plate

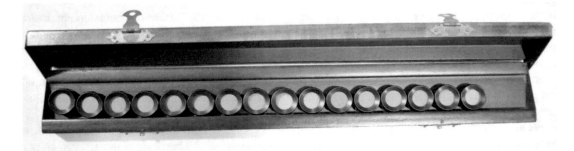

Fig. 4.8 Farnsworth Panel 15-D test with the colour tablets arranged in the right order

fatigues the patients which in turn can make the patient response inconsistent. The 15-D test is easier to do and has only 15 tablets of different hue the patient has to arrange in a series (Fig. 4.8) so that the change in colour/hue is very gradual. The sensitivity of this test is poor, around 50% only.

Another test uses standard pseudo-isochromatic plates. SPP 1 for red green defects and SPP 2 plates for blue yellow defects (tritan). These plates also have dots like Ishihara's charts. The two series plates have a sensitivity and specificity of over 85%. Test like Ishiharas and 15-D hue test have a sensitivity of below

50%. The specificity of these tests however is high. This means with the latter tests we can miss out the patient who has a problem but if a defect is detected then the chances that there is a real problem is high.

In optic nerve diseases, it is worth asking the patient to compare a red coloured object in the temporal and nasal half of the field and see if the colour appears drained out in one half of the field.

Colour vision is tested most commonly as part of screening to recruit for armed forces or other similar jobs requiring distinction of colours. In the ophthalmic clinics, it is done to reconfirm a failed screening test. Testing for colour deficiency is useful for evaluating compressive or inflammatory lesions of the optic nerve. In patients with poor vision and those with nystagmus colour vision testing is used to figure out the underlying aetiology. If the problem is due to an underlying heredomacular degeneration, the patient will have no colour perception.

4.8 Tests for Malingering

When patients come with complaints of decreased vision and no obvious cause for the decreased vision can be found, one has to think of amblyopia or malingering. Malingering becomes more of a possibility if the decreased vision is bilateral and of recent origin. In trying to uncover malingering, the idea is to look for inconsistencies in response from the patients and outsmarting the patient!

If the patient claims loss of perception of light, it is not difficult to make a diagnosis of malingering. In patients with bilateral vision loss, the menace reflex is an objective way to see if the patient can see. One can throw a sudden punch at the patient's face stopping short at the level of the eye to see if the patient blinks or move back in fear. A brisk pupillary reaction will also rule out any real pathology in these patients. The way patient navigates in the clinic will give a clue to visual potential of the patient. Unilateral sudden loss of vision due to no organic cause can be diagnosed with the help of a normal pupillary reaction.

It is only when patients complain of partial decrease in vision that a diagnosis of malingering can be difficult. Here one has to look for inconsistencies in patient's response to individual letters of different sizes and languages presented using the projector chart. When projectors are not available, after going down to the last line the patient can read, the patient should be moved closer to the chart to see if the patient can read the smaller letters, if not then he is probably malingering.

Tests for vision though often done by the optometrist is crucial for making diagnosis and has to be repeated by the physician in case of any doubt.

Evaluating Refractive Error and Prescribing Glasses

5

An important part of examination of the eye in many general ophthalmology clinics is to decide on the power of the spectacles the patient requires in case the patient has a refractive error. In health systems where the optometrist do not have a significant presence it is the Ophthalmologists who prescribe the glasses. Prescribing glasses is not just science but also an art. It needs a certain amount of experience and an understanding of the plasticity of the human brain.

If patients have problems with vision and visual assessment reveals vision worse than 6/6 or 20/20 which improves with pinhole, then one should consider refractive error as a diagnosis and proceed to evaluate the power of the correction required.

5.1 History and Preliminary Examination

5.1.1 History

A patient requiring glasses will usually complain of decreased vision for distance or near or both. Some may complain of eye strain or headache with prolonged visual task. Patients should be asked the circumstances under which they noticed the decreased vision. The age of the patient, history of using glasses in the past, any issues with the previous glasses, profession and requirements of vision are all necessary before prescribing the glasses. A patient in his 40s has to be checked to see if there is any near vision problems. A patient less than 40 presenting with near vision problems may be having hypermetropia. A person who has to do his near work in the upper part of his field like a dentist will need the near segment above rather than below! A person who could not tolerate glasses has to be handled with special care and past problems analysed to ensure he does not have similar problems again. A family history of refractive errors can point to the type of refractive error the patient may have and the potential reason for the same. Patients should be asked about a history of diabetes. Diabetics with uncontrolled sugars should be refracted only after the sugar is controlled for a week at least so that the hydration of the human lens that occurs with hyperglycaemia does not affect the refraction value. History of diplopia (intermittent or constant), past history of trauma to the eye, treatment for squint, lazy eye, etc. should be asked for when relevant.

5.1.2 Spectacle Power Evaluation

If the patient is wearing glasses, one needs to check the power and type of glasses the patient is

© Springer Nature Singapore Pte Ltd. 2020
T. Kuriakose, *Clinical Insights and Examination Techniques in Ophthalmology*,
https://doi.org/10.1007/978-981-15-2890-3_5

wearing. The glass power can be checked by neutralisation of the patient's lenses with an equal and opposite power lens from the trial set. Objects viewed through a plus lens appear to move against the movement of the lens and vice versa for minus lens. There will be no movement if spectacle lens is exactly of the same power as the neutralising lens from the trial set. While neutralising, care should be taken to place, the centre of the trial lens on the optical centre of the spectacle lens. The presence of astigmatism can be detected by rotating the lens in the antero-posterior axis. Astigmatic lens will cause elongation or compression of the image. With astigmatism both axis should be neutralised separately. Incorporation of a prism in the glass can be made out by looking at the figure of a cross. If the cross cannot be centred on the lens and appear shifted, then there is a prism incorporated into the lens. The direction of shift gives the direction of the prism.

The optical centre of the glasses is made out easily by looking at the reflection of the ceiling light on the lens. The point where the reflection from the anterior and posterior surface of the lens coincides gives the optical centre of the lens. A lensometer if available gives the optical centre and the power of the lens in a very short time.

5.1.3 Examination

After the vision examination (Chap. 4), one can do a cover test to look for any phorias or tropias, and this will also help with the muscle balance test done at the end of the refraction routine. One can also shine a torch in the eye to get a view of the anterior segment to see if there are any corneal opacities or there is an intra-ocular lens inserted.

It is best to start the refraction (process of giving correction) with an objective assessment of the refractive error. Retinoscopy or one of the automated refractometers can be used to get an objective assessment. A streak retinoscope is the most useful equipment to do a manual objective assessment of the refractive power.

5.2 Retinoscopy or Objective Refraction

Streak retinoscope is essentially an equipment that throws light into the patient's eye (Fig. 5.1) and at the same time allows the examiner to see the reflexes from the eye to study its character. It has a single filament bulb that can be moved closer or further away from a plus lens to give, convergent, parallel or divergent rays of light. The light is reflected of a mirror with a peephole to throw light into the patient eye. One could ask, does not the Ophthalmoscope also do the same thing? The best analogy to understand the difference between ophthalmoscopy and retinoscopy is the analogy of a room with a key hole. Retinoscopy is only concerned with the light from the room coming out of the keyhole observed from afar, whereas ophthalmoscopy is looking into the room through the key hole for details.

The character of the light reflected from the retina gives us an idea of the refractive error the patient has. In the present day, retinoscopy should only be done with the streak retinoscope invented by Jack Copeland as it not only gives an idea of the spherical error but also the cylindrical error and its axis. Here the light source, a single filament bulb gives light which is like a slit. The filament of the bulb can be rotated 360° by turning a sleeve on the scope. This light illuminates a vertical strip of retina which then acts like a light source.

The physics of retinoscopy is described well in most standard books of optics and refraction and will not be described in detail here. Reading the physics from any standard book on the subject will help one understand the concepts described here better. To understand the physics, one need **not** think about the light being thrown into the eye as it confuses students. With respect to light thrown into the eye, one needs to focus only on the plano (parallel rays)/convex (divergent) mirror light going into the eye. The concave mirror (convergent rays) light only has a historic significance and came into being because candles were used as a light source in the beginning. Light reflected by plane mirrors with a central

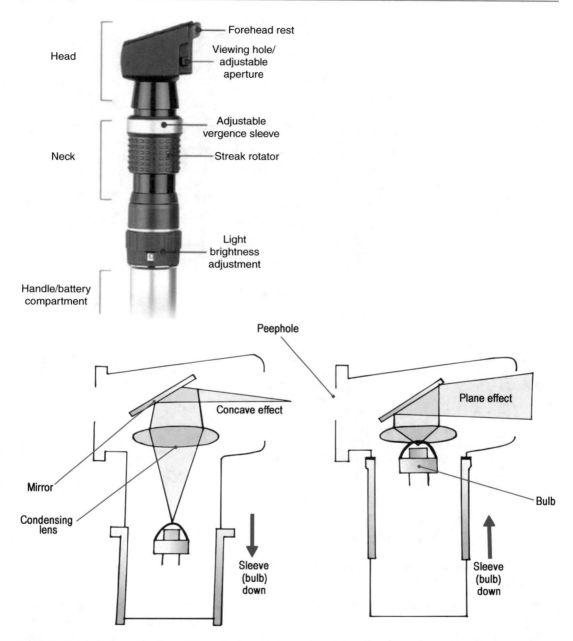

Fig. 5.1 Retinoscope and section of the retinoscope demonstrating its optics to show the position of the bulb to get convergent and divergent rays of light

peephole was weak and one needed concave mirrors to focus more light into the pupil. A dilated pupil likewise also allows more light into the eye. Optically, the concave mirror mode adds nothing to the practice of retinoscopy except for the fact that the directions of the light reflected from the eye is reversed because the position of the incoming light is reversed. It is therefore best to ignore the existence of this option in the retinoscope and ensure that the sleeve of the retinoscope is always

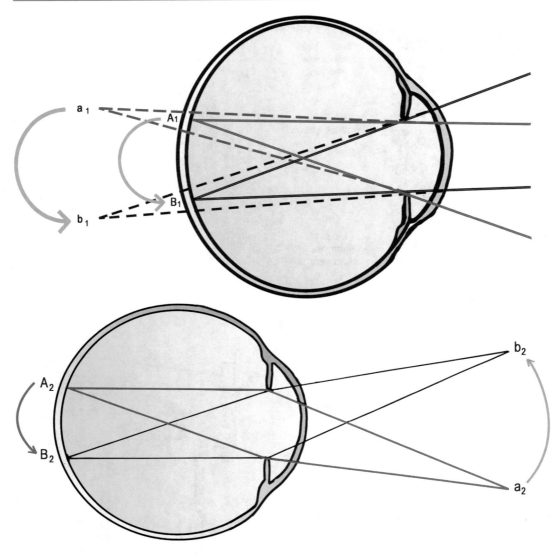

Fig. 5.2 The ray diagram for 'with' a_1 to b_1 and 'against' a_2 to b_2 movement of light in hypermetropia (with movement) and myopia (against movement)

kept in the plano or convex mirror mode while doing retinoscopy.

Now ignoring how the light reached the retina, consider the retina as a source of light (due to reflection of light thrown into the eye) and try to understand the with and against movement from that point. From the diagrams (Fig. 5.2) it will be obvious how as the illuminated retinal area moves from A to B its reflex moves with the light source in hypermetropia and against in myopia. The light thrown into the eye which also falls on the iris and lids is called the **face light** (Fig. 5.3). The part that falls in the pupillary area

goes on to illuminate the retina and reflected back as the **retinal reflex**. The movement of the face light is compared to the retinal reflex in retinoscopy. The retinal reflex that comes through the pupil appears as a bright streak (Fig. 5.3). If the face light and retinal reflex move in the opposite direction, then the patient has a myopic refraction of more than -1 D when the examiner is doing the retinoscopy at 1 m distance from the patient. If the movement is 'with', then the refractive error of the patient is hypermetropia, or myopia less than 1 D. In the practice of retinoscopy, if an against movement is observed,

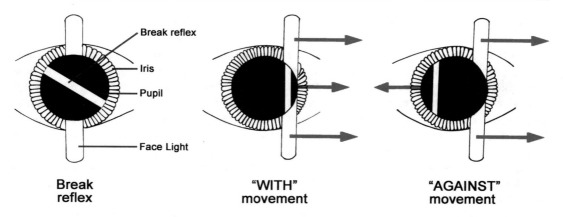

Fig. 5.3 Retinoscopy showing break reflex and with movement and against movement of the retinal reflex

increasing minus lenses are placed before the eye till the end point is reached. For 'with' movement plus lenses are put likewise. The end point is when all the light reflected from the retina gets focused at the point (**far point**) where the examiner is sitting and examiner appreciates the on/off phenomenon. Here all the light from the patient's retina either falls at the pupil of the examiner ('on' phenomenon seen as fully illuminated pupil) or outside it ('off' phenomenon, pupil is fully black) with slight movement of the retinoscope. At the end point, the refractive power of the patient with lenses in the trial frame if any is the dioptric value of the far point. That is if patient is sitting 1 m from the examiner, then the end point is seen when the patient's refractive power is –1 D myopia. If the examiner is sitting at 66 cm (arm length), then the patient's refractive power is –1.5 D myopia (1/0.66) when the examiner gets the on/ off reflex or the end point reflex.

The speed of movement of the reflected streak light, its brightness and width gives an idea of the quantum of the refractive error that needs to be corrected. The further a moving object is from the eye, the slower it appears to move. That is why the moon and the stars appear stationary even though they are moving at great speeds in space. Likewise, the higher the refractive error the further is the far point of the reflected light from the examiner and so movement appears slower. As one approaches the neutral point the speed is so high, it is difficult to make out if it is

a with or against movement. The with movement in hypermetropia is easier to make out because the far point in hypermetropia is further away from the examiner compared to myopia.

As mentioned earlier at the end point, the entire pupil fills up with light. As you go further away from the end point, i.e. when the refractive error gets bigger the width the light reaching the examiner becomes less. The same goes with brightness. As the refractive error increases, since the amount of light reaching the examiner's eye is less and the reflex starts becoming dimmer. It is easy to mistake very dim reflexes as media opacity in patients with high refractive error and one should use a +10 and −10 D lens to see if the reflex intensity increases, unravelling a high refractive power. Thus, the speed of movement of the reflex, its width and brightness give an expert retinoscopist an idea of the quantum of refractive error and will require lesser trial and errors before the end point is reached.

In myopic patients, one could get an idea of the refraction by moving closer to the patient while doing the retinoscopy and see at what point they can appreciate an end point. The distance from the patient at which the end point is reached is an indicator of the refractive error of the patient. For example, if the end point is reached when the examiner is at 25 cm from the patient then the patient has a refractive error of −4 D. The streak light from the retinoscope allows one to refract the different axis of the eye by rotating the axis of the light to the desired angle.

5.2.1   The Practice of Retinoscopy

Retinoscopy is best done with a trial frame and working lens. Working lens is a plus (convex) lens which when placed in the frame gives the end point retinal reflex (on/off) when patient is emmetropic instead of the patient's refraction being −1 or −1.5 D myopia. If examiner is sitting at 1 m, then a +1 D lens is used, at 66 cm, a +1.5 lens is used. The presence of the trail frame and working lens facilitates the use of cylindrical lenses for retinoscopy.

Ideally, the patient should be refracted in a dark room with the patient being asked to look at a dim red light at the plane of the vision charts. This enables the patient to relax his accommodation during the retinoscopy. Cycloplegics or dilated retinoscopy is best avoided unless there is an indication to do so. The non-central reflexes from the aspheric peripheral areas of the dilated pupil confuse the examiner in deciding on the end point. Refracting only the central pupillary area in a dilated pupil can be difficult and unless there are indications for it, retinoscopy is best done with undilated pupils.

Like ophthalmoscopy one should use one's right eye to refract the right eye of the patient and vice versa. This ensures that the light reflected from the macular region is refracted for both eyes.

With the trial frame and working lens in place, throw a vertical streak of light into the patient's eye and move it side to side over the iris. Observe the movement of the reflected light with respect to the face light. Now rotate the streak 90° and move the streak light vertically up and down. If there is difference in the character and movement of the light in the two axes, then astigmatism should be suspected. If the face light and the reflected light are not aligned in the same axis and one observes a break phenomenon (Fig. 5.3), it means that the principal axis is not in the 90/180 axis. The face light axis should then be turned to align with the reflex to remove the break phenomenon and retinoscopy performed in the new axis. Reducing the streak light width by sliding the sleeve into concave mirror mode and seeing what axis the light coincides with the axis

marking on the trial frame gives a good idea of the axis of cylinder.

The more myopic or less hypermetropic axis is neutralised first with appropriate spherical lens. By this strategy what will remain after neutralising one axis is the 'with' movement in the axis 90° away. It is easier to work with, 'with' movements than against. This is not the same as using concave mirror mode to convert an against movement to a with movement. The remaining axis to be corrected can be then neutralised with plus cylindrical lenses kept in the axis noted before.

The end point (neutralisation point) in retinoscopy is a zone of confusion and one need not always get the 'on/off' phenomenon. Quite often, one sees the fully lit pupillary reflex splitting like a stage curtain in the centre rather than going off suddenly. Therefore, it is best not to waste too much time trying to find an exact end point if it is not obvious. At the end point, moving your ahead towards the patient gives with movement and moving back gives an against movement. The zone between a with movement and against movement is the end point. No study has shown that the agreement between retinoscopy (objective refraction) and subjective refraction is good enough to be prescribed directly. In addition, the inter- and intra-observer agreement of retinoscopy is poor. Therefore, time is better spent doing a subjective refraction (described later) rather than trying to find an exact end point with the retinoscope.

Once both axes have been neutralised, removing the 'working lens' should give the **objective refraction** power of the patient. The vision will be good if the retinoscopy value is the same as the real power the patient requires. Since this is seldom the case what follows after this is the refinement of the objective refraction or doing the **subjective refraction**. The subjective refraction done following retinoscopy is different from the classical subjective refraction described in specialised textbooks. In the latter case, the effort is to find patient's power without the help of a retinoscope. This is time-consuming and seldom done nowadays. In this book, subjective refraction will be refinement of the power got by retinoscopy or from one of the many auto-refractometers.

5.3 Subjective Refraction

The subjective refraction is done one eye at a time. With the objective refraction lenses in place first the patient is asked to read as much as he can with one eye occluded. Instead of occlusion there have been suggestions to use a +1.5 D lens to fog the fellow eye during subjective correction. One then proceeds to refine the spherical power of the glasses. For this, a +0.5 and −0.5 D lens is placed in front of the trail frame alternatively and patient is asked with which lens he sees better. Patient can be asked if 'A' is better or 'B' is better. If patient says +0.5 D or A is better, it means the hypermetropia is under corrected and a +1.0 D lens is added to the spherical power. Again a +0.5 D and a −0.5 D lens is put alternatively in front of the eye and the process repeated again till the patient says that neither of the glasses is significantly better. Patient can be asked to look at a letter preferably an 'O' letter on the line above the best corrected vision for this refinement. Once the spherical power is refined then the axis of cylinder is corrected.

Refinement of cylinder is done using a lens called Jackson's cross cylinder which is a cylindrical lens having equal and opposite power kept at 90° to one another (Fig. 5.4). A 0.5 cross cylinder will have a power of +0.5 D cylinder power in one axis and a −0.5 D cylinder in the axis 90° to it. The lens is mounted on a frame with a handle. The cross cylinder works on the principal that when there is a mismatch between the axis of one cylindrical power (patient's residual power) and another cylinder (cross cylinder) the axis of the new cylindrical power will be far away from the existing power deteriorating the vision significantly.

When refining the axis of the cylinder, the cross cylinder is placed such that its cylindrical axis straddles the axis of the cylindrical lens in the trial frame. To do this, the handle of the cross cylinder lens is kept in line with axis of the correcting lens. When the handle of the lens is rotated, the axis of the cross cylinder exchange places. The patient is asked to compare the vision in the two positions and asked to report which is better, A or B. If a minus cylinder is kept in the trial frame, the axis of the correcting cylinder is moved towards the minus axis of the cross cylinder position where vision is better. This movement of axis is continued till patient says both axis of the cross cylinder are equally bad. The power of cross cylinder used; 0.25, 0.5 or 1 cylinder depends on the potential vision of the patient. If the vision anticipated is 6/6 or better, then a 0.25 cross cylinder can be used as the patient will be able to make out the subtle changes caused by a 0.25 cylinder.

After refining the axis, power of the cylindrical lens should be refined. This is done by aligning the axis of the cross cylinder to the axis of the lens on the trial frame. If the +0.5 cylinder part of the cross cylinder is initially aligned to the axis of the lens in the trial frame, by rotating the handle or flipping the cross cylinder the minus axis will align. Again the patient is asked to choose between the two positions. If a plus cylinder is in the trial frame and patient says placing the minus cylinder feels better, it means there is an overcorrection and power of the plus lens in the trial frame has to be reduced by 1 D and test done again till the patient says that with either position of the cross cylinder the vision is equally bad and what is in the frame is ideal. If the cylindrical

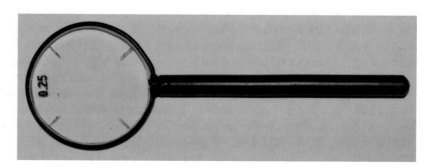

Fig. 5.4 Jackson's cross cylinder to refine axis and power of the cylinder during subjective refraction

power has been changed significantly, then the spherical power will change again. So at the end, after refining the axis and power of the cylinder one should refine the spherical power again if there is over 0.5 D change in the cylindrical power.

A **duo-chrome test** is done after refining the sphere and cylinder. For duo-chrome test, the patients are shown letters in red and green colours and asked which is better. Due to the prismatic effect of lenses on light rays, the red colour is focused further from the lens. As myopia is being corrected, the red letter comes to focus on the retina before the green or blue colour. Since under correction is better in myopes, one can err on the red letter being clearer than the green. Both colours being equally good is also an acceptable end point. In hypermetropia, as opposed to myopia since the aim is to give as much correction as possible it is better to err on keeping the red letters clearer with duo-chrome testing if not equal clarity of both colours.

Subjective refraction and duo-chrome testing are done uni-ocularly. With the correcting lenses in place when both eyes are opened patients usually express a 'ha' feeling appreciating the visual experience with both eyes open. This is because with both eyes working together the visual experience is much better than either eye used alone. Instead of appreciation if the patient expresses unhappiness or doubt when both eyes are open, then one should suspect a problem with binocular interaction and should proceed with the test of binocular balancing and muscle balance. During the time of training, it is a good practice to do binocular balancing and muscle balance for all the patients being refracted. As one becomes experienced, binocular balancing and muscle balance test need not be done for every case as the pre-test probability of having any of these issues is very low if the patients are happier when both eyes are open after subjective refraction.

Binocular balancing is done to uncover any compensatory accommodation the patient is using in one eye that will cause a stress in the long run. The assumption is that the patient may read the smallest letter with the help of generated plus power due to accommodation and this

accommodative effort may be different in each eye when tested separately. The simplest way to uncover the accommodation is to fog one eye by using a +1.5 spherical lens and put a +0.5 D lens in the fellow eye. If the patient's vision has not deteriorated with +0.5 D lens, it means he has relaxed the accommodation being generated internally and this should be given. Same should be done for the other too and this process is continued till the patient accepts the maximum plus. Since this is a laborious process, there are projection charts and screens with letters polarised in different axis. A polarising 'clip on' glasses with both eyes having lenses polarised at right angles to each other is placed before the trial frame and patient is asked if there is a difference in the clarity of letters in the two charts projected simultaneously. If there is no difference, then both eyes are balanced. If one eye is blurred, then plus lens is added to that eye till it is as clear as the other.

When there is significant phoria on cover test or patient is complaining of double vision or worsening of vision when both eyes are open, a **muscle balance test** should be done. Non-specific symptoms and worsening of vision when both eyes are open are again indications for muscle balance test. To do muscle balance for distance, the patient should be asked to look at a distant white spot of light in a dark room. The red Maddox rod available in the trail set is now placed in front of one eye with its lines running horizontally. The patient is asked if he can see a red vertical line. Once the patient appreciates the red line the other eye is opened and the patient is asked the relation between the red vertical line and the white spot. If the red Maddox rod light passes through the white spot of light from the fellow eye, it means there is no horizontal muscle imbalance. If it does not coincide, it means there is a deviation and horizontal prisms depending on the deviation is placed in front of the eye without Maddox rod till the red line intersect the white light. In esophoria/esotropia, the white spot of light will be on the same side as the eye (uncrossed diplopia) and a base out prism has to be used to bring the white light to coincide with the red Maddox rod light. If the Maddox rod is now rotated by 90°, the red line will be horizontal and the white light should again cut it. If not, vertical prisms should be added till there is coincidence. If the white light in the left eye is above the right eye red light (hypotropia of left eye), then the prism should be placed base up in the trial frame. The general rule is that the apex of the prism faces the direction of the deviation of the eye. If a patient is suspected to have horizontal and vertical misalignment, then the horizontal deviation is corrected first with prisms. After this, if required, the vertical deviation can be corrected. Here one eye can be given vertical prism and the other the horizontal. With high prism values, the prisms can be distributed between the two eyes.

After subjective refraction in each eye, patients who have astigmatism that is not in the vertical or horizontal axis should be asked to look around to see if the floor and its edges look normal. If it appears slanting and troubling to the patient, it may be best to move the axis of the cylinder to the nearest vertical or horizontal axis at the cost of some degradation of vision. In patients who are already wearing glasses one should be very careful when changing the axis of the cylinder. It is best to keep the axis unchanged if possible, as the brain gets used to the existing meridional magnifications.

Once muscle balancing is done; for patients requiring presbyopic correction, plus lenses are placed in both eyes and the patient asked to read the near print at the distance he is most comfortable. If there is no history of surgical interventions or trauma, one could give similar plus addition lenses in both eyes simultaneously and check for differences between the two eyes by occlusion. If there is a difference in clarity, then additional powers may have to be given in one eye.

The prescribed glasses need not have the same power one gets after subjective refraction. One may want to undercorrect a myope even further. A hypermetrope may be given an additional plus for the accommodation to relax. Whenever this is done, the patient should be told the reason for doing it, failing which they will be unhappy with the prescription.

The final prescription is given after taking the whole patient and his visual needs into consideration. This need not be the values got after subjective refraction.

Inter-pupillary distance is usually measured by the optician before they make the glasses. The doctor should know how this is measured. To measure the inter-pupillary distance, one can use the corneal reflex of both eyes or the position of the medial limbus in one eye and lateral limbus in the other eye. The optician rule or a transparent scale is kept against forehead of the patient and patient asked to look at the distance. With the patient looking straight ahead, the 0 of the scale is aligned to medial limbus of the right eye using the examiner's left eye. Now, with the examiner's right eye the scale mark which aligns with the lateral margin of the left eye limbus is marked. Similarly, the pupillary reflex of both eyes can also be used as landmarks to make the measurement.

Further Reading

Elkington AR, Frank HJ, Greaney MJ. Clinical optics. 3rd ed. Oxford: Blackwell Publishing; 1999.

The Slit Lamp Examination

6

A slit lamp is a combination of a light source and a microscope. The slit lamp is currently the most important instrument one needs for a proper clinical examination of the eye. If we understand this biomicroscope and its working, one will be able to put it to optimal use and improvise along the way for our clinical examination.

6.1 The Instrument

A slit lamp is the combination of a light source and a microscope. In histopathology, we slice the tissue with a microtome so that light passes through the thin layer of tissue we are interested in and images/reflections from the surrounding tissue do not distort these images. Since most of the tissues in the eye are transparent, with the slit lamp, a thin slit of light (hence the name of the instrument) illuminates only a thin section of the tissue. Reflections from this tissue seen from the side enable us to get optical cross-sections (as opposed to microtome sections) of the tissue which then can be viewed with the microscope of the slit lamp. Slit lamp examination is therefore also called **biomicroscopy**. Theoretically, if we could have a powerful and very thin beam of light; with a very powerful microscope that does not touch the eye we could see cross-sections of the eye much like a pathologist would be able to! The cross-sections also enable us to localise the depth of the lesion which is not possible with spot illu-

mination like the torch. The light of the slit lamp is made into a slit by moving a light stop in front of the light source. The width of the slit can be varied by moving the stop in and out of the path of the light. The light acts like a spot illumination if the stops are moved out completely. When the light housing and the microscope is in the same axis without any angle separating them, it is called co-axial viewing. Here one cannot get a cross-section of the tissue illuminated due to lack of a viewing angle. Retro-illumination is however possible.

Slit lamps having the above features are manufactured by different manufactures; each with their own variations of the control knobs and other features. The Haag-Streit slit lamp model (Fig. 6.1) is what is used here as the prototype for descriptions in this book. Whatever model one uses the clinician should be aware of the controls and functions of the slit lamp one is using to get the maximum benefit from it.

In most of the slit lamp models, besides the width of the beam, the height of the beam can also be altered with the help of another stop. The height of the beam can be read out from the scale on the light housing above the 'filter selector switch' (Fig. 6.1). Lesions up to 8 mm can be measured using this scale. The axis of the slit beam is vertical normally, but this can be made horizontal by turning the top part of the light housing by 90° in the vertical axis. Horizontal measurement of lesions can be made by turning the housing and then measuring.

© Springer Nature Singapore Pte Ltd. 2020
T. Kuriakose, *Clinical Insights and Examination Techniques in Ophthalmology*,
https://doi.org/10.1007/978-981-15-2890-3_6

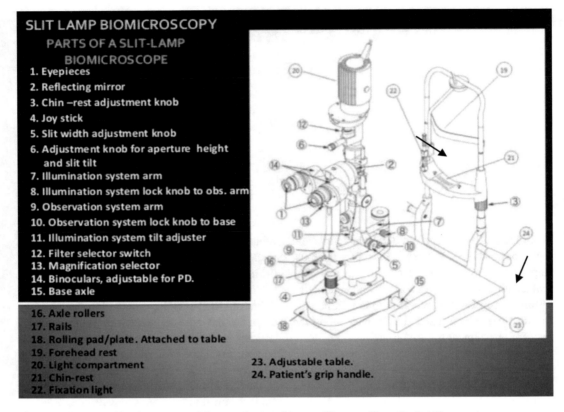

SLIT LAMP BIOMICROSCOPY
PARTS OF A SLIT-LAMP BIOMICROSCOPE

1. Eyepieces
2. Reflecting mirror
3. Chin –rest adjustment knob
4. Joy stick
5. Slit width adjustment knob
6. Adjustment knob for aperture height and slit tilt
7. Illumination system arm
8. Illumination system lock knob to obs. arm
9. Observation system arm
10. Observation system lock knob to base
11. Illumination system tilt adjuster
12. Filter selector switch
13. Magnification selector
14. Binoculars, adjustable for PD.
15. Base axle

16. Axle rollers
17. Rails
18. Rolling pad/plate. Attached to table
19. Forehead rest
20. Light compartment
21. Chin-rest
22. Fixation light
23. Adjustable table.
24. Patient's grip handle.

Fig. 6.1   Slit lamp with microscope and the examination chin rest. (Courtesy Haag-Streit AG)

The light beam and the microscope have a common axis on which they can rotate independent of the other around the eye. This mechanical coupling helps to ensure that the light falls at the same place the microscope focuses. There is an angle gauge at the base of this rotating axis below the 'illumination system arm' that gives the angle between lighthouse and microscope. To get good cross-sectional view, the light housing and the microscope should be about 45° apart. However, there is no hard and fast rule for this and the lesion decides the angle at which it is best seen. The light hits the eye from one side and illuminates a slit cross-section of the structure of interest say the cornea (Fig. 6.2). The cross-section is viewed by the microscope from the opposite side to see the optical section. If the viewing angle is small, then the ability to see from the side is also decreased. Limited independent movement of the lighthouse alone (without moving the lamp arm) is possible in the vertical axis. This independent

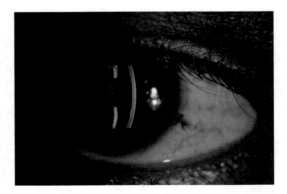

Fig. 6.2   Slit illumination of the cornea with light coming from left side of the patient

movement of the lighthouse enables us to have a different viewing angle.

The play of light and shadows in different viewing angles, as the light moves gives us clues to the pathology seen. This is **dynamic slit lamp biomicroscopy** and is more useful than fixed angle viewing to pick up subtle lesions, especially in the cornea. The joystick of the slit lamp enables us to move the whole slit lamp assembly forward, backward and from side to side.

At 5° angular separation of the light housing and the microscope, there is a clique sound to enable the examiner to set the viewing angle at this point. This viewing angle helps the light reach the deeper structures like the posterior vitreous and the retina without the light being cut out by the pupillary margin and at the same time giving a slightly off, co-axial viewing.

The beam of light can also be moved slightly on either side from the area of interest to enable viewing of structures with scattered/internally reflected rays from the off axis light. The whole light housing can be tilted anteriorly so that light appears to be coming from inferior to the viewing axis. This is useful to examine the posterior vitreous. When examining the posterior vitreous, due to the restriction of the pupil size the lighthouse cannot be moved beyond 5° off axis if light and the line of view of the microscope have to reach the posterior pole. Tilting the lamp housing forward can be done to give additional 'off axis' viewing in the vertical axis.

The light housing also has filters, whose colour highlights features of the tissue depending on its light absorbing and reflecting characteristics. The filters can be moved into place with the appropriate knobs on the machine. The 'red free' filter which has a greenish colour highlights the red (blood vessels) by appearing as black against a green background. Red-free light is also useful to study the nerve fibre layer of the retina. The nerve fibre layer reflects red-free light well and gives a bright fibrillary appearance when the nerves are intact compared to areas with unhealthy nerve fibres which appear dark.

The grey filter in the light housing reduces the glare for the patient and for the examiner and delineates lesions better if there is associated glare-related noise.

The cobalt blue light is used when using the fluorescein stain. Fluorescein stain absorbs high energy blue light which stimulates the electron to go into a higher unstable orbit. When the electrons fall back to its stable orbit, it emits light of

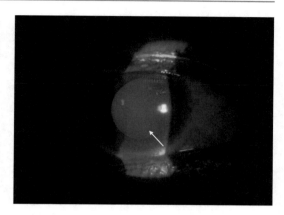

Fig. 6.3 Circular iron line on the cornea delineated as a dark area—white arrow

lower energy (green) that is seen as fluorescein staining which is bright green in colour. The colour also depends on the dilution of the dye. Concentrated dye looks blackish brown, as it gets diluted it becomes progressively reddish brown, green and yellow colour. This is the basis for the Seidel test to look for leaking aqueous.

The cobalt blue light is also used to delineate the iron lines of the cornea like Fleischer ring seen in keratoconus. The iron line looks dark against the blue background of the reflected light (Fig. 6.3).

The slit lamp also has a provision on it to fix the applanation tonometer to measure intraocular pressure. Though not used nowadays, this same provision is used to attach a corneal thickness measuring apparatus (optical pachymeter). Various types of laser delivery units can also be attached to the slit lamp for treatment.

6.2 Setting up the Slit Lamp

6.2.1 Microscope Setting

The light coming out from the microscope eyepiece of the slit lamp is parallel. That means, the examiner should look as though one is seeing distant objects rather than something close to you. If the examiner is emmetropic, then the eyepiece power is set at zero in both eyes. If not, one should use their distant correction glasses or set the eyepiece power of the microscope to the refractive error of the examiner by rotating the eyepiece to the required power marked on the eyepiece. Astigmatism cannot be corrected however. Once the eyepiece power is set, the distance between the eyepiece is set to get a binocular single vision (BSV) and stereopsis. To get BSV, a paper with a dot on it (or any appropriate target like the palm of the hand) is kept in front of the eyepiece at the chin rest. One eye is closed and with the other eye make sure the dot on the paper is in the centre of the field. Now close the viewing eye and open the fellow eye to see if the dot is in the centre of that eye field as well. If not, the eyepiece is moved in or out till the spot comes to the centre. Now open both eyes to check for diplopia. If there is no diplopia, then the eye is having BSV. For the more experienced examiner, the appreciation of stereopsis while adjusting the distance between the eyepieces gives the end point.

6.2.2 Checking Parfocality

To ensure that the light focus from the lighthouse intersects the point of focus of the microscope, the two are mechanically coupled around one axis. However, it is not necessary that the focal point of the light from the slit lamp (the point where the slit is the sharpest) is at the same point as the focus of the microscope. The microscope is said to be parfocal if both points are the same. To check the parfocality, the manufacturer gives a rod that is fixed in a slot above the illumination system arm (Fig. 6.1). The thinnest slit possible is projected on to the flat surface of the rod; once the slit is the thinnest the examiner views the slit through the microscope to see if it is well focused. If the slit is not in focus, then one should change the power of the microscope eyepiece by turning the eyepiece, one eye at a time till both eye sees it in focus.

Once the microscope magnification (set at the minimum to start with), binocularity and parfocality are set then one is ready to examine the patient. It is also important that one familiarises oneself with all the knobs so that they can be adjusted even while the examiner's eye is focused on the patient.

6.2.3 Unlocking the Slit Lamp

The slit lamp should be kept in a locked position at the end of an examination so that the microscope and light housing do not hit the head rest or move around while cleaning the room and equipment. To lock the slit lamp, tighten the screw on the horizontal steel bar (base axle) (Fig. 6.1) on which the whole assembly moves on the table. Before examination the screw should be loosened to ensure that the base of the SL is moving freely on the base plate with the help of the joystick. The examiner's chair should be at the right height and intensity of the light for examination should not be kept at the highest when one does the examination.

6.3 Examination of the Eye

Slit lamp examination is done after taking the history and examining the ocular motility, lids, adnexa and anterior segment with the torchlight. The pupil examination is best done before the slit lamp examination. One should resist the temptation of doing a slit lamp examination directly without an initial torchlight examination of the face and the eyes. Important features like a squint or a proptosis will be missed with a slit lamp. If a corneal pathology is not suspected, then a drop of local anaesthetic can make the examination more comfortable for the patient. The slit lamp examination is best done with the room dimly lit or darkened for better appreciation of the pathology. The lights must be turned off if one is checking for cells and flare in the anterior chamber. Fluorescence is also better seen with dim light.

Seat the patient in such a way that his chin rests comfortably on the chin rest, and the eye is at the level of the black line marked on the vertical support of the chin rest frame. The height of the chin rest can be changed by turning the chin rest adjustment knob on the chin rest frame (Fig. 6.1). The forehead of the patient should rest against the headband of the chin rest to get a clear view of the area examined. For patients who tend to take back their forehead, a bystander or a physician assistant can help keep the head in place.

The patient should also be told that what is being done is examining the eye with a special light and magnification to get a better view into the eye. Patients are anxious when with a doctor; informing them what you are about to do will make them relaxed and more cooperative for the examination. In some patients who are sensitive; the bright light of the slit lamp induces a sneeze reflex (**photic sneeze reflex**) mediated by the trigeminal nerve. This should not startle the examiner nor upset him that the patient sneezed. The clinician should be aware and the sneeze reflex usually stops after one or two sneezes. Rarely, some patients keep sneezing intermittently during the examination.

6.3.1 Examination Using Focal/ Diffuse Illumination

Using the focal illumination is like a refined torchlight examination. The 'light stops' both vertical and horizontal are fully open and a spot of light illuminates the area of interest. The magnification is kept at minimum so that large areas can be seen at a time. If the glare is too much, one can use the grey filter to see the details better. As you observe through the microscope, progressively scan through the lid margins, ocular surface and then the anterior segment. During the examination, one should also have an idea as to what one is looking for. Common sense would dictate that one would see a lesion automatically if it is there. This however is not true. It is easy to miss lesions if you are not looking for them. Some of the more subtle lesions are not seen due to the reflections of the focal illumination.

6.3.2 Examination Using Sclerotic Scatter

Some lesions like subtle corneal oedema and opacities may not be detected by direct illumination. To see these lesions clearly, light is shown at the limbus with the lighthouse kept as far apart from the microscope as possible. One can decouple the lighthouse from the microscope to move

the light 'off' centre by turning the knob above the illumination system tilt adjuster (Fig. 6.1) and rotating the lighthouse. When the light is shown at the limbus of the cornea or away from the area of interest, the light passes through the cornea by total internal reflection and is also scattered by its stroma. Subtle lesions like corneal oedema and opacities are seen best against this lighting.

6.3.3 Examination Using Slit Illumination

Once a lesion is detected the illumination is made into a slit so that one can make out its cross-sectional characters like its depth, height, extent, etc. This is especially useful for lesions in the transparent structures like the cornea and lens. The slit also reduces the reflection from surrounding structures thereby enhancing the view of the area of interest. Doing a **dynamic biomicroscopy** by moving the slit across the anterior segment sometimes shows up lesions that may not be appreciated by fixed viewing. The wider the angle between the light beam and the microscope better is the cross-sectional view. An angle of 45° is ideal for most examinations. To look at the more posterior structures like the lens and vitreous the angle between the microscope and the lighthouse needs to be reduced so that the light does not get cut by the pupillary borders. Thick slit sections also can be useful in some situations.

6.3.4 Examination Using Indirect Illumination

This strategy is used to examine corneal lesions. Most of the information got by this can be gleaned while doing a dynamic biomicroscopy also. Here the lighthouse is decoupled from the microscope and moved slightly away from its line of sight as mentioned above. The scattering of light from the adjacent tissues and the light reflected from the deeper iris make some subtle opacities clearer.

6.3.5 Examination Using Retro-Illumination

Keeping the lighthouse and the microscope at 0°
separation or in the same line (co-axial illumination) makes the reflected light come directly back
into the examiner's eye. To perform retro-
illumination, the light is thrown into the pupillary
area near its margin. The light enters the pupil,
hits the retina and choroid and gets reflected back
giving the pupil a red glow. In the background of
this red glow, one can see opacities in the media
as blackish discoloration. It also gives an idea as
to how much light is blocked by the opacity. This
is especially useful for assessing posterior capsular opacities and corneal opacities. The reflected
light from the fundus will also reveal trans-
illumination defects of the iris (Fig. 6.4). In
lightly pigmented race trans-illumination defects
may also be seen in conditions like pseudo-
exfoliation syndrome and pigmentary glaucoma.
To look for patency of peripheral iridectomy in
coloured race, peripheral iris trans-illumination
is sometimes better seen when the angle between
the microscope and the light housing is kept at 5°.
When light is shown on the iris, lesions can be
seen on the cornea against the reflected light from
the iris.

6.3.6 Examination Using Specular Reflection

At the interface of media of different refractive
indices, light gets reflected and follows the laws
of reflection studied in physics. The air-tear film
interface and cornea-aqueous interface are two
smooth surfaces where images formed by reflections can be observed. Reflections from the tear
film can be easily seen as a multi-coloured oily
layer (due to meibomian secretions) when the
angle of incidence is equal to the angle of observation. At the cornea-aqueous interface the corneal endothelium is not seen so easily because
the reflected light is just about 20% of the incident light. To appreciate the endothelium clearly,
one should first use the highest magnification
possible. Specular view of the endothelium is a

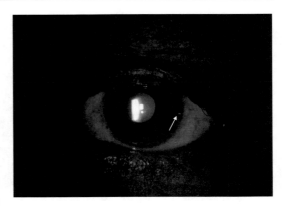

Fig. 6.4 Trans-illumination of the iris seen on retro-
illumination in a patient with peripheral iridotomy—white
arrow

uni-ocular phenomenon. To increase magnification, one can change the eyepiece of one eye to
the ×16 eyepiece. With the light kept at an angle
of 60° and the slit beam made to about 4 mm in
height and 1 mm in width the light is shown on
the eye. When the light is shown on the cornea,
one can see the cornea and iris illuminated. One
can also see the reflection of the bulb of the slit
lamp in an adjacent area. Focusing on the deepest
layers of the cornea, the slit beam is now moved
till it coincides with the reflection of the bulb on
the cornea. At this stage, the endothelial cell
mosaic will come into view as a bright reflected
image (Fig. 6.5). To see the cells more clearly,
one can rotate the ×16 eyepiece till the endothelial cell mosaic is seen clearly. The edges of the
cells appear as dark lines because the light
reflected from here does not come back to the
eye. The density of the cells, its shape and pleo-
morphism should be observed.

6.3.7 Examination of the Anterior Chamber

The space between the cornea and the iris is optically transparent as there is nothing particulate to
reflect the light. However, when there is inflammation of the iris, proteins and cells leak into the
anterior chamber and this can be appreciated
with the slit lamp. The light reflecting from the
protein shows the path of the light much like the

Fig. 6.5 Specular reflection of the endothelium showing a slit lamp-magnified view of the endothelium seen in the reflection

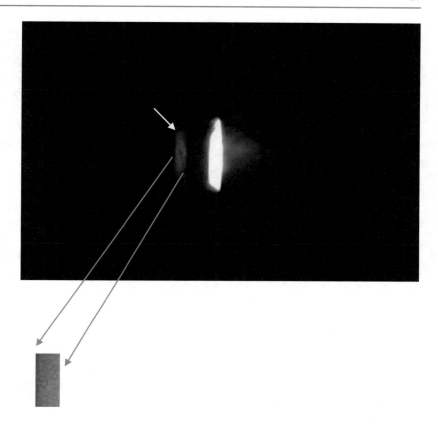

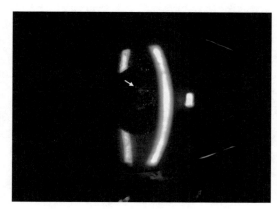

Fig. 6.6 Pigments seen in the path of the slit beam in the anterior chamber (white arrow)

Table 6.1 SUN grading of cells and flare in the anterior chamber using the 1 mm beam of a slit lamp

Grade	Cells	Flare
0	<1	None
+0.5	1–5	
+1	6–15	Faint
+2	16–25	Moderate
+3	26–50	Marked
+4	>50	Intense

Slit lamp beam field size: 1 × 1 mm²

light beam of the car at night on a dusty road. This is called **flare**. **Cells** which are much larger reflect the light and can be seen as white dots moving around in the AC. Vitreous strands and pigments in the anterior chamber can also be seen in the slit beam (Fig. 6.6). Since the aqueous move in the AC due to thermal currents, the cells can also be seen to be moving up near the cornea and in the reverse direction closer to the iris. Flare and cells are best seen with the room totally dark so that extraneous light does not remove the contrast. The light is kept at a 0.2 mm circle size and the illumination is kept at the brightest. Depending on the amount of cells and flare in the anterior chamber, it can be recorded as shown in Table 6.1. For this classification, a 1 mm circular pencil of light is used. Pigments or blood can be seen as coloured spots in the anterior chamber. If there is excess of cells in the anterior chamber, it settles down at the bottom of the anterior chamber and is called **hypopyon**. Similarly, if blood collects it is called **hyphaema**.

The distance between the cornea and the iris gives an idea of the depth of the chamber and if it is regular, etc.

6.4 Slit Lamp Examination in Difficult Situations

For the big-chested patients, it is difficult to get the head close to the chin rest. The height of the chair can be increased in these cases and patients are asked to lean forward so that the chest do not come in the way. For patients with a stiff neck like in ankylosing spondylitis, the chin rest is done away with by lowering it fully and only the headband is used to rest the forehead. The slit lamp can also be brought forward much more than normal to get a view. Details on how an infant is examined by a slit lamp is given under examination of the child. The flying baby position is used to examine a baby.

Though not ideal, a portable slit lamp can be used for the patients who cannot sit at the slit lamp for examination.

The slit lamp though a wonderful machine in itself may have a limited role in the near future with the availability of cheaper OCT machines. OCT is a better in vivo microscope than the slit lamp. The day may not be far off when every Ophthalmologist will have an OCT machine with an image enhancing camera in their examination room. The slit lamp then may become the screening tool! The day may not be far off when after the initial assessment, photographs of the areas of interest and OCT cross-sections of the various structures would be taken as part of the routine evaluation by the clinician. This will also be part of the EMR with clinician's comments or labels on it. Of course, the history will still need to be taken!

6.4.1 Examination Using Lenses

Contact and non-contact lenses are used in conjunction with the slit lamp to see areas that cannot be seen just with the slit lamp. Its use will be discussed in the appropriate sections of this book. Gonioscopy lenses to see the angles and three mirror lenses to see the fundus are the usual contact lenses used. The 78 D (dioptre) and 90 D lenses are non-contact lenses used to see the fundus. Before using the lenses, tell the patients what you are going to do and the reason for doing it. When possible, it is better to do non-contact lens examination of the fundus before the contact lens examination so that the retina can be seen clearly.

To reiterate, slit lamp examination should be done in conjunction with the torchlight. The latter gives an over-view of both the eyes. Slit lamp shows the details. Slit lamp examination is a must and the expense of the equipment cannot be a reason for not doing this examination in any hospital setting. In remote areas with very poor medical facilities and for beside consultation, the torchlight with a magnification like a loupe may have a role.

Diseases of the lids and adnexa is not uncommon and can present in unexpected ways to the outpatient clinic of an Ophthalmologist. Orbital involvement is rare and examination strategy is different. The obvious function of the eyelid for a layman would be the protection of the globe. While protecting the eye from too much light and injury is important, the eyelid has a big role to play in maintaining good vision by way of ensuring adequate resurfacing of the cornea with tears and maintaining the tear drainage by pumping tears out of the eye. By making the palpebral fissure into a thin slit, a near pinhole effect is produced and one can improve the vision in ametropia.

The tear production is sub-served by the lacrimal glands. The passage of tears from the eye to the nose via the canaliculus, nasolacrimal sac and ducts is facilitated with the help of the pump mechanisms.

The orbit encases the eyeball, muscles moving the globe, fat, nerves and blood vessels. The eyeball which literally floats in the orbit to enable quick eye movements is protected by the orbit like a jewel!

7.1 Applied Anatomy of Orbit

The orbit has bony outer wall except anteriorly to keep the eyeball protected. In addition to the eyeball, the orbit has muscles, fat, fascia, nerves,

blood vessels and most of the lacrimal apparatus. The orbit is made up of multiple bones that is also a part of the cranium and facial bones. Each orbit is pear shaped with the optic nerve canal being the stalk. The anterior part of the bony orbit which is open is covered by the orbital septum and the eyelids. The anterior opening is about 40 mm wide and 35 mm high. It is 40–45 mm deep. The orbital volume in an adult is about 30 cc. It is much smaller in a child and grows along the growth of the eyeball. Absence of the eyeball stunts the growth of the orbit.

Table 7.1 gives the names of bones that form the four walls of the orbit. The **superior orbital fissure** separates the superior wall from the lateral wall in the posterior part and is connected to the middle cranial fossa (Figs. 7.1 and 7.2). The **inferior orbital fissure** separates inferior wall from the lateral wall posteriorly and is connected to the pterygo-palatine fossa and infero-temporal fossa. At the apex of the orbit in the sphenoid

Table 7.1 Orbital walls and the bones constituting them

Wall	Bones forming the wall
Medial	Ethmoid, lacrimal bone, frontal process of maxilla, sphenoid body
Inferior (floor)	Orbital plate of maxilla, zygomatic bone, orbital bone of palatine
Lateral	Zygomatic bone, greater wing of sphenoid
Superior (roof)	Orbital plate of frontal bone, lesser wing of sphenoid

© Springer Nature Singapore Pte Ltd. 2020
T. Kuriakose, *Clinical Insights and Examination Techniques in Ophthalmology*,
https://doi.org/10.1007/978-981-15-2890-3_7

Fig. 7.1 Left orbit showing the structures passing in and around the superior orbital fissure. *LPS* levator palpebrae superioris, *SR* superior rectus, *SO* superior oblique, *MR* medial rectus, *IR* inferior rectus, *LR* lateral rectus, *III*$_{sup}$ superior division of oculomotor nerve, *III*$_{inf}$ inferior division of oculomotor nerve, *IV* trochlear nerve, *VI* abducens nerve, *SOV* superior ophthalmic vein, *n* nerve

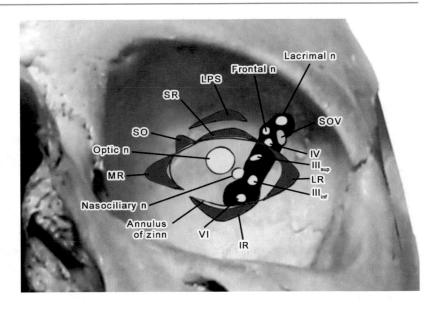

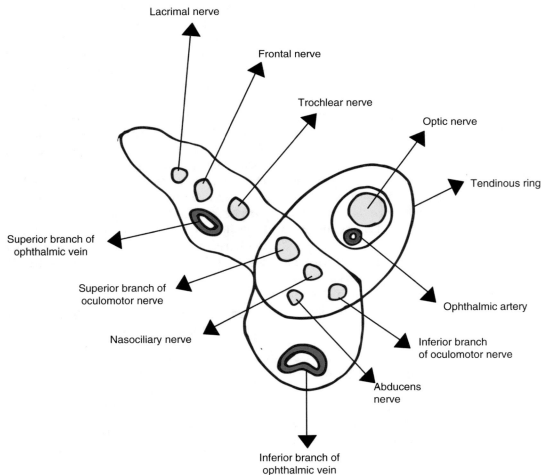

Fig. 7.2 Pictorial representation of the right orbital apex

bone lies the **orbital canal**. Most of the nerves and blood vessels supplying the eye and the orbit come through the orbital apex via the optic canal, superior orbital fissure and inferior orbital fissure (Figs. 7.1 and 7.2). The infra-orbital nerve from the maxillary division of the trigeminal traverses the floor of the orbit in its canal to come out on the anterior surface of the maxilla 5 mm below the rim to supply the cheek. The bones of the orbit are covered by periorbita that is continuous with the covering of the bones outside the orbit. The periorbita can temporally halt infections and infiltrative tumour coming into the orbit from surrounding tissues. It gives rise to the orbital septum in the front; the **common tendinous ring** posteriorly from which the recti originate; encloses the lacrimal sac and also form the tissue over which the superior oblique passes in the trochlea. The medial walls of the two orbits are parallel to each other, and the lateral wall is at 45° to the medial wall.

All the four recti muscles of the eye originate in the common tendinous ring and pass forward to insert on the globe. These muscles along with the inter-muscular septum form the **muscle cone**. Important blood vessels and nerves, second cranial nerve (CN), third CN, branches of fifth CN, sixth CN and ciliary ganglion lie within the muscle cone. Fourth CN and branches of nasociliary nerve travels outside the cone.

The superior, medial and inferior orbital walls are related to the frontal, ethmoidal and maxillary sinuses, respectively. Diseases in the sinus especially the ethmoid which has a thin bone separating it can affect the orbit. The orbit opens posteriorly via the optic canal, and superior orbital fissure to the cranial cavity. Anteriorly through the nasolacrimal fossa it opens to the nasal cavity.

7.1.1 Orbital Spaces

For diagnostic and surgical purposes, the space behind the orbital septum within the bony wall is divided into subperiosteal space, peripheral or extraconal space, central or intraconal space and sub-tenon's space (Fig. 7.3). The intra- and extra-conal spaces are connected at the apex. The space in front of the orbital septum between the septum and the lids is called the pre-septal space.

The **subperiosteal space** lies between the periosteum and the bony orbit and tries to restrict the spread of infection and tumours. Dermoid cyst, haematomas, mucocoele, subperiosteal abscess, bone tumours, etc. are seen in this space.

The space between the periosteum and the recti muscles bound anteriorly by the orbital septum is called the **peripheral or extraconal space**. Lymphomas, capillary haemangiomas, lacrimal gland tumours and pseudotumours are the more commonly seen tumours in this area. In addition to the forward push, depending on the location, lesions in the above space cause a shift of the globe to a side.

The space within the four recti muscles bound anteriorly by the insertion of the tenon's capsule is the **intraconal space**. Cavernous haemangioma, neurofibromas, lymphomas, meningiomas and optic nerve gliomas are some of the lesions seen here. Though masses in the intraconal space can shift the globe sideways, they are more likely to produce an axial (forward pushing) proptosis.

Lymphatic drainage if any of the orbit has not been defined.

The space between the orbital septum and the lid tissue is the **pre-septal space**.

7.2 Applied Anatomy of the Lid

The eyelids are a mobile curtain to protect the eyes when not in use. The space between the upper and lower lids is called the palpebral or **inter-palpebral fissure** (IPF). The IPF is widest in the centre in the orientals but more medially in the other races. The adult IPF is about 26–30 mm long and 8–11 mm in width in the widest portion.

The eyelid is complex in its structure and function. A good understanding of its anatomy will help in diagnosing the underlying pathology. Unlike cataract one has to analyse the signs and symptoms to understand the disease process. The role of gravity has to be kept in mind when analysing the reasons for the observed pathology.

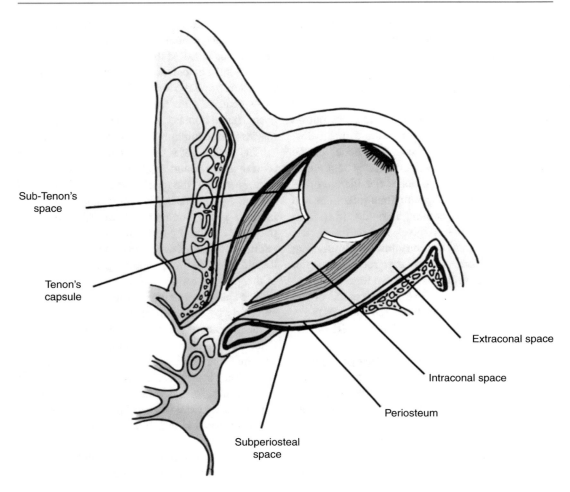

Fig. 7.3 Surgical spaces of the right orbit

The upper lid is much wider than the lower lid and does bulk of the corneal covering when the eye is closed. The lower lid moves up only about 2 mm on lid closure. In addition, due to the **Bell's phenomenon** (the upward rotation of the globe during lid closure), the lower lid does not really play a part in covering the cornea when the eye is closed. The lower lid is however important in tight lid closure of the eye, protecting the lower conjunctiva and for the drainage of tears.

The multilayer arrangement of the lid is obvious on looking at its cross-section (Fig. 7.4). The **skin** of the lid that extends till the lid margin is the thinnest in the body and enables quick stretching during lid closure. There is no subcutaneous fat in most human races. The other parts of the body having a near similar skin to the lid for grafting are the prepuce, labia, supra-clavicular area and back of the ear. The skin of the lid has fine hair with sebaceous glands. In the upper lid, fine strands of the levator palpebrae superioris (LPS) tendon get inserted into the skin; mainly in the region of the lid crease and below in front of the tarsal plate. In the oriental races, the skin insertion of the LPS is much lower down in front of the tarsal plate.

Just beneath the skin is a loose areolar **connective tissue layer** that can collect fluid easily and make the eyelid look puffy. It has only fine blood vessels and no fat.

Deeper to the connective tissue is the layer of **orbicularis muscle** arranged circularly in multi-

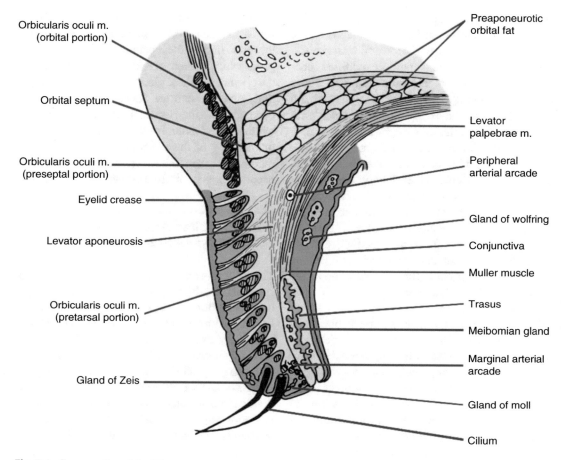

Fig. 7.4 Cross-section of the lid

ple layered rings around the eye. It can be considered as three parts functionally. The **orbital part** of orbicularis muscle extends from above the eyebrows to the region of the sulcus of the upper and lower lid. This muscle comes into action when one wants to voluntarily close the eye tight.

From the lid sulcus to the lid margin lies the **palpebral part** of orbicularis. These muscles originate from the medial palpebral ligament traverses laterally in an arch over both upper and lower lid to attach to the lateral palpebral fibrous raphae lying over the lateral palpebral (canthal) ligament. These ligaments are part of the system by which the upper and lower lids are anchored on to the medial and lateral margins of the orbit in such a way that it apposes to the globe well. The palpebral muscles sub-serve the spontaneous and forced lid closure. A roll of muscle extends to

the margins of the lid and is called the **muscles of Riolan**. These fibres have an extra function of keeping the lids well apposed to the globe. The grey line on the lid margin overlies this muscle.

The third functional portion of the orbicularis muscle passes deep in front and behind the lacrimal sac (**lacrimal part**) to act as a pump to suck fluid into the sac from the ocular surface and pump it out into the nose. The orbicularis muscle is supplied by the temporal and zygomatic branches of the facial nerve.

Between the orbicularis muscle and the tarsal plate is a **layer of fibrous tissue** that has the larger blood vessels and nerves. In the upper lid, slips of the LPS attach to the anterior surface of the tarsal plate.

The **tarsal plate** is a 1 mm thick and about 29 mm long dense sheet of fibrous tissue which acts like a shield and gives the lids its shape. The upper tarsal plate measuring 10 mm at its broadest area is double the size of the lower lid tarsal plate. Within the tarsal plate is multiple modified sebaceous glands or **meibomian glands**. These glands numbering about 40 in the upper lid and 30 in the lower lid are vertically oriented with their openings at the lid margin. The meibomian glands open in a row at the lid margin between the posterior lid border and the grey line in front. It can be seen clinically as dots on the lid margin. These glands produce a lipid secretion that forms the superficial layer of the tear film and prevents its evaporation. The tarsal plate is attached to the orbital rim both medially and laterally by the medial and lateral canthal ligament. The ligament especially **the posterior slip of the medial canthal ligament** keeps the lid well apposed to the globe.

On the superior margin of the upper tarsal plate is attached the sympathetic muscle fibres (**Muller's muscle**) that originates from the under surface of the levator palpebrae superioris (LPS). In the lower lid, this muscle arises from the lower lid retractors and inserts on the lower margin of the inferior tarsal plate. The lower lid retractor has a role in keeping the lower lid vertical.

Posterior to the orbital part of the orbicularis muscle is the **orbital septum** which extends from the orbital rim to the LPS aponeurosis. Laterally, the palpebral part of the lacrimal gland lies in front of the LPS. Behind the orbital septum lies the **orbital fat**. The orbital septum has weak areas medially and laterally through which orbital fat can prolapse especially in older people.

The posterior most layer of the lid is the **conjunctiva**. The conjunctiva is tightly adherent to the tarsal plate. Above the tarsal plate, up to the fornix it is loosely adherent with loose fibrous tissue.

7.2.1 The Lid Margin

The anterior part of the lid margin has lashes arranged in 2–3 rows. The hair follicles here are associated with sebaceous (**Zeis**) glands and sweat (**Moll**) glands. Posterior to the lash line running from medial to lateral end is a **grey line** which

corresponds to the position of the muscles of Riolan and an avascular plane deeper. Posterior to the grey line is the opening of the meibomian gland which is seen as multiple dots. In line with the openings of these glands medially is the **upper and lower punctum**. These punctums are the openings of the lacrimal canaliculus located within a small mound or the **lacrimal papillae**. At the opening of the meibomian glands in the lid margin, the keratinised epithelium of the skin becomes non-keratinised conjunctival epithelium.

7.3 Applied Anatomy of Levator Palpebrae Superioris

The LPS muscle arises from the lesser wing of sphenoid at orbital apex directly above the origin of the superior rectus (SR) muscle. Both muscles have the same embryological origin. The muscle travels anteriorly between SR and the roof of the orbit till superior suspensory ligament (**Whitnall ligament**) posterior to the orbital septum (Fig. 7.4). At the Whitnall ligament, the muscle divided into an anterior aponeurotic portion and a posterior superior tarsal (Muller) muscle. The tendinous part bend downward to the lid. Part of aponeurotic fibres insert on to the anterior surface of the tarsal plate and part goes through the orbicularis muscle to insert on the skin at the superior lid sulcus. The Muller's muscle inserts on the upper border of the tarsal plate. The muscle belly measures about 40 mm and the aponeurotic portion measures about 15 mm. The LPS elevates the upper lid and is innervated by the superior division of the third CN.

7.4 Applied Anatomy of the Lacrimal System

7.4.1 Lacrimal Gland

The main lacrimal gland is situated in a fossa located in the upper outer quadrant of the orbital wall. A fibroadipose tissue separates the frontal bone from the gland. The gland is divided into the main **orbital part** and **lacrimal part**. The lateral edge of the levator aponeurosis demarcates the two parts. Eversion of the upper lid enables us to see the lacrimal portion of the gland. The lacrimal gland is an exocrine gland and produces the aqueous portion of the tears. Fine ducts from the main gland, about 12 in number pass through the lacrimal part of the gland along with their own ducts to drain into the upper outer fornix and can be seen clinically with a slit lamp. In order to avoid damage to these draining ducts, it is the orbital part of the lacrimal gland that is usually biopsied.

7.4.2 Lacrimal Drainage

Secretion from the main and accessory lacrimal glands along with the mucin and lipid compo-

nents form a thin layer on the ocular surface to both lubricate and form a uniform refracting layer. The tear passes along the margin on the upper and lower lid margin to reach the medial canthal region where it forms a tear lake. Tears from here then pass through the lacrimal punctum, canaliculi, common canaliculus, nasolacrimal sac, nasolacrimal ducts (NLD) and into the inferior meatus of the nose (Fig. 7.5). Developmentally, the lower end of the NLD opens up at birth or a little later. At times, this distal canalisation gets delayed and do not canalise. This is the reason for the congenital NLD blocks, most of whom will resolve without surgical intervention. The puncta is apposed to the globe to facilitate passage of tears into the canaliculus. With the closure of the eye the lacrimal part of the orbicularis muscle which attaches to the lacrimal sac opens the sac. This pulls in the

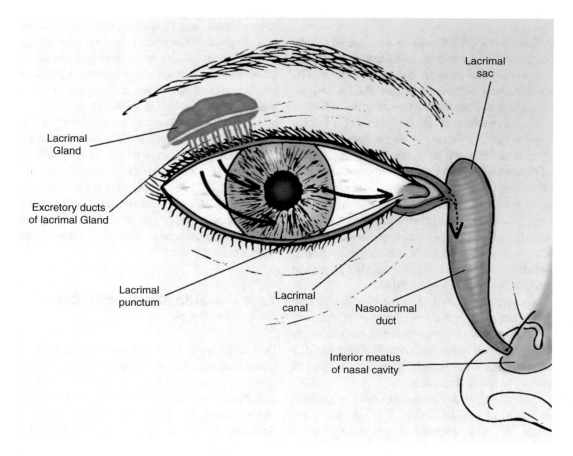

Fig. 7.5 Tear production at the lacrimal gland, its passage on the ocular surface and drainage into the nose

fluid from the canaliculus. When the eye opens, the sac collapses and fluid is pushed to the NLD from the sac. Valves prevent tears going back to the eye. When the eye opens, the canaliculus stretches, pulls in the fluid from the lacrimal lake. Thus, there is a pump mechanism that is helped by the orbicularis muscle to push the tears out from the eye.

7.5   Examination of the Orbit

In most of Ophthalmology, we can see the pathology directly with our eyes. Examination of the orbit is different and is like examining the abdomen. This is the closest an Ophthalmologist will come to a general surgeon!

7.5.1   History

Patients with orbital disease may present with, the patient or an acquaintance noticing that the eye is becoming more prominent. In patients with sudden onset of proptosis, one should enquire about trauma, headache, humming sensation in the head and redness, all suggestive of a carotid cavernous (CC) fistula. In all patients including those with unilateral proptosis, history suggestive of thyroid-related illness, both hypo- and hyperthyroidism should be explored. Patients should be asked about tolerance to heat and cold, lethargy, diarrhoea, palpitations, weight loss or gain, etc. History of diabetes and hypertension should also be asked. The former can suggest a fungal infection. Spontaneous CC fistula may be seen in atherosclerosis and hypertension.

History of discomfort in the eye, eye feeling gritty, etc. can occur due to dry eyes related proptosis and increased exposure. Double vision can occur in some gaze positions if the pathology affects the globe or muscle movement and patient should be quizzed about it.

Variability of the proptosis with the position of the head (orbital varices increase when the head is down like when bending to pick up things) may give a clue to the diagnosis. If the patient is complaining of pain, the character of the pain,

severity, pain in the surrounding areas, etc. should be explored. Infections, inflammation and malignancies produce pain.

In conditions associated with trauma, the exact mode of trauma is important. If the trauma is with a sharp object or flying missile, penetration or even perforation of the orbit is a possibility. A retained intra-orbital foreign body should also be ruled out. A patient with a non-healing skin wound on the lids with or without discharge is very strongly suggestive of a retained foreign body in the orbit. History of bleeding from the nose may suggest a sinus wall fracture, infection of the sinuses, nasopharyngeal carcinoma or a pathology in the nose causing the orbital problem.

In patients presenting acutely, history of infections in other parts of the body especially sinuses should be asked for. Patients should be asked about fever, pain, tenderness running nose, blocked nose, etc. History should also be taken rule out possibilities of malignancies or swellings in other parts of the body. Patients should be asked about loss of weight and appetite, previous treatment for malignancies, recently noted swelling in the body including the breast.

History of decreased vision, the way it was found out, progression if any should be explored.

The family album scan or (**family album topography**) **FAT scan** is a review of the patient's old photographs to compare the present state of affairs with the past. Sometimes, the so-called recent onset proptosis can be seen in the 20-year-old photograph the patient has, thus avoiding any further investigations.

7.5.2   Local Physical Examination for Proptosis

One could argue that in the present day of electronic imaging, clinical examination has a limited role. There are three reasons why it is still important. Firstly, one can order the appropriate imaging modality based on the clinical findings. Secondly, to interpret the image one needs the clinical data. Finally, the most important and may be the only reason in future is the clinician's intellectual stimulation and the challenge of solving the clinical problem. The thrill one gets in making a correct clinical diagnosis is unique and can be addicting!

Unaided vision, best corrected vision and colour vision should be taken for all patients.

The first thing to do in a patient with orbital problem is to stand back and look at the face as a whole to get a feel of how the orbits are set in the facial bones and compare one with the other. Look for facial dysmorphia and asymmetry. Patients with proptosis due to craniostenosis have typical facial features. A swelling in the temporal fossa could be due to sphenoidal meningioma.

When patient complaints of prominence of eye, the first question to answer is if it is unilateral or bilateral. In either case, the next question to answer is if it is pathological or a **pseudo-proptosis**. Pseudo-proptosis is when the proptosis is due to an ocular cause like a long eyeball rather than an orbital cause. It can be difficult sometimes to distinguish prominent eyes from bilateral proptosis and one has to go by other symptoms and findings. The easiest and simplest way to make out asymmetry in antero-posterior position of the eye is to do the Nafziger's test. To make out unilateral proptosis or enophthalmos one needs to first stand behind the patient and look over the forehead to make out which eye is more prominent. The lids are elevated by the examiner's fingers, and the patient is asked to look at the distance. As one moves the head forward over the patient's forehead, one looks to see which cornea meets the examiner's eye first (Fig. 7.6). The cornea of the more prominent eye will be seen first.

In unilateral proptosis, one should ask oneself if we are looking at the proptosis of one eye or the enophthalmos of the other eyes or even a combination of the two. This is especially important in patients with trauma. Besides blow-out fractures of the wall of the orbit, enophthalmos can be seen in patients with fibrotic malignant secondaries from the breast.

If proptosis is suspected, the next step is to see what type of proptosis it is. Is the eye coming straight out, axial proptosis or is it coming out and shifted to a side non-axial proptosis? By

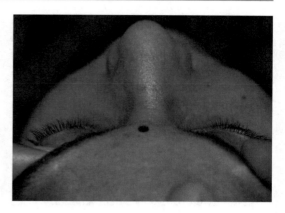

Fig. 7.6 Nafziger's test to check for asymmetry in the prominence of the two eyes (normal patient)

itself this differentiation has no value. Its importance is only in trying to guess what the aetiology may be. In axial proptosis, the push of the eyeball is uniform from all sides like in a diffuse infiltrative disease of the orbit like idiopathic orbital inflammation (pseudotumour), IgG4 disease, etc. or the push directly from behind the globe like an intraconal mass, e.g. cavernous haemangioma and optic nerve glioma.

Eccentric or non-axial proptosis can be due to a push by a mass from the opposite side, e.g. a proptosis that is pushing the globe 'down and in' can be due to a lacrimal gland tumour, an eye shifted up can be due to maxillary carcinoma. Non-axial proptosis can also be due to pull from the same side, e.g. a blow-out fracture of the inferior wall can pull the eye downward. Depending on the presentation and history, one should be able to figure out which of the two mechanism is in action.

That the proptosis is axial or non-axial is made out first by a visual impression of the eye positions. It is then confirmed by asking the patient to look at the distance (not at the light) and a light shown in the eye. The torch is positioned in such a way that the corneal light reflex falls on the centre of one eye. Now the reflex on the fellow eye is noted. The proptosis is axial if the corneal reflex is in the centre of the pupil in the fellow eye too. The degree of eccentricity/displacement can be measured by the vertical and horizontal scales of an optician's rule

(Fig. 7.7). The horizontal displacement is measured by measuring either the unilateral pupillary distance from the nose or the distance from
the centre of the nose to the medial limbus. The
measurement of vertical displacement is even
more subjective. The optician's rule is held horizontally (can be subjective) such that upper
reflex lines up with the corneal reflex. The displacement of the fellow pupillary reflex down-
wards is then measured on the vertical scale of
the optician's rule.

The amount of displacement anteriorly in an
axial proptosis can be measured by various specialised rulers available for the same. By itself
these exophthalmometers do not have any diagnostic use. Its main value is in follow-up of proptosis. Asymmetry of more than 2 mm between
the eye should raise suspicion of either proptosis
of the more prominent eye or enophthalmos of
the fellow eye. The inter-observer variability in
the measurement of exophthalmometer is so
much that comparing the reading of two observers to make clinical decisions should be avoided.
To minimise intra-observer error in exophthalmometers like Hertel's ophthalmometer, the
inter-orbital distance (**bar reading**) should be
noted and the same distance used in subsequent
measurements. For this reason, the bar reading is
also recorded each time the readings are taken
(Fig. 7.8). The exact way to take the reading is
given in the booklet that comes with the meter.
Essentially, the scales are kept against the zygomatic bones (lateral orbital rim) on each side and

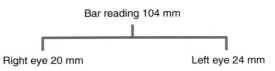

Bar reading 104 mm

Right eye 20 mm   Left eye 24 mm

Fig. 7.8 *Recording of proptosis using a Hertel's
ophthalmometer*

the antero-posterior position of the corneal tip
read off a scale without parallax. The mark on the
scale corresponding to the tip of the cornea gives
the reading. The two eye scales are mounted on a
graduated bar that gives the distance between the
side scales (Fig. 7.9).

Before examining the eye itself, one should
look at the lid position to see if it is retracted like
in thyroid eye disease (TED) or if the lid is boggy
and S shaped suggestive of neurofibromatosis or
if there is drooping of the lids due to a ptosis.
Normally, the lid is 2 mm below the upper limbus. If the upper sclera is seen when the patient
looks at a distance, it is suggestive of a lid retraction. The lower lid may also have a scleral show
in lid retraction. The lower lid is normally at the
level of the lower limbus of the cornea. In marked
proptosis, the eye may be pushed forward so
much that one can have a scleral show all around
the cornea without lid retraction. Associated with
lid retraction, there is usually a lid lag too and
this should be checked (see below).

Postulated reasons for lid retraction are excessive action of the Muller's muscle due to hypersensitivity to adrenalin. It may also be due to the
hypertrophy of the inferior rectus causing a
downward put of the eyeball. To counteract this,
the superior rectus along with its agonist the LPS
have to overact causing lid retraction.

Lid lag is seen in patients with TED. To examine lid lag, the patient is first asked to look at the
top of the wall on the opposite side of the room.
Next, the patient is asked to follow a horizontally
kept pen or finger as it moves slowly from top to
bottom. If lid lag is present, the lid will not follow
the globe smoothly (made out by the increasing
distance between the lid margin and the upper
limbus) and drops down in steps. The hold-up is
due to the hyperaction of the Muller's muscle
which does not relax so easily. Lids should be
inspected for any scarring to rule out other causes

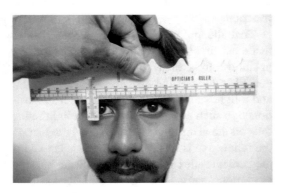

Fig. 7.7 Measuring the vertical shift of the globe using
the corneal reflex and optician's rule

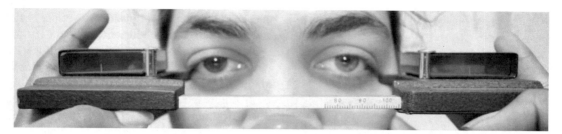

Fig. 7.9 Hertel's exophthalmometer

of retraction. The lid retraction need not be symmetrical in TED.

When inspecting the lid if ecchymosis is noted, it could be due to conditions like leukaemia or neuroblastoma. However, simpler conditions like a markedly inflamed chalazion, pre-septal cellulitis, etc. should be ruled out before chasing the less common exotic diagnosis. As a rule in clinical medicine, think of the simpler more common conditions first. Eczematous lesions could be due to lymphoma (mycosis fungoides).

Once the lid is examined, attention is drawn to the eye. Ocular motility should be examined in both eyes (see Chap. 8) to look for reduction in eye movement. Both ductions and versions should be checked. While checking for versions, patient should be asked about diplopia and if present an effort should be made to quantify the extent of the field of single vision. If limitation of eye movement is noted, one needs to differentiate between a paralysis and restriction. A force duction and force generation test (see Chap. 8) will distinguish the two.

The conjunctival surface of the globe should be inspected to look for localised or generalised congestion; any mass under the conjunctiva, dilated blood vessels, tenderness, etc. Congestion over the insertion of the recti muscle may be due to TED or parasitic infection. Scleritis which can cause proptosis can have conjunctival congestion with tenderness at the fornices. Posterior scleritis may show no congestion but will have pain and tenderness. The cornea and the conjunctiva should be examined for evidence of dryness related to exposure. On staining with fluorescein or lissamine green (see Chap. 9) punctate stain-positive areas can be seen in the inter-palpebral

area or inferior cornea due to dryness-related epithelial cell damage.

Relative pupillary defect should be looked for as this may be the only indication of involvement of the optic nerve in patients with mucormycosis, TED, etc. (see Chap. 11).

Applanation tonometry (see Chap. 13) both in the straight gaze and up gaze should be done when one is examining a patient with TED. A difference of more than 6 mm suggests significant globe compression.

7.5.3 Orbital Tonometry

Once intraocular pressure is measured, in patients with proptosis or suspected proptosis orbital tonometry is done to look for resistance on retropulsion. Here the patient is asked to close both eyes and look forward. With the fingers on the temporal fossa on both sides of the patient (Fig. 7.10), the thumb is used to press on the eyeball over the lids on both sides. The resistance on both sides is compared. If the resistance on one side is increased, it suggests extra tissue in that orbit. In pseudo-proptosis, the resistance will be the same in both eyes. One can also compare the resistance to retropulsion with a normal patient in cases of bilateral proptosis. If the position of the tumour is to a side, then one may not appreciate an increase in orbital pressure.

While checking for resistance if the patient winces, it suggests that there is tenderness and inflammatory conditions like scleritis should be suspected.

To rule out a reducible mass like orbital varices, continuous pressure is applied on both eyes

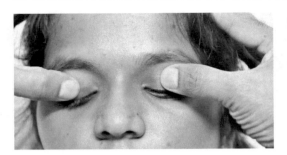

Fig. 7.10 Orbital tonometry to look for differential resistance on retropulsion of both the globes simultaneously

for about 2 min and released quickly. If the proptosis slowly increases, it suggests filling of the varices.

7.5.4 Palpation

If increased orbital pressure is suspected, one should palpate to see if a localised mass can be felt. If the mass is obviously seen through the lids, then the first thing to determine is the plane of the swelling. A pre-septal swelling may be mistaken for a mass in the orbit. Mass in front of the septum will become more prominent if the orbital septum is stretched. To stretch the orbital septum, pull the upper lid down and lower lid up. The lid is pulled by holding the lid margin and lashes. If the mass becomes less obvious on stretching the septum, then the mass is orbital and behind the septum.

Mass in the anterior part of the orbit can be palpated between the orbital bony rim and the globe. The little finger (with no nail jutting out) is the thinnest 'palpator' available easily and both hands should be used depending on the ease of insinuation. After telling the patient what one is going to do and asking him to inform you in case there is pain, the little finger should be insinuated as deep as you can into the orbit between the globe and the orbital rim. The finger is moved from side to side. Normally, there is nothing that one can feel. If the finger does feel something, the examiner should look for the following characters of the mass. Is the mass firm, hard or soft? Hard tumours could suggest malignancy. Is the mass fixed or mobile? The antero-posterior and side to side movement should be

checked out by trying to push the swelling back and forth and side to side. One should try to make out if the mass is well defined or diffuse. A lymphangioma may not have a well-defined margin. Size or shape of the swelling cannot be made out as one will not be able to palpate the entire swelling. Mass posterior to the equator of the globe is difficult to localise with palpation.

To check for the reducibility of the mass, all four fingers except the thumb is used to press the globe backward over the closed lid. Pressure is maintained for about a minute and then let go. If there is no change in the globe position, then the mass is not reducible. In conditions like AV malformations and haemangiomas, the proptosis increases slowly on removal of pressure. If one observes closely, one may even be able to make out this increase with each systolic pulsation. Comparison with the fellow eye will help us appreciate the increasing proptosis better. Pulsation may also be felt over the temporal fossa if the mass is extending into the fossa.

During the compression with the four fingers, one should also pay attention to see if there is any pulsation of the globe. High flow vascular lesions may give a pulsatile proptosis. Alternatively, it may be a transmitted pulsation from the cranium due to a defect in the walls of the orbital cavity as seen in neurofibromatosis or encephalocoele. Mild orbital pulsations can be picked through the exaggerated pulsation of the mires when applanation tonometry is done.

In patients who give a history of intermittent proptosis, one needs to check for onset or increase in swelling with Valsalva manoeuvre. To check this, first familiarise the patient with this manoeuvre. Then the patient is told to do the Valsalva manoeuvre by closing the mouth and nose and blowing out. Doing the Valsalva manoeuvre with the patient bending over slightly, the proptosis can be observed better.

Auscultation of the orbit is useful to make out the bruit in cases of high flow CC fistulas. The bell of the stethoscope is used to pick up this flow bruit. Like other clinical examinations, one should familiarise oneself with the normal noises one hears in an orbit before trying to pick up pathology. Bruit may also be heard by keeping the stethoscope on the mastoid process.

In cases of trauma, sensation of the cheek below the lower eyelid should be examined to rule out injury to the infra-orbital nerve, typically seen in blow-out fractures of the orbit. In malignant lacrimal gland tumours, the skin over the lateral part of the upper lid may be anaesthetic due to the infiltration of the nerves by the tumour.

A crackling feeling under the skin (crepitus) around the orbit or on the lids suggest air in the soft tissue. The crackling feeling is due to air bubbles moving within the areolar tissues and the bubbles breaking up. This is seen in sinus fractures when air escapes from the sinus into the soft tissues especially when one blows the nose to clear blood collected in the nose. All patients with suspected orbital wall fracture has to be palpated to look for crepitus. If crepitus is felt, patients should be instructed not to blow their noses as it would push more air from the sinus into the soft tissue, which in turn can increase the chance of infection of the subcutaneous tissue.

Examination of the eye may give clue to the diagnosis of orbital disease. Nodules on the iris suggest phacomatosis that can cause optic nerve glioma or neurofibroma of the orbit. Iris nodules are seen in histiocytosis group of disorders and these can infiltrate the orbit too. A pupil examination will reveal involvement of the second, third CN and sympathetic nerve supply. Enophthalmos with pupil constriction and ptosis would suggest a sympathetic nerve involvement (Horner's syndrome).

Fundus examination should be done in all cases suspected with orbital pathology. Disc oedema may be seen when the posterior scleritis patch abuts the optic nerve. Cupping of the disc with glaucoma may be associated with TED. Optic atrophy can be seen in meningiomas and optic nerve gliomas. The periphery of the fundus should also be looked at carefully. Intraconal mass may indent the globe giving us a clue to the location of the mass. A melanoma or retinoblastoma can spread into the orbit and can be the cause of the proptosis. Compression of the ophthalmic artery at the orbital apex can cause a central retinal artery or vein occlusion.

Finally, examination of a patient suspected with an orbital pathology is not complete without a systemic examination and examining the mouth, nose and the sinuses. One should also look for lymph nodes in other areas if lymphoma or secondaries is suspected. Nodules on the body and cafe-au lait spots are suggestive of phacomatosis.

At the end of the examination, one should ask oneself if the following questions have been answered. Is there a real proptosis? Is it an enophthalmos of the fellow eye? Are there any local and systemic symptoms and signs associated with proptosis? Is the eye in danger of secondary effects? What is the cause of the proptosis? Depending on the age and sex of the patient, the structures involved, a list differential diagnosis should be made. It does not matter if the final diagnosis after imaging and biopsy does not figure in your list!

7.6 Examination of Anophthalmic Socket

Examination of an empty socket due congenital maldevelopment or surgical removal of the globe is necessary to follow-up on the original pathology and manage problems due to prosthesis.

Since anophthalmia can be very depressing for the patient, one should be sensitive during the history taking and be positive about the anophthalmic status. The important points to know in the history are the reason for anophthalmia, the time since first surgery, the use of prosthesis and current problems with it if any. Discharge, discomfort in the socket, prosthesis coming out spontaneously, unhappiness due to the cosmesis are some of the problems patients have and should be explored.

The lid should be first inspected to see if there is any inward or outward turning of the lid margin. The length of the palpebral fissure should be compared to the fellow eye, a shorter length suggest contraction of the socket. The lid should be pulled outward to see if it is very lax or tight. The lids should be held apart and the socket inspected to see if there are any discharging sinuses, ulcers, exposed implant or if there is excessive scarring. Fluorescein stain can be used to examine the socket as conjunctival ulcers are better delineated with stain. An assessment of the socket size should be made, especially the status of the inferior fornix that tends to scar over time and become shallow.

In patients with a history of orbital implant or a tumour in the orbit or eye; the empty socket should be palpated with the little finger. Effort should be made to locate the implant or look for any recurrence of the tumour. A drop of local anaesthetic makes the palpation more comfortable. The glove covered little finger should press the conjunctiva against the orbital wall to make out any firm to hard mass. Fingers can also be run against the fornices and orbital walls to feel for scar tissue and also to assess the size of the socket.

In patients with prosthesis, one should look to see the symmetry between the normal eye and prosthesis in terms of the lid position, conjunctival colour, iris colour and the size of the cornea by looking at the patient from a distance of 60 cm or more (the distance closer to which a casual acquaintance is unlikely to come). If patient has been given glasses, the same examination should be done with the glasses on, as the glasses may have been given to increase the cosmetic appeal. The position of the prosthetic eye should be assessed using the Krimsky method (see Chap. 8) of shining a torch into both the eyes and looking for the corneal reflex on the prosthetic eye. If the corneal reflex is not central, then the prosthesis is deviated. In a patient with shallow fornix, the whole prosthetic may be tilted backward. Finally, ask the patient to follow the torch with the good eye and look for movement of the prosthesis medially, laterally and in the up and down directions. This gives us an idea of the mobility of the prosthesis and hence the cosmetic appeal.

7.7 Examination of the Lids and Periorbita

The lids in addition to giving protection are intricately linked to keeping the ocular surface healthy. Symptoms other than cosmetic requirements are due to the anterior segment dysfunction resulting from the lid disease. A patient coming with redness of the eye with apparent pathology in the eye may have its origin in the lid like a molluscum contagiosum which may not be obviously seen.

7.7.1 History

Patients with lid problems complain of ocular discomfort, decrease in vision, watering (epiphora), redness of the eyes and feeling of foreign body sensation or irritation, etc. Some patients come with complains of pain and/or swelling of the lids. Like other history taking; characteristics of the pain should be enquired. For swelling of the lids, in addition to the onset, one should also ask for variability of the swelling during the day. Swelling of lids due to anasarca is more in the morning.

7.7.2 Examination

Normally, the lid is well apposed to the globe with the lashes turned outward. The lashes do not turn grey usually. There is no discharge on the lids and the eye is white. The IPF on both sides is the same width and patient tolerates light well. The eyebrows on both sides are symmetrical and at the same level. The punctum of the upper and lower lid is turned posteriorly facing the medial tear lake. The punctum lies flush with the globe like the rest of the lid margin and is not congested.

The examination of the lids is first done with the torchlight and then with the slit lamp. Before the detailed examination of the individual lid, one should look at all the four lids in general. Normally, the medial canthus is slightly lower than the lateral canthus. The distance between the medial canthi should be noted to ensure it is not unusually wide (**telecanthus**), the length of the palpebral fissure should be symmetrical. One should also observe the lid closure to see if it is effective and the blink rate about 15 times a minute. When measuring the blink rate, patient should not be aware you are observing the blink rate as that can affect it.

With the torchlight the apposition of the posterior lid margin across the full length of the lid is noted. Sometimes, one area may be not apposed to the globe, and this is enough to disrupt the tear outflow pathway. The lash line is noted to see if lashes and lids are turned outward (**ectropion**) or inward (**entropion**). Entropion should be differentiated from **trichiasis** or misdirected lashes rubbing the cornea and **distichiasis** or extra row of lashes growing from the meibomian opening and rubbing the ocular surface. This is done by looking at the posterior lid margin which will be just apposed if there is no entropion. Sometimes, the trichiasis or distichiasis can itself cause a spastic entropion. Trichiasis and distichiasis is better appreciated with slit lamp as some of these fine misdirected lashes can be missed with torch-light examination.

It is good to remind oneself when evaluating lid position that the lid is held in position by interaction of forces exerted by the medial and lateral canthal ligament, the capsule-palpebral ligament, gravity, the tone of the orbicularis, LPS and inferior rectus muscles. The lid tissues themselves and the surrounding tissue can affect the position of the lids. Besides making the diagnosis, the aim of the examination should also be to analyse which of these forces or lack of it are responsible for the altered lid position. This understanding is useful for the targeted management of these patients.

The laxity of the medial and lateral palpebral ligament is checked by pulling the centre of the lid away from the globe. If the lid can be pulled out more than 1 cm, then the lid tissue especially the medial and lateral palpebral ligament is very lax. On leaving the lid (**snap back test**) if it snaps back quickly it means the orbicularis muscle has good tone. If the tissue goes back slowly, then the muscles have also lost tone due to either paralysis or age-related atrophy. The medial palpebral ligament laxity can also be checked by pulling the medial part of the lid outward with finger and observing how far laterally the lacrimal punctum goes. Normally, the punctum would move up to the medial limbus. If it reaches the middle of the cornea when the patient is looking straight ahead, then the ligament is very lax. The position of the inferior edge of the lower lid tarsal plate should be examined. In entropion if the tarsal plate is turned in with the inferior edge of tarsal plate pointing anteriorly and up it means that the lower lid retractors are lax. The strong action (spasm) of the marginal orbicularis muscle pushes the upper tarsal margin in. In ectropion, if the lower lid is lying flat with the conjunctival side of the tarsal plate facing up and inferior tarsal margin pointing posteriorly, it again means the lower lid retractors are lax. Here the orbicularis muscle and the palpebral ligaments are lax and the tarsal plate falls outward due to gravity. In spastic entropion, however, the orbicularis muscle especially the marginal muscles (muscle of Riolan) are very active and move the lid inward. The upper lid does not show spastic entropion because the globe is in contact with most of the upper tarsal plate and opposes the inward push of the tarsus by the orbicularis. The gravity also aids the position. When upper lid entropion is noted, it is invariably due to a contracture of the posterior lamellae (tarsal plate and conjunctiva) of the lid. With ectropion the anterior lamellae (skin and orbicularis muscle) will be shortened.

Ectropion and entropion of upper and lower lid can be due to the scarring of the tarsal plate or surrounding tissues due to trauma or chronic inflammation/infection like trachoma. In entropion, the inner layers of the lid are scarred and one should evert the lid to see if the tarsal plate is scarred and bowed in. In ectropion, the outer layers like the skin on the lids may be scarred, pulling the lid out.

When patients have watering of the eye, the position of the lacrimal punctum should be examined to ensure it is apposed to the globe.

In patients with irritation and redness of the eye, lid margin should be carefully examined with slit lamp for inturned and abnormal lashes, encrustations due to infectious blepharitis, dandruff like material on the lashes seen in seborrhoeic or squamous blepharitis. In between the lashes, one should also look for umbilicated nodules seen in molluscum contagiosum and louse (phthiriasis palpebrarum). The latter is seen in very young or very old unhygienic people. The lid margins should also be inspected for any notches in the margin that could be congenital or trauma induced. If a notching is suspected, the patient should be asked to close the lid lightly to see if there is any exposure of the ocular surface.

The posterior lid margin is examined for meibomianitis or posterior blepharitis by pressing the lower lid against globe with the thumb and the index finger. After warning the patients of mild pain and discomfort, the lid is bend on itself (Fig. 7.11) and the two folds of lid squeezed against each other. The meibomian opening is looked at to see if any paste-like material comes out. Normally, there is very little material that comes out. In meibomianitis, there will be a lot of oily secretion or inspissated paste-like material that may come out. Frothy secretion on the lid margins may also be seen in this condition. Dilated capillaries on the posterior lid margin along with prominent opening of the meibomian gland is also suggestive of meibomian gland disease. White lashes (**poliosis**) and loss of lashes (**madarosis**) should also be looked for and may add weight to a diagnosis of chronic ulcerative blepharitis.

Patients who come with complaints of pain and swelling of the lid should be examined for small pustules near the anterior lid margin suggestive of hordeolum externum or stye. Inflamed chalazion (hordeolum internum) can also present with pain and swelling. In the early stages of the disease, a chalazion may not be obvious due to lid oedema and has to be kept in mind when seeing patients with painful lid swellings. Chalazion normally appears as a swelling in the tarsal plate

with some mild pain and discomfort. Due to associated oedema, these lesions are sometimes better felt than seen. To feel the chalazion, slide the index finger on the tarsal plate from one end to the other to see if one can feel a bump. If older patients give a history of a similar swelling being incised once, a meibomian cell carcinoma should be suspected.

Older individuals, especially those with fairer skin, may come with reddish swellings on the skin of the lids or surrounding areas. This should be examined like any mass in general surgery. The size, shape, edges, surface, consistency, fluctuation, plane of swelling, adherence to adjacent structures, etc. should be noted. A clinical diagnosis is made based on the findings of the examination. The lymph nodes draining the lids, namely pre-auricular and submandibular nodes should also be palpated to look for lymph node involvement.

Yellowish plaques seen usually on the medial aspect of the lids (Xanthelasma) may be suggestive of a hyperlipidaemic state. Rarely, it can be seen laterally too (Fig. 7.12).

When examining a patient with suspected lid oedema, one should rule out prolapse of orbital fat through weak areas of the septum. The orbital fat has a lumpy feel. Lid oedema is more when the patient lies down for some time, e.g. in the morning. In orbital fat prolapse, the swelling is constant. The lid folds like do not get obliterated with orbital fat prolapse. In young patients with recurrent lid oedema

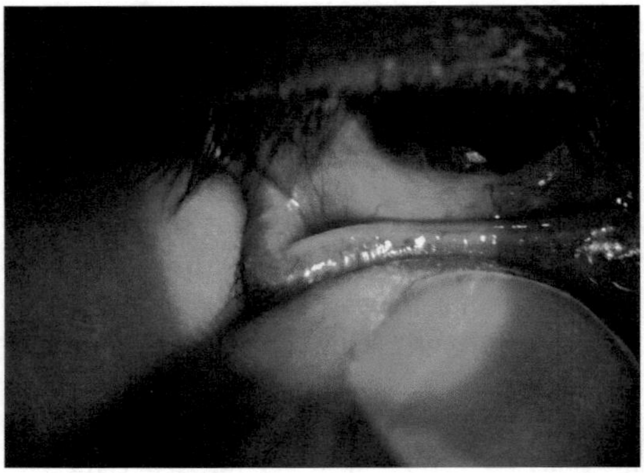

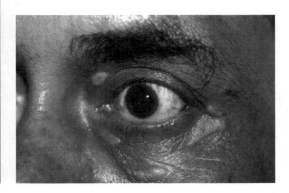

Fig. 7.11 Bending the tarsal plate on itself to express meibomian secretions

Fig. 7.12 Xanthelasma seen at the medial and lateral aspect of the lids

(**blepharochalasis**), one may find excess of fine upper lid skin hanging over the upper lid crease. As opposed to this in old age, one can get **dermatochalasis**, where again the upper lid skin is lax and hangs over the lid.

When a patient comes with a lid injury, after getting the history on the mode and other characteristics of the injury, patient should be examined to see the extent of lid injury. It is advisable to wear a glove when examining bloody wounds to avoid contracting any blood bore infections. The examination should be directed to answer the following questions. (1) Is the tarsal plate involved? (2) Is it a full thickness tear? (3) Is the canaliculus torn and if so at what point? (4) Is there missing tissue? (5) Is the medial palpebral ligament (especially the posterior lip) and lateral palpebral ligament torn? (6) Is the attachment of the LPS muscle to the lid affected? (7) Is the globe intact? (8) Is there a possibility of a foreign body in the orbit? Local anaesthetic drops on the injured tissue can make the examination less painful. At the time of surgery, under anaesthesia a second examination should be done before repair.

In patients who will require skin grafts on the lid to correct the lid condition; examination of the donor site for the skin should be done. The pre-puce, supra-clavicular area and the post-auricular areas are the common sites from where skin is harvested because it is only at these sites the skin resembles the lid skin.

7.8 Examination of Ptosis

Blepharoptosis or ptosis (Fig. 7.13) is the drooping of the upper eyelid. It can be unilateral or bilateral. Examination of ptosis requires a separate checklist that needs to be ticked!

Clinical evaluation of ptosis should attempt to answer the following questions during the workup. Is there a ptosis? Which eye is the ptotic eye? Is it unilateral or bilateral? How long has the ptosis been there? How much is the ptosis? Does ptosis affect vision? Is there a compensatory brow lift? What is the cause of the ptosis? Is the LPS involved? How much is the LPS action? Is there an associated systemic or local eye disease?

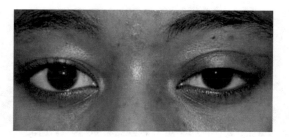

Fig. 7.13 Mild ptosis of the left eye with narrower palpebral fissure

What was the previous surgical intervention if any? What should be the management strategy?

7.8.1 History

In the history, finding the duration of ptosis can sometimes be the challenging. In adult patients with mild ptosis of recent onset, one should rule out if it is a congenital ptosis. Patients seek help because they or an acquaintance suddenly notice the asymmetry in the inter-palpebral fissure (IPF) height. In these situations, it is useful to look at the old photos of the patient and more often than not they will show pre-existing asymmetry. With ageing a congenital ptosis can get exaggerated due to failure of the compensatory mechanisms. A history of variability in the ptosis during the day or with time is useful to make a diagnosis. Ptosis that gets worse during the evening may have myasthenia gravis (MG). Ptosis that is getting progressively worse over time may be due to progressive external ophthalmoplegia. A family history of ptosis suggests a hereditary cause including congenital ptosis. History of double vision should be taken. Diplopia can be seen in MG and conditions where the other ocular muscles are involved like in third nerve palsy. Visual defects if any should be asked for. Systemic problems like weakness of muscles, heart problems, swellings in the neck, etc. should be looked into to explore the possibility of diseases like MG, myotonic dystrophy and malignancies. Patient should always be asked a history of previous medical or surgical interventions that may have been an effort at treating the problem or is the cause of the current problem. History of constant rubbing of eyes due to allergic conjunctivitis in young patients can also be a cause of ptosis.

7.8.2　Examination

First the patient's face is inspected from a metre distance to see if the level of the lids and brows are at the normal levels. The forehead area should be inspected for excessive wrinkles suggestive of a compensatory lift of the eyebrows. Swellings of the lid or scars if any should be noted. Differentiating a true ptosis from a **pseudoptosis** can be difficult sometimes. Asymmetrical lid retraction and mild proptosis may give the appearance of a ptosis in the fellow eye. If one eye is hypertropic and is the fixating eye, then the fellow eye may appear ptotic because the hypertropic eye will move down to take fixation bringing down the fellow eye with the lid. Enophthalmos, phthisis bulbi, etc. can produce drooping of the lids due to lack of support of the normal globe. In older people, the skin over the lids become lax and hang over the lid crease to give an appearance of ptosis.

Once the obvious causes of pseudoptosis are ruled out then the next question to answer is, are both eyes are involved? Often when ptosis is detected in one eye, the fellow eye is ignored. If the more ptotic eye is the fixing eye, it will appear that the fellow eye is normal as the lid in the fellow eye is elevated more than it normally would due to the extra innervation needed to lift the fellow ptotic eye. Only on occlusion of the more ptotic eye will the ptosis in the fellow eye be revealed. Sometimes, a compensatory brow lift will mask the ptosis.

Once true ptosis has been established its likely aetiology should be established. The anatomical causes of ptosis are myogenic (congenital ptosis), neurogenic (e.g. third CN palsy), aponeurotic (e.g. senile ptosis), traumatic (due to mixture of reasons) and mechanical (lid oedema or tumour). The following examinations should help make the distinction.

The measurements in a patient with ptosis is useful to quantify the problem, do the follow-up, make a diagnosis and plan the treatment.

Since the lower lid position also affects the IPF (inter-palpebral fissure) size, the distance between the pupillary reflex and the upper lid margin called margin reflex distance (**MRD1**) is a better measure of ptosis. The measurement is zero if the lid margin is at the level of the pupillary reflex. If the lid is lower than the pupillary reflex, then the reading becomes minus. Here the amount of lid that has to be lifted to reach the zero position is measured. Normally, the MRD1 is 4 mm. The **MRD2** measurement from the corneal reflex to the lower lid is not a useful measurement.

Cosmetically what matters is the inter-palpebral fissure measurement, so that should also be measured and is the distance between the upper and lower lid margin at the level of the pupillary reflex when the eye is looking straight ahead. It is normally around 10 mm. One could argue that, is not the difference in the IPF measurement between the two eyes be enough to give the amount of ptosis. This is not enough as lower lid position can affect the IPF measurement. The value of the amount of ptosis is important because it is an indicator of the LPS pathology. Four millimetres or more of ptosis or severe ptosis means the LPS has few normal muscle fibres and is mostly fibrotic. Moderate or 3 mm ptosis means there is an equal mixture of fibrous tissue and muscle fibres. In 2 mm or less mild ptosis, then there is a significant amount of muscle fibres in the LPS. The IPF can also be measured with the chin up position and the eye looking down to the floor to see how it compares with the straight ahead position. If the IPF is wider in the ptotic eye compared to the normal eye in the looking down position, it is suggestive of a congenital ptosis. The fibrotic congenitally malformed LPS does not lengthen enough thus increasing the IPF on down gaze. In aponeurotic ptosis, the ptosis gets worse on looking down and can even occlude the vision.

The measurements are best taken with a transparent millimetre scale kept against the forehead to negate the action of the frontalis muscle which can life the brow and thus indirectly lift the lid (Fig. 7.14). Parallax should be avoided when taking the readings. The left hand can hold the scale against the forehead such that the zero mark is aligned with the lid margin. The light is shown with the right hand if no other light source is available and the position of the pupillary reflex on the scale is noted.

In races that have an upper eyelid crease the distance between the lid margin and the crease should be measured in both eyes. The normal lid crease is about 9 mm from the lid margin. If the upper lid crease is abnormally high in the eye with ptosis, it suggests the LPS that is normally inserted lower down is disinserted and shifted up causing an **aponeurotic ptosis**. The lid crease position of the fellow eye is used when planning the lid crease incision during surgery.

The action of the LPS should be measured both to make a diagnosis and plan the surgery. Since the brow elevation can contribute about 2 mm to the lid elevation, its action should be nullified when measuring the LPS action. To isolate the action of the LPS muscle, the brow is fixed by pressing the examiner's fingers against the forehead (Fig. 7.14). Care should be taken not to slide the fingers up and down on the forehead during measurements as that can affect measurements. After fixing the brow the scale is kept vertically between the thumb and the index finger, the patient is asked to

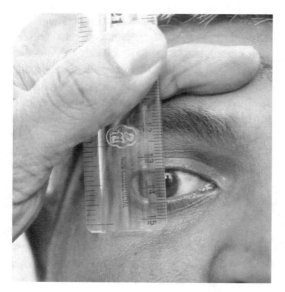

Fig. 7.14 Placement of measuring scale on the forehead for ptosis measurement. The brow is fixed with the index finger during the measurements

look down at the floor of the room. The position of the upper lid margin is noted on the scale. The patient is then asked to look up to the ceiling and the new position of the lid noted. A movement over 15 mm is normal. If the movement is less than 4 mm, it means there is really no useful functional LPS muscle that can be made more effective by muscle resection. In congenital ptosis, the LPS action is significantly reduced. In aponeurotic ptosis, the LPS action is not affected and is well over 15 mm. In babies who will not cooperate for measurements, an estimate of the LPS action can be got by everting the lid. If the lid straightens out by itself when the baby opens the eye, it means that the LPS action is good.

In aponeurotic ptosis, due to the disinsertion of the tendon, the supra-tarsal part of the lid becomes thinner and in lightly pigmented patients the corneal outline can be seen through a gently closed eye. The cornea will not be seen in darkly pigmented people.

When contemplating surgical correction, **Bell's phenomenon** should be checked. The upper lids of both eyes should be held slightly above the normal position, and the patient should be asked to close the eye forcefully. If the cornea rotates up and is covered by the lid, the patient has a good Bell's phenomenon and it means that the chance of the eye being dangerously exposed after corrective surgery is less. If the Bell's phenomenon is not good, then an under correction may be preferable.

In all patients with ptosis, the extraocular movement should be examined both for making the diagnosis and planning the treatment. Ptosis associated with third CN palsy will affect the other ocular movements. In aberrant regeneration of the third CN after trauma, the ptotic lid may open up on adduction. Since the superior rectus develops with the LPS, congenital ptosis may be associated with eye elevator palsy. Both eyes may be affected in double elevator palsy.

The pupils should be examined in patients with ptosis. Ptosis associated with miosis in dim light may be due to Horner's syndrome. If the pupil is dilated in bright light, then the ptosis is due to third CN palsy. Traumatic ptosis may be associated with a dilated pupil and a sphincter rupture.

In **mechanical ptosis,** the lid will be oedematous or thickened due to inflammation or mass lesion. It is the weight of the lid that causes the drooping here. Contact lens wear causing giant papillae can also cause ptosis. The lid should therefore be everted to examine for papillae.

In patients suspected to have MG, the patient can be asked to look up continuously for 5 min at least. If the lids start to come down while looking up, then it is suggestive of MG. The continuous stimulation depletes the acetylcholine stores. Conversely, if the eye is kept closed for 5 min with or without an ice pack (a plastic cover with ice **cubes**) kept on the lid, the ptosis will improve by over 2 mm in MG. The **ice pack test** is supposed to have a sensitivity of over 75% and specificity of over 90%.

In **Cogan lid twitch sign** described in MG, one sees a twitch in the lid margin as the patient follow a finger moved from down position to up. This is not a very specific sign and seen in many other conditions including normal people.

7.8.3 Difference Between Ptosis and Spasm of Lids

In **blepharospasm** the IPF appears narrow and should not be mistaken for ptosis. In conditions where the blepharospasm is secondary to an ocular condition like a corneal ulcer the underlying condition gives the clue. In essential blepharospasm, however, the eye will be white. In blepharospasm, the lower lid will be in a higher position than normal. The brow which shows a compensatory elevation in ptosis will show a depression in spasm because the orbicularis muscles around the brow is also in spasm. Twitching of the lid skin may be noted in essential blepharospasm.

7.9 Examination of the Lacrimal Drainage System

Since the production of tears is intricately related to the health of the ocular surface, evaluation of tear production is dealt with in the examination of the ocular surface. Deficiencies in the drainage of the tears can also cause patient discomfort.

7.9.1 History

Babies with lacrimal drainage system block are brought with complaints of discharge from the eye with or without watering. If the discharge is bilateral, one should rule out conjunctivitis before entertaining a diagnosis of bilateral nasolacrimal duct (NLD) block. As against the standard teaching mothers of children with NLD block invariably say the discharge has been there from birth. Some babies are brought with complaints of swelling at the medial canthal ligament suggestive of a mucocoele.

In adults, the common complaint when the tear drainage is blocked is of excessive watering in one eye. There is usually no other associated symptoms like irritation of the eye, decrease in vision, etc. If the epiphora is intermittent, then a drainage obstruction is less likely. Some patients may complain of recurrent redness of eye medially (**lacrimal conjunctivitis**) with some discharge. Patients may present for the first time with acute pain, redness and swelling over the medial canthal region suggestive of **acute dacryocystitis**. Syringing of nasolacrimal duct should be avoided in the acute stage. Some patients present with complaints of painless swelling (distended nasolacrimal sac) in the medial canthal region that may or may not be reducible with pressure on the swelling. If it is reducible, it means there is a functional block of the nasolacrimal duct and the mucous that collects in the sac can be pushed into the nose with pressure. Patient should be asked about any history of blocked nose or bleeding from the nose. Past history of facial trauma may predispose to a nasolacrimal duct block. Patients should be asked about chronic use of topical drops that may close the punctum and canaliculus. The nature of discharge if present should be explored. Mucoid discharge suggests NLD block. Discharge with granules that may be coloured suggest canaliculitis due to nocardia/actinomyces infection.

Watering of eyes can be due to multiple reasons and blocked tear drainage system is only one of them. All causes of excessive production of tears must be kept in mind though not necessary to rule out if history does not suggest any cause for the same.

Dry eye may paradoxically cause watering (**pseudoepiphora**) in a white eye like that seen with blocked ducts. This watering is due to the reflex tearing in response to the drying.

7.9.2 Examination

In babies with discharge and watering of eyes, the conjunctiva should be checked to see if there is any redness or foreign body. Congenital entropion with inturned lashes medially rubbing the ocular surface should be ruled out. On palpation, there may be a swelling at the medial palpebral ligament area. In lightly pigmented children, the lacrimal sac swelling may have a slight bluish colour due to the vessels around the sac. The swelling may be cystic and tense. Sometimes, pressure over the swollen sac in a downward direction may be curative as the pressure of the collected mucous breaks open the last part of the NLD that is yet to be canalised in cases of congenital NLD block. In children, the patency of the lacrimal drainage system is tested by doing the **dye disappearance test**. Here fluorescein strip dipped in saline is touched on the lid margin in both eyes. A drop of paracaine before putting the fluorescein reduces the stinging. After 5 min, the cobalt blue light of the indirect ophthalmoscope is shown on both eyes to look for differential retention of the dye. Normally, very little dye is visible after 5 min. Trying to recover the dye from the nose with a cotton bud is traumatic for the child and adds no diagnostic value. Trying to recover the dye from the nose is only useful in children who are crying incessantly during the testing. If dye is present in the tears, it means there is a hold-up in the drainage system. In babies if there is hold-up of dye, the eye should be examined with the slit lamp to look for the patency of the punctum. If the punctum is patent, then the NLD is at fault and is yet to canalise. With the slit lamp one should also look at the skin around the sac to see if there is fistula draining

out. Rarely in children, NLD block is associated with a draining fistula in the region of the sac.

In adults with watering, one should rule out lid and ocular surface causes for excessive tear production. Inspection of the lids may show matting of lashes into 4 or 5 bunches in patients with NLD block. Pressure over the lacrimal sac area may cause regurgitation of the mucous material into the eye via the punctum. In atonic sac, there is no physical block in the ducts but the pump mechanism is not effective to push out the discharge into the nose. Here pressure on the sac will empty the contents of a tense sac into the nose.

With slit lamp the punctum should be examined first. The punctum will be found at the medial end of the tarsal plate in line with the openings of the meibomian glands. The punctual opening should be obvious and white in colour. Pouting of the punctum with redness suggest canaliculitis. The punctum may be absent or very small in some patients and may be the cause of the epiphora. Like in a child, dye disappearance test can be done for adults too and is better than syringing of the ducts to assess a block both functional and structural in the system.

Regurgitation on pressure over the lacrimal sac (ROPLAS) is a simple way to rule out block in the NLD if the sac collects mucous. Here with the patient on the slit lamp the area just below the medial palpebral ligament overlying the lacrimal sac is pressed with the index finger to see if there is any mucous regurgitating back into the upper or lower punctum (Fig. 7.15). If there is regurgi-

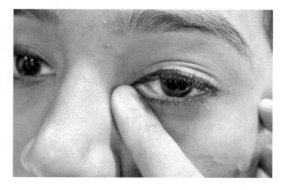

Fig. 7.15 Placement of index finger to give pressure for ROPLAS test. The punctum is exposed to look for mucous regurgitation

tation, the test is positive and this means there is a block in the NLD. In patients with atrophic sac and blocked NLD, this test is not useful because there is not enough collection of mucous for it to regurgitate.

Syringing of the ducts can be done as a clinic procedure and is useful to localise the site of block once the dye disappearance test shows a hold-up of dye. Here saline is taken in a 5 cc syringe. Under topical anaesthesia (using multiple topical drops of proparacaine), a blunt lacrimal cannula fixed on to this syringe is guided past the punctum into the vertical part of the canaliculi which is about 2 mm long. If there is difficulty in passing the cannula through the punctum, then a punctual dilator is used to dilate the punctum. When the resistance at the end of vertical part of the canaliculus is felt, it is turned at right angles into the horizontal portion of the canaliculi and passed medially to the medial canthal area for about 10 mm. Normally, the cannula will go past the common canaliculi into the nasolacrimal sac where the cannula will hit the medial bony wall of the sac. At this point, the cannula is withdrawn slightly and saline injected into the sac. If the NLD is patent, the fluid will go into the nose and patient will be able to feel the saline in the throat. If there is a common canalicular block, some fluid may come out from the upper punctum if the lower punctum is used for syringing. If while passing the cannula, the tip does not go beyond the common canaliculus region and the examiner cannot feel the bony hard touch of the medial wall of the sac, a canalicular or common canalicular block is suspected. If the cannula does not reach even up to the medial canthal region, then a canaliculus block should be suspected and the other punctum should be canulated. The feel of the blocked common canaliculus area is described as a soft touch, as opposed to the hard touch of the bone.

If blood regurgitates through the opposite punctum while syringing, one should suspect a sac malignancy or a rhinosporidial infection. If one gets a gritty sensation while passing the cannula through the canaliculus, then an Actinomyces canaliculitis should be suspected. The regurgitating fluid here should be sent for culture to confirm the diagnosis. Pressure on the canaliculus with a cotton tip applicator may show regurgitation of pus in canaliculitis.

Examination of Ocular Motility and Squint

Examining ocular motility and interpreting the findings by far is the most challenging and fascinating part of clinical Ophthalmology. It challenges one to think all the time while eliciting and interpreting the findings. There is so much in our nervous system that is still not understood clearly. The visual system and its controls are no exceptions. This uncertainty should be accepted and taken as a challenge rather than be put off by it. Most of us like 'certainty' in life which is the exception rather than the rule. An understanding of the physiology of ocular motility will go a long way in doing a good clinical examination and coming to sensible conclusions.

It is presumed that the reader of this book has had an exposure to human anatomy and physiology during the undergraduate course. A brief revision of the anatomy and the physiology is in order because information evaporates easily or gets buried in the more recently acquired knowledge. The physiology is dealt with in greater detail because an understanding of physiology helps interpretation of the clinical signs better.

8.1 Applied Anatomy and Physiology

The movement of each eye is controlled by a set of six extraocular muscles (Fig. 8.1). These muscles work together or against each other in an eye and also with the fellow eye to maintain the required eye position. These muscles and its control systems enable one to stabilise images on the retina and also track objects in the field of vision. Besides the extraocular muscles, we have three intraocular muscles—ciliary muscle, constrictor and dilator muscles of the iris. These three intraocular muscles help in focusing the image and control the light entering the eye.

The eyeball literally floats in the soft tissue of the orbit enabling it to move in three axes within the orbit (Fig. 8.2). The eye moves up and down in the X axis, medially and laterally in the Z axis rotates inward and outward in the antero-posterior Y axis. To understand the function of the extraocular muscles, one should be aware of the position of the insertion and effective origin of the muscle and its relation to the axis of rotation of the eye. The superior oblique muscle though originating from the posterior part of the orbit passes through the trochlea near the anterior border of the orbit before inserting on to the globe. The trochlea thus becomes the **effective origin** of the muscle in order to understand its function. The superior oblique muscle gets inserted in the upper outer posterior quadrant of the globe as opposed to the other recti muscle which gets inserted into the anterior half of the globe. The extraocular muscles may have more than one function (e.g. abduction and intorsion) in moving the eye. Depending on the position of the eye, the effectiveness of these functions vary and this can be worked out depending of the effective origin and insertion of the ocular muscles. The superior and inferior recti are at an angle of about 90° to their synergistic muscles inferior oblique and superior rectus,

© Springer Nature Singapore Pte Ltd. 2020
T. Kuriakose, *Clinical Insights and Examination Techniques in Ophthalmology*,
https://doi.org/10.1007/978-981-15-2890-3_8

Fig. 8.1 Extraocular muscles with its origins outside the eyeball and the insertion on the globe

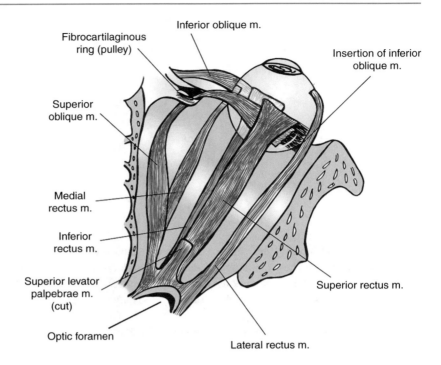

Fig. 8.2 The three axes in which the eye moves within the orbit

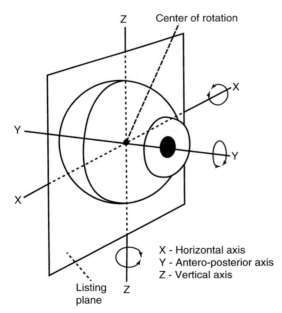

rectus has to be checked in isolation, the patient should be asked to look up and out. The muscles and its functions when the eye is in the primary position and its nerve supply is listed in Table 8.1. The tertiary action is not tested clinically. Instead of trying to memorise the action of each muscle, the clinician is advised to mentally work out what would happen to the globe if these muscles contract. This mental exercise would also help one to understand the rationale of testing the action of these muscles and interpret the movements that occur when they are dysfunctional. The number of muscles and its elaborate control systems exist so that the image of interest of the outside world is focused on the fovea of the retina in both eyes simultaneously. In its intended mode of action, this then gives us a single binocular vision with the ability to perceive depth or stereopsis.

When the two eyes are able to put the image of the object of regard on the fovea simultaneously, it is call **orthotropia** (straight direction). When the same image falls on both the fovea, the brain is able to fuse the two images so that we perceive it as a single object in space with respect to us. In addition to seeing it as a single object, a third dimension or depth is added to the image by

respectively. What this means is that the action of the two muscles can be isolated when the eye is abducted (recti action only) or adducted (oblique action only). So if the elevation action of superior

Table 8.1 Extraocular muscles, their actions and nerve supply

Extraocular muscle	Muscle action (primary)	Muscle action (secondary)	Muscle action (tertiary)	Cranial nerve (CN) supply
Medial rectus	Adduction			Third CN or oculomotor nerve
Inferior rectus	Depression	Adduction	Extorsion	Third CN or oculomotor nerve
Inferior oblique	Extorsion	Elevation	Abduction	Third CN or oculomotor nerve
Superior rectus	Elevation	Adduction	Intorsion	Third CN or oculomotor nerve
Superior oblique	Intorsion	Depression	Abduction	Fourth CN or trochlear nerve
Lateral rectus	Abduction			Sixth CN or Abducens nerve

Fig. 8.3 Orthotropic eye with the visual axis intersecting at the point of regard located in the centre of the field in each eye

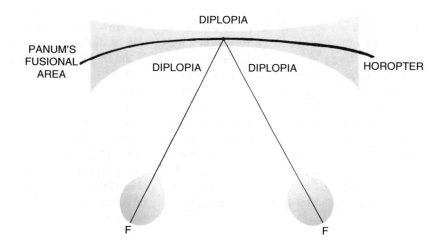

the brain. This is called stereoscopic vision and has its origins in the slightly dissimilar images seen from two different angles by the two eyes kept apart in the orbit. If the neural circuitry for stereopsis is not developed, then binocular single vision does not give the experience of the third dimension. In fact, there is a significant proportion of the population who do not experience stereopsis in its full glory. Lack of stereopsis, however, is not a big disadvantage because one can use monocular clues to assess depth.

The monocular clues to assess depth include—contour overlay (objects in front will cover those behind), shadows and play of light on the objects (shadow of an object on the screen is only possible if there is a gap between the two), known size of objects (objects appear smaller as it moves further away), motion parallax (when fixating on a point, objects further away will move

with the head and those closer against) and aerial perspective (atmosphere, changes appearance of objects depending on the distance of objects away from us).

If the visual axis does not meet at the point of regard when both eyes are open (i.e. one eye is deviated), it is called a **squint** or **strabismus** or **tropia**. If the non-fixing eye is deviated out, it is called exotropia, inward deviation is call esotropia, upward deviation is hypertropia and downward deviation is hypotropia.

When the eyes are straight or orthotropic and the image of the object of regard falls on the fovea, our brain assumes the object is in front, in line with forehead. This localisation of the object in space with respect to oneself is called egocentric (self-centred) localisation. Fovea thus sees the centre point of the field (Fig. 8.3). Images falling nasal to the fovea will be localised temporal to the point of regard. Similarly, those falling nasal, superior and inferior to fovea will be projected temporal, inferior and superior to the object of regard. When the eye is foveating on an object, points around it in space projects to points around the fovea in either eye. The point on the retina of either eye which receives light from a single point in space is called the corresponding retinal points (Fig. 8.4). As a corollary, only when corresponding retinal points are stimulated by an object, the images will be fused by the brain to be perceived as one. If images of an object fall on non-corresponding retinal points, then it will be perceived as double by the brain. The two foveae of either eye are corresponding retinal points. Fovea has a **retinomotor** value of zero. This means the eye does not have to make any movement to put the object of regard on the fovea. As one moves away from the fovea, the retinomotor values of the retinal point increases. This means larger excursions of the eye have to be made to bring objects falling on that part of the retina to the fovea. In Fig. 8.4, point touching the green line will have a higher retinomotor value that point touching the yel-

low line. The retinomotor value can be in terms of the degrees the eye has to move to fixate from that point and gives us an idea of the concept. In this figure, the eye is cross-sectioned from temporal to nasal part in both eyes. Point (touching the purple line) on the nasal side of the retina of the right eye corresponds to the point (touching the purple line) on the temporal part of the left eye. In the up-down direction, however, the corresponding points will be either above or below the fovea in both eyes as both eyes have to move in the same direction to fixate on an object above or below the fovea. Motor fusion (to avoid diplopia) is the exclusive function of extrafoveal retinal periphery and it is the sensation of diplopia due to the extrafoveal location of the image that induces the eye movement.

The loci of points in space formed by the intersection of projected lines from the corresponding retinal points of the retina is called a **horopter** (Fig. 8.4). Points on the horopter will appear single when the subject is fixated on the centre of the horopter. In practice, however, it is observed that images that fall in a limited area around the corresponding retinal points can also be fused by the eye. This area on the retina projected in space is the **Panum's fusional area** (Fig. 8.3); though not depicted in the figure this fusional area is three dimensional. This area is smallest at the point of fixation and becomes larger as one goes to the periphery. This stands to reason because the receptive fields increase in size as one goes into the periphery. In other words, as one goes into the retinal periphery more number of rods and cones connect to one ganglion cell. This retinal disparity tolerated by brain is in fact essential for stereopsis or three-dimensional viewing. Placing the image of the point of regard at the fovea of the two eyes so that it can be fused is the most important driver to keep eye straight. If the visual axis of the two eyes does not intersect at the point of regard, it is called squint or strabismus.

In strabismus or squint, in one eye the fovea gets the image from the object of regard. The image of the same objects falls elsewhere in a non-corresponding part of the retina in the fellow eye. This image then projects the object elsewhere in space depending on the turn of the eye

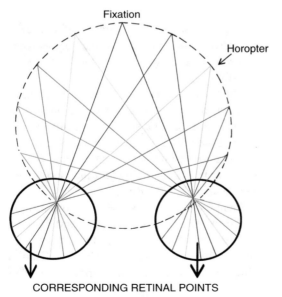

Fig. 8.4 Horopter—Locus of points formed by projection from the corresponding retinal points on the retina when the eye is fixed on a target

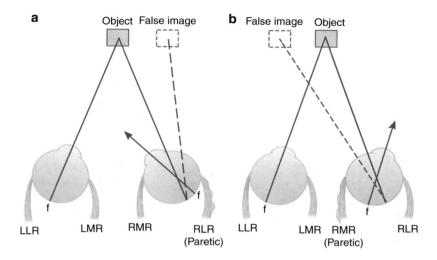

Fig. 8.5 Uncrossed diplopia in esotropia (**a**) and crossed diplopia in exotropia (**b**)

and the patient experiences diplopia or double vision. If the squinting eye is turned inward or esotropic, then the second image falls on the nasal half of the retina which projects the image on to the same side as the squinting eye and one gets an **uncrossed diplopia**. In outward turning or exotropia, the opposite happens and one gets a **crossed diplopia** (Fig. 8.5).

In the fovea of the squinting eye, the image of another point in space which is not the point of regard gets imprinted. The two different images on the fovea thus cause confusion, and there is retinal rivalry. The brain seems to compensate for the retinal rivalry more easily than the diplopia as patients with recent onset squint complains more about diplopia rather than confusion. Confusion is more of a problem when the quality of image (size, shape, etc.) of the same object is different in both the fovea (e.g. unilateral cataract).

In long-standing squint, the double image is compensated in two ways. In children where the nervous system is still plastic, the dissimilar images both at the fovea and the periphery is **suppressed** by the brain centrally. Long-standing suppression prevents the neural connections from developing and the eye becomes **amblyopic** (decreased vision without any clinically obvious ophthalmic pathology). The other compensatory mechanism is to change the retinomotor value the retinal elements and the zero retinomotor value of the fovea is taken by the area where the image of the point of regard falls. Along with the new fovea all other points also change their retinomotor value. This compensatory mechanism is called **anomalous retinal correspondence**. Since the non-foveal area does not have the retinal structure (higher concentration of cones with a very small number of cones being connected to a single ganglion cell) that enable high visual acuity, the new area of the retina with the retinomotor value of the fovea does not have the same vision as the normal fovea. In adults since central suppression is not possible due to the lack neural plasticity the diplopia persists, some patients however learn to ignore the troubling second image.

Even when the eyes appear to be fixed, there is a constant firing of impulse to all the muscles giving rise to a fine flicker movement. The position of the eye in the obit results from the interactions of all the muscles acting on it.

Yolk muscles or agonist muscles are the pair of muscles from both the eye which act together to achieve a similar purpose. The medial rectus of right eye and the lateral rectus of the opposite left eye are yolk muscles which enable the person to look to the left. **Antagonist muscle** is the eye which sub-serves the action opposite to the agonist muscle. The lateral rectus muscles of the same eye are the antagonist muscles of the medial rectus (Table 8.2).

Eye movements and imaging follow a certain pattern and these patterns have been described as laws though they are different from the laws one is used to in Physics.

Table 8.2 Showing examples of some yolk and antagonist muscles in different directions of gaze

Action required	Agonist muscles		Antagonist muscles	
	Right eye	Left eye	Right eye	Left eye
Moving eyes to the right	Lateral rectus	Medial rectus	Medial rectus	Lateral rectus
Moving eyes to the left	Medial rectus	Lateral rectus	Lateral rectus	Medial rectus
Moving the eyes down and right	Inferior rectus	Superior oblique	Superior rectus	Inferior oblique
Moving eyes up and to the right	Superior rectus	Inferior oblique	Inferior rectus	Superior oblique
Moving eyes straight down	Inferior rectus, superior oblique	Inferior rectus, superior oblique	Superior rectus, inferior oblique	Superior rectus, inferior oblique

Donders' law states that for each position of the eye the retinal meridians of the eye are fixed. It does not matter how the eye reached this position, i.e. came from lateral, medial or superior position, the orientation of the retinal meridians will be the same.

Sherrington's law of reciprocal innervations states that when the agonist muscle acts the antagonist muscle is inhibited.

Hering's law of equal innervation states that the yolk muscle of both eyes gets equal innervation impulses.

When there is an object on the left side of the face, shifting gaze to that object on the left entails lesser movement of the left eye compared to the right eye. Here it would appear the innervations to left eye should be lesser than the right eye. In reality what happens is more complex. The movement of the left eye due to equal innervations to the left eye lateral rectus is inhibited by the medial rectus of the left eye once foveation occurs.

As mentioned earlier, the positioning of the eyeballs is a result of interplay of all the muscles and is much more complex than what the above laws dictate. The above laws are just guidelines to help one understand eye movements and explains the findings seen when examining patients with ocular motor pathology. In conditions like congenital fibrosis syndrome, Duane retraction syndrome the above rules of innervations do not hold and it is now being recognised that there are central innervation abnormalities responsible for the findings seen in these patients. The clinicians therefore should not restrict themselves with the above laws or assumptions when trying to decipher unusual eye movement abnormalities.

8.2 Normal Eye Movements

A good idea of normal eye movements and its variations are needed to assess patients with ocular motility problems. Classically, the extent of ocular movements is checked in the seven diagnostic positions (cardinal positions) of the eye. Figure 8.6 shows the normal eye positions in each of the positions of gaze.

Normally in the primary position, both eyes should be looking straight at the point of regard. They should be equally prominent with no proptosis or enophthalmos of either eye. The position of the upper lid (upper lid margin is 2 mm below the upper limbus) and lower lid (lower limbus at the lower lid margin) should be the same in both eyes. The palpebral fissure width should be comparable in both eyes. Up to 1 mm difference in the palpebral fissure width is not uncommon in normal people. When the patient looks into the examiner's eyes, both eyes will appear to look in the same direction in a person with no squint. The corneas of both eyes should be stationary with very little noticeable eye movements.

There are three types of broad eye movements one can examine in evaluating eye movements. These are ductions, versions and vergence.

Ductions are uni-ocular eye movements with the fellow eye occluded so that the effect of the occluded eye does not dictate the movement of the tested eye. This is evaluated by asking the patient to follow a target that is moved from the centre to the periphery in all directions of the

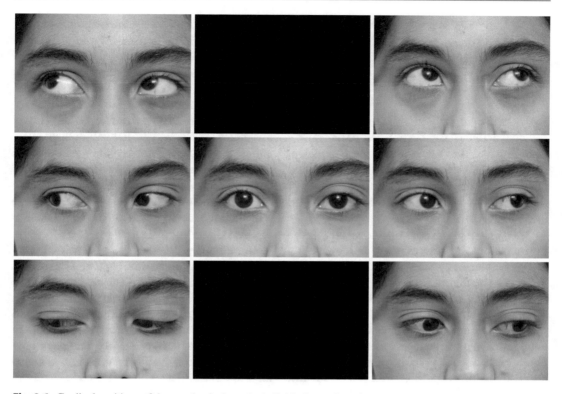

Fig. 8.6 Cardinal positions of the eye that isolates the individual muscle action

gaze testing position. Adduction is the movement of eye medially towards the nose. In a fully
adducted eye, 2 mm of the corneal limbus should
be hidden within the canthus. Alternatively, one
third of the medial part of the cornea should just
cross the lower punctum.

Abduction is moving the eye laterally. In
normal people when the eye is fully abducted
the lateral limbus will just touch the lateral canthus. There will be no scleral show. However,
in patients with prominent eyes and in patients
over 70 years one may see a millimetre of bare
sclera between the lateral canthus and cornea. If
this scleral show is symmetrical, then one can
be even more confident that it is only a variation
of normal. **As a general rule, clinical findings
acquire significance only in the overall context
of an underlying symptom or sign one is trying
to evaluate.**

Since the upper and lower lids move along
with elevation and depression, one does not have
fixed landmark on the lids to evaluate these move-

ments objectively. Comparing with the other eye
is one alternative. The normal position of eye in
the remaining four diagnostic positions is again
not well defined for the same reason. By repeated
examination of normal patients, one will get a
visual impression of the normal range of movement in these eyes.

The up, down and side to side movements of
the eye can also be assessed using the limbal test
of **Kestenbaum**. To assess the extent of movement, a plastic ruler is used. After aligning the
patient's eye with the examiner's eye (i.e. right
eye of patient with left eye of the examiner) to
avoid parallax, adduction, abduction, elevation
and depression can be evaluated. The plastic
ruler is kept bisecting the pupil vertically (for
vertical eye movements) or horizontally depending on the movement being measured. In normal
adduction when the scale is kept horizontally, the
lateral limbus of the eye moves 10 mm medially
when the eye is fully adducted from the mid position. Likewise, there is a 10 mm movement of

Table 8.3 Normal range of abduction, adduction, elevation and depression using a scale

Abduction	9–10 mm
Adduction	9–10 mm
Elevation	5–7 mm
Depression	9–10 mm

the medial limbus in abduction and 10 mm downward movement of upper limbus for depression. For elevation, the movement is about 5–7 mm (Table 8.3). These measurements are difficult to do especially when the lids cover the upper and lower limbus.

Though in most clinical situations one is looking for underaction of eye movements, overaction of eye movements are important when relevant and should be looked for.

Versions are movements of both eyes together in one direction. This is tested with both eyes open and the range of movements is similar to ductions. Again the patient is asked to follow an object that is moved from the primary position to all positions of diagnostic gaze. **An important instruction to be given to the patient is ask him to report to the examiner if he perceives double vision (seeing the object as two) at any point during examination.** Patients may report double vision in subtle movement deficiencies where the limitation of movement may not be obvious to the examiner. The upper lid can be held up to assess movement if needed especially if the lid positions are not equal on either side or there is significant overaction of a muscle in the up gaze. Versions are better to detect subtle limitations in movement because when checking duction's excessive impulse may be sent to see the objects in periphery. In versions usually the better eye will decide the nervous input and hence the weaker muscle will lag behind. One needs to be aware that in the extremes of lateral gaze position, the nose blocks the adducted eye and the patient will have a uni-ocular vision through the abducted eye with a break in fusion. Besides the ranges of movement, one should also look for any lag in the start of the eye movement (seen in weaker muscles) or any sudden change in speed of movement suggestive of a release from a resistance or encountering a resistance (seen in adhesion syndromes).

In patients with freely alternating esotropia, there exists a condition called **cross fixation**. Here, since there is no fusion and abduction is not a preferred movement for these patients, they just switch fixation when looking laterally. For example, when a patient is looking to the right the esotropic left eye fixates on the object of regard. As this object is moved to the left half of the field, at around the midpoint the esotropic right eye takes over fixation and follows the object. It will thus appear like the lateral rectus is paralysed in both eyes if one did versions alone. Occluding one eye will elicit the lateral rectus movement in the fellow eye.

Before doing versions, it is also a good practice to identify the **dominant eye** if possible. The dominant eye can be made out by asking the patient to look at a distant object with both eyes. Then ask him to hold a pencil in front of him so that the eye, pencil and the distant object is in one line. Now ask the patient to close one eye at a time and look at the alignment. The eye that is aligned more closely with the pencil is the dominant eye. In right-handed people, the right eye is usually the more dominant eye. The dominant eye can also be made out by asking the patient to look at an object being brought close to the nose of the patient. At one point, the fusion will break and one eye will diverge. The eye maintaining fusion is the dominant eye.

If the dominant eye is a mildly paretic eye, patients will fixate with the paretic eye and will appear normal. The non-dominant eye following Hering's law will then show overaction or underaction and confuse the clinician not aware of this. For example, in a right superior oblique palsy if the right eye is the dominant fixing eye then the left eye will be hypotropic in primary position. If left eye is the fixing eye, then the right paretic eye will appear hypertropic.

Vergence is simultaneous movement of both eyes in the opposite direction. Moving both eyes towards the nose is convergence and is observed when looking at close objects. The nearest point one can converge on is called the **near point of convergence**. It is about 10 cm normally and is much closer than the near point of accommodation. Normally, convergence movement does not occur in isolation. To see near, besides convergence, the eye needs to accommodate to see things closer. In addition, there is pupillary constriction. Ciliary muscle contraction which facilitates accommodation and pupil constriction is mediated by the parasympathetic nerves of the third nerve. The combination of convergence, accommodation (due to ciliary muscle contraction) and pupillary constriction constitute the **near reflex**.

8.3 Examination of Ocular Motility

8.3.1 History

For emphasis, it needs to be mentioned again that history is important to make a clinical decision. A good number of patients with ocular motility problems are children. In the history, one should enquire about the prenatal period, history of prematurity, development history, trauma, neonatal illnesses and behavioural issues. All these have an association with ocular motility problems. Since squint can run in families, besides a family history of squint, family history of wearing glasses, wearing patches and having eye surgeries may be suggestive of interventions for squinting eyes. If patient gives a history of double vision, one needs to clarify what the patient actually means. Sometimes, even blurring of vision in one eye is termed as double vision. If patient complains of diplopia, he should be asked about the relationship between the two images. Are they situated side by side or up and down? Patient or the mother should be asked about the intermittency of the symptoms. Myasthenia gravis is a classical condition where the diplopia may be more prominent in the evenings. If the mother/primary carer says the child squints sometimes and you cannot make out any squint even after repeated examinations, it is best to believe the mother and keep the child under follow-up. It may be useful to get past photos of the patient to see when the problem started. Past photo may show that a squint noted recently was always present. In children, it may be worthwhile examining the child while the history is being taken from the parents and the child is not the centre of attention.

8.4 Examination of the Eyes

Visual assessment is an integral part of examination of squint and its assessment is difficult in children. Details of evaluation of vision are given in Chaps. 4 and 16. What is important to ascertain especially in children is to see if there is a difference in vision between the two eyes. Resenting closure of the good eye or a constant squint in one eye is suggestive of poor visual acuity in that eye. When examining vision in one eye (by occluding the other eye), look for latent nystagmus (oscillatory movements manifesting only when one eye is occluded) which can reduce vision when one eye is occluded. In these cases, a plus three-diopter lens should be used instead of an occluder.

Refraction should be part of the ocular motility examination especially in children. Uncorrected refractive error can be the cause of squint or amblyopia. Correction of refractive error is an integral part of the treatment. It was traditionally thought that all children were hypermetropes and emmetropisation occurred with the growth of the child. There are authors who think up to 25% of new-borns may be myopes and they too undergo emmetropisation. Refer to Chap. 14 for doing refractions in patients with squint.

The eye examination starts with how the patient walks into the room and his head posture while navigating around. Look to see if there are any dysmorphic facial features which could be indicators of abnormalities in the orbit too. Attention is then drawn to the palpebral fissure. Look for any ptosis or pseudoptosis (due to a hypotropia rather than a lid problem). Pseudoptosis will correct itself if the affected eye is made to fixate by occluding the fellow eye. Look at the level of the canthi to see if they are at the same level. In patients with ptosis, ask the patient to clench or move the jaw to see if the ptotic lid moves up to rule out Marcus Gunn jaw-winking. In infants observe the child while sucking the bottle to look for lid movements.

Mothers can come complaining their baby has a squint because the eyes appear drawn inward due to a large nasal bridge. Pulling up the skin at the base of the nose will remove a pseudo-squint (Fig. 8.7). A cover test is needed to confirm a **pseudo-strabismus**.

The eye position is judged grossly by the position of the cornea. **Visual axis** or the line connecting the fovea to the point of regard decides the direction of the globe. The angle between the line connecting the centre of cornea to the point of regard or **pupillary axis** and the visual axis is called angle kappa (Fig. 8.8). If the angle between these two lines is large, then one can get a false appearance of squint. In high myopes, the visual axis is temporal to the pupillary axis (negative angle kappa) and the eye will look deviated inward. If the visual axis is nasal to the pupillary axis (positive angle kappa), the eye will appear to be deviated out. A positive angle kappa is supposed to make a person more pretty! In conditions where the macula is drawn temporally, one can get a large positive angle kappa and the eye will appear as though it is exotropic. One should therefore be aware of the effect of angle kappa when evaluating patients with squints. Cover test (described later) when applicable is the best method to detect and quantify squints.

Before we proceed to examine a patient with squint, one should be clear about the objective of the examination. There are many clinical examina-tions described in the evaluation of a patient with squint. There are also equipment available to examine patients with squint. The plethora of 'toys'/equipment available to examine a patient with squint confuses the ordinary Ophthalmologist. So much so, many develop a block when confronted with a patient having squint.

The important questions to be answered with respect to diagnosis and management are: **Is there a squint? How much is the deviation? What is the function of the various extraocular muscles? Is there any fusion or potential for fusion? What suppression mechanism if any is present?** Answers to the above questions will give us the diagnosis, the management strategies and the prognosis for cosmetic and visual improvement. Simple tests are enough to answer these questions and one may not need to resort to all the tests described and get confused in the process.

8.5   Assessment of Vision

Assessment of vision (see Chap. 4) is done one eye at a time and with both eyes open. The latter is more useful in children. A cycloplegic refraction (with atropine in pigmented eyes or cyclo-pentolate) is a must in children (see Chap. 5) to uncover all the accommodation-related refractive changes. This is especially important when evaluating children with esotropia and hyper-metropia. Cycloplegia is also important if the accommodation in children is giving varying values. When possible all tests for squint should only be done with the refractive correction if any in place as that is the only way to control accommodation (i.e. both eyes will use the same

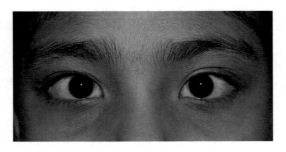

Fig. 8.7 Pseudo-esotropia (cover test will not show any deviation)

Fig. 8.8 Angle Kappa

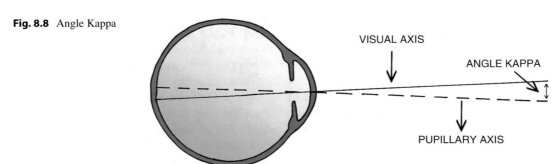

accommodative effort when seeing a distant or near target) during the examination.

8.6   Cover Tests

As mentioned fusion (combining the images of the two eyes to give the sensation of one object) is the biggest incentive to avoid squint. The stronger the fusion mechanisms better is the person's ability to overcome inherent deviations of the eye. Looks can be deceptive when assessing squint. Small angle squint may not be apparent even to a trained person. The only way to make sure there is no squint (i.e. visual axis is meeting the point of regard) is to check for the same, one eye at a time. This is done by the cover test. Before covering either eye, one should look to see if the eyes are apparently straight or not, for in patients with weak fusion mechanisms, breaking the fusion mechanism by covering one eye will cause a squint, the patient cannot overcome easily. Knowing if the patient has fusion, however weak it may be, can be useful in the management of strabismus.

To look for manifest squint or strabismus, patient is asked to look at a distant accommodative target like a 6/9 (20/30) letter if there is visual potential. An accommodative target controls accommodation. If the patient presents with spectacles, the glasses should be put on when doing the cover test and can then be repeated without it later. In patients who are presenting with spectacles, ensure that the glasses do not have any prism incorporated in them as it can give false readings. For the management of squint, a cycloplegic refraction should be done and the cover tests repeated with the best corrected glasses. This standardises the accommodation.

The eye which is thought to be fixing is now covered with an opaque or translucent occluder (Fig. 8.9) and the suspect eye is observed. The examiner's hand which has spaces between fingers if used as an occluder can give wrong findings. If the visual axis of the suspect eye is meeting the fixating letter, then the eye will not move. However, if the image of the letter was not at the fovea of the examined eye the eye will

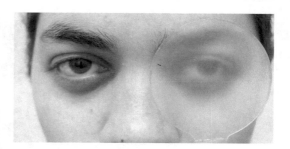

Fig. 8.9 Translucent occluder covering the eye enables one to track the eye movement behind the occluder

move to align it to the fovea. This re-fixation movement of even two prisms can be observed by the trained examiner. If there is no re-fixation movement, both eyes are opened and the eye that was open is now covered to look for re-fixation movement in the fellow eye. This is called the **cover test**, done to detect **manifest squint** or **tropias**. The movement of the eye or degree of squint can be measured in '**degree of an arc**' or '**prism diopter**' and is measured using prisms or an equipment called synoptophore (discussed later). One degree is approximately equal to two-prism dioptre. If on cover test there is no re-fixation movement of the observed uncovered eye, one can ensure that the uncovered eye is fixing on the target by gently moving the chin from side to side and ensuring the eye is fixing and following the target. Now continue to observe the eye while uncovering the fellow eye. In small tropias sometimes the eye movement that occurs when the observed eye relinquishes fixation, in favour of uncovered fellow eye is easier to make out than the re-fixation movement during the initial cover test. The eye movements that may be seen in different types of tropias when the cover is shifted to the fellow eye is shown in Fig. 8.10. In this figure, 1, 2, 3 is for orthotropic eyes and shows no movement, 4 shows outward movement in esotropia, 5 shows inward movement in exotropia, 6 shows downward movement in hypertropia and 7 shows the opposite movement in hypotropia.

The *cover uncover test* is done to look for **latent squint** or **phorias** and **intermittent squints**. Phorias and intermittent squints are ocular deviations compensated by fusion and thus

Fig. 8.10 Possible eye movements in common tropias during cover test

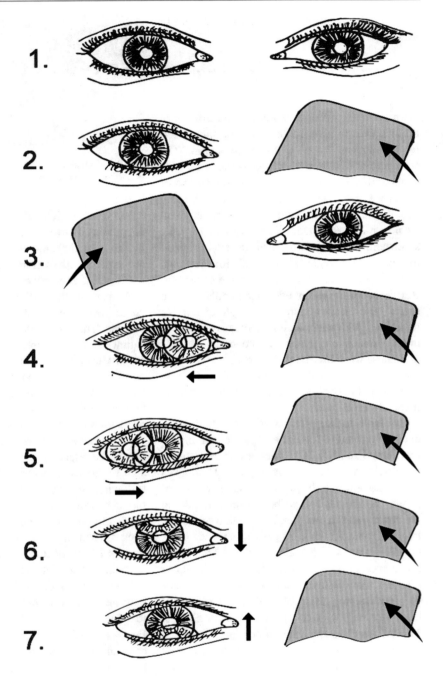

1.

2.

3.

4.

5.

6.

7.

can be hidden. This test therefore also helps us evaluate the fusional mechanisms. The breaking down of compensatory mechanisms when one eye is occluded and the ability to re-compensate when occlusion is removed forms the basis of this test. Here the assumption is that a manifest squint has been ruled out and if present this test does not give added information. Again the patient is asked to look at the distant or near accommodative target. One eye is now covered and patient's attention drawn to the target again. Now the covered eye is opened and the examiner looks at the eye under cover to see if the straight position was maintained or it makes a re-fixation movement to take up fixation. If there is a re-fixation movement of the eye under cover when the occluder is removed, then there is a latent squint that made the eye deviate away from the straight position. If a translucent occluder is used, then as the eye is covered the eye under cover can be seen to deviate in cases of phoria. In some patients with poor fusion, the re-fixation movement may not occur spontaneously and will be seen only when the eye that was not occluded is occluded. In some patients with phoria, the eye under cover may not deviate spontaneously. Occlusion alone may not be enough to move the eye away from the direction it has been looking. In such a case after occlusion the chin of the patient should be moved gently from side to side. The doll's eye movement behind the occluder will change the direction of the eye and the lack of fusion stimulus will keep the eye deviated and reveal a latent squint if present.

In patients who have intermittent squint' the fusion reflex is not very strong and they may not make an effort to fuse all the time. These patients manifest the squint when tired or are daydreaming. Squint in these patients may be made out transiently when the patient is thinking and looking at a distance to answer your questions. Intermittent exotropia or outward movement is more common than intermittent esotropia. Cover uncover test can bring our intermittent squint.

Once a latent (phoria) or manifest (tropia) squint is detected the next step is to measure it. An **alternate cover test** or **prism cover test** is done to measure the squint. Here patient is asked to fixate at a distant or near target depending on what the objective of the test is. The occluder is then moved from one eye to the other while the patient is fixating at the target. The re-fixation movement of the uncovered eye as the fellow eye is covered is observed. Here prisms of increasing powers (designated in prism dioptres) are placed in front of the eye with the better vision and alternate cover test done till there is no re-fixation movement seen. For a patient with right esotropia, the patient is asked to look at a distant accommodative target say 6/9 letter. Prism is placed in front of the left eye with its base towards the temporal side and the right eye is covered. Now transfer the cover from the right eye to the left eye to observe the re-fixation in the right eye. The power of the prims is increased till there is no re-fixation movement or the direction of the re-fixation movement changes. For exotropia, the prism is placed with the base inward. Loose single prisms of different powers or prisms of increasing powers stacked in frame is available to neutralise the tropia. The position of the prism with respect to the plane of the eye can change the measurement value. Loose prisms should be placed such that the side facing the eye is parallel to the eye. The stacked prism is placed parallel to the face (Fig. 8.11).

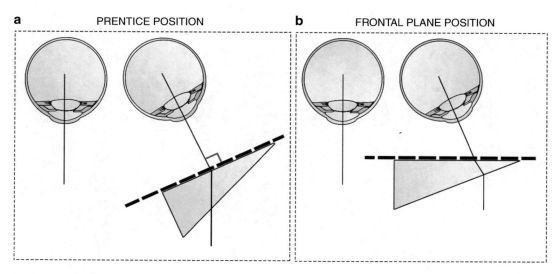

Fig. 8.11 Direction of prism to be placed in front of each eye; (**a**) when using loose prism and (**b**) when using stacked prisms

Adding two prisms if needed during examination is not straightforward. So if more than one prism is required, to get the adequate strength it is best to place them separately in front of both eyes. For example, 10 ΔD base out in RE and 10 ΔD base-out left eye if 20 ΔD base out is needed for one eye.

Concomitant squints are those that have the same angle of deviation for both eyes in all directions of gaze. Childhood squints usually fall into this category where the pathology is not due to a muscle or peripheral motor nerve pathology. In **non-comitant squints,** the angle of deviation differs depending on the eye occluded and the direction of gaze. It is therefore important to measure the angle of squint in different directions of gaze so as to reveal the nature of the squint and its pathology.

In concomitant squints, one can get changes in magnitude when it is associated with conditions like **A or V phenomenon**. In V exotropia, the divergence increases in the up gaze giving a V pattern. In A exotropia, the divergence increases in down gaze. This difference in the angle of squint here has to be taken into consideration when correcting squint so the eye is straight with bi-foveal fixation in most directions of gaze.

8.6.1 Measurement in Different Directions of Gaze

To measure the angle of deviation in different directions of gaze, moving the distant fixation target or the position of the examiner is difficult in a clinic situation. To overcome this, the face of the patient is turned keeping the fixation target the same (Fig. 8.12). To do the alternate cover for right gaze, the face should be turned to the left. Patient should be binocular and both eyes of the patient should be able to see the target when the face is turned for cover test. If the face is turned too much, the nose acts as an occluder! A near target can, however, be moved easily and the patient can be asked to hold an accommodative target and move it to different position of gaze while the examiner does the prism cover test.

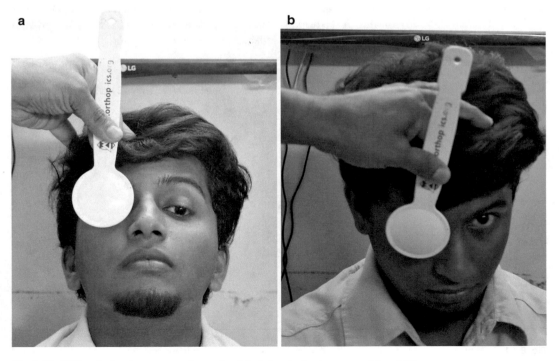

Fig. 8.12 Tilting the head to measure the angle of deviation in the down gaze (**a**) and (**b**) up gaze

8.6.2 Limitations of Cover Test

Cover test has limitations, and one should be careful when interpreting the results. If the patient's fixation is not good either because the vision is not good or the child is frightened and uncooperative, the results can be variable. If patient has eccentric fixation, then the re-fixation movement if any will not be a true reflection of the position of the eye.

Rebound saccades are seen in some patients during neutralisation. Here during the neutralisation, the re-fixation saccade does not stop as soon as foveation occurs. The eye overshoots and comes back to the fixation. Making out the end point can be difficult here.

8.7 Cover Test in Special Situations

Children may be intimidated when the occluder is brought near their eye. In these situations, one can do an indirect cover test where the occluder is kept far from the child between the child's eye and the fixation target. One can also use the thumb to occlude the eye while steadying the child's head with the rest of the hand (Fig. 8.13).

Translucent or Spielman occluder is used to assess the behaviour of the eye behind the occluder (Fig. 8.9). Here the patient will not be able to see enough with the occluder to fuse. When either of the eyes in a child with esotropia is covered with a Spielman occluder, the eye will straighten out if the esotropia is induced by accommodation and the accommodation is relaxed by getting the child to look at the distance.

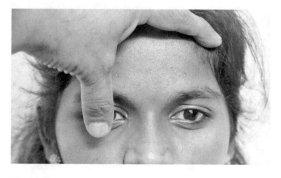

Fig. 8.13 Using the finger as an occluder, especially useful in children

8.7.1 Measuring Combined Deviations

When patients have a combination of a horizontal and vertical deviation, the horizontal deviation is first neutralised with the prisms placed horizontally in front of one eye. Keeping the horizontal prisms in place, the vertical deviation is then neutralised by placing the prisms over the fellow eye.

8.7.2 Measuring Cyclotorsion

Maddox rod can be used to measure cyclorotations of the globe that occur due to oblique muscle dysfunction. Unlike what is mentioned in Chap. 5 here two maddox rod glasses are placed in the trial frame with the rods kept vertically in front of each eye and the patient is asked to look at the white spot of light. If there is cyclotropia along with vertical deviation the two red lines produced by the maddox rod will not be parallel but at an angle to each other. The amount of angulation can be read of the trial frame after turning one maddox rod till the two images are parallel. An equipment called synoptophore or major amblyoscope can also be used for this purpose.

8.7.3 Four Prism Base-Out Test

This test is done mainly to assess suppression, and hence amblyopia in patients suspected to have a microtropia or a small angle esotropia. When a patient comes with complains of decreased vision in one eye often noticed accidently and there is no ocular cause one can find, amblyopia should be ruled out. Cover test may reveal a small esotropia. It is easy to miss the small flick on cover test, and a 4 prism base-out test helps in these situations. This is done by placing a 4-dioptre prism base out in front of the eye with the normal vision and the fellow suspect eye observed. In a normal person fixating at a distant target when a 4 ΔD prism is placed base out in front of one eye, the image on the fovea is shifted temporally and the eye has to move inward to re-fixate on the object. This causes the fellow eye to move out due to simultaneous innervation. This, however, causes the image to

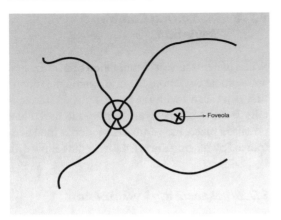

Fig. 8.14 Area of suppression in small angle esotropia (microtropia)

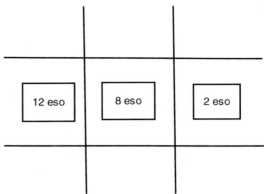

Fig. 8.15 Depicting deviations in prism diopters in a patient with right lateral rectus palsy

fall out of the fovea in the fellow eye and a small corrective movement is made to re-foveate and get the single vision back. In patients with small angle esotropia (microtropia), there is a small area of suppression nasal to the fovea (Fig. 8.14). In a patient with a suspected microtropia of the left eye, the shifted image in the left eye on bringing in a 4 ΔD base-out prism in front of the good right eye does not fall outside the suppression area. The initial lateral movement that occurs in the left eye with the movement of the right eye produces no re-fixation movement as there is no incentive for re-foveation. Lack of re-fixation movement confirms the presence of a suppression area and possible amblyopia in the left eye.

8.8   Documentation

To record findings, besides photography in different directions of gaze, different strategies have been used. Figure 8.15 depicts one method of recording deviation in relevant directions of gaze when doing a prism cover test for a patient with an isolated right lateral rectus palsy. For patients with diplopia, Hess charting can be done if the special charts and charting paper is available (not discussed here).

When one does not have the time to measure formally, underaction of a muscle can be graded from 0 to −4. For recording underaction, −4 can be no action at all and 0 is considered normal full

range of movement. −2 is when the cornea can be brought to the midline by the paretic muscle. For overaction, authors have suggested 0 to +2. +1 being mild overaction and +2 being gross overaction. A scale of 2 may be better for overaction as it serves no clinical purpose to divide it further. Figure 8.16 shows the recording of a patient with an underaction of lateral rectus and overaction of superior oblique.

8.9   Corneal Reflex Testing

8.9.1   Hirschberg Test

In patients who do not fix on a target or who have poor vision in one or both eyes, the position of the reflex of a light source on the cornea will help the assessment of deviation. The **corneal reflex test** or **Hirschberg test** (named after one of the first people who described it) looks at the position of first Purkinje image (corneal reflex) of a light source on the cornea. If the corneal reflex is in the centre of the pupil in both eyes, then the eye is straight or **orthotropic**. If the position of the reflex is shifted nasally in one eye and is in the centre in the fellow eye, the patient has an exotropia in the eye where the reflex is shifted medially. The fixating eye is the one with the reflex in the centre. Likewise, in esotropia the reflex is shifted laterally, in hypertropia the reflex is shifted down. One millimetre of shift in the reflex from the cen-

Fig. 8.16 Gross representation of movement defects in a patient with abduction deficit and a right superior oblique palsy. *ET* esotropia, *HT* hypertropia

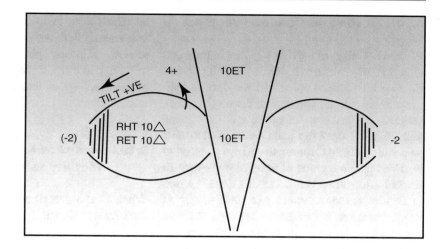

tre could mean a deviation of 7–12°. This large variation is due to the difference in the position of the landmark and the difference in the interpersonal assessment of these reflexes. Keeping this limitation in mind, as a rough indicator, corneal reflex at the border of a 3.5 mm pupil suggest a 15° deviation (1° is equal to 2-prism dioptre). A reflex at the limbus suggests a deviation of 45° or more of deviation. Assessment of the position of the reflex for finer assessments is made even more difficult in pigmented race as the delineation of the pupil and the brown iris is difficult when you are at a distance to assess the reflexes.

8.9.2   Krimsky Test

In eyes not able to fixate (blind or otherwise), Krimsky measured deviation using prisms and the corneal reflex. Here increasing strengths of the prism is placed in front of the good eye till the reflex of the cornea is centred in the blind eye. The power of the prism required to centre the reflex gives the amount of deviation. The examiner should sit in front of the deviating eye to avoid parallax. Unlike prism cover test, here the prism in placed in the opposite direction. In esotropia, the prism is kept base in. The difficulty in seeing the target through a prism, more so when assessing the reflex with a distant light source and the other factors mentioned before make the measurement less accurate than the prism cover test. However, it is still useful when one eye cannot perceive light or has very poor vision.

8.10   Diplopia and Other Eye Movement Testing

When a patient complains of double vision, the first thing to do is to confirm if the symptom is really diplopia. As mentioned previously, patients have different understanding of diplopia. Sometimes, patients with unequal vision in both eyes feel they have diplopia. Others complain of diplopia when the quality of image is not the same in both eyes. Once it is confirmed that patient does indeed have diplopia then he should be questioned about the position of one image with respect to the other. Side by side (horizontal deviation) or up and down (vertical deviation) or a combination of both. It is difficult for the patient to make out which image belongs to which eye. If a red glass (from the trial set) is placed in front of the right eye and patient asked if the red image is on the right side (uncrossed diplopia) or the left side (crossed diplopia) of the central image one can get an idea of the muscle involved. Uncrossed diplopia suggests esotropia because here the second image falls nasal to the fovea which is then projected temporally. Provided the paretic eye is not the fixating eye (due to dominance) the distance between the two images is maximum in the direction of action of the paretic eye. This can be confirmed with the prism cover test.

8.10.1 Testing Versions and Vergence

Version is both eyes moving together in the same direction (e.g. dextroversion or looking to the right with both eyes open) and vergence is both eyes moving in the opposite direction (e.g. convergence). When examining the eye movements with both eyes open in a patient suspected to have an ocular motility disorder, the primary objective is to compare the globe position of one eye with respect to the other. Version testing done as a part of central nervous system examination (CNS) is to check the coordination between the two eyes or the ability to initiate version through the higher centres that is being tested for. The pursuit movement part of the version testing is done with the examination of ocular movements.

To check for versions ask the patient to look up, down, left, right on voice command. As mentioned previously one can also ask the patient to follow the examiner's finger. See if there is a lag in movement of either eye or there is a difficulty in looking to any particular direction. Next, the examiner should hold out the index finger of both his hands on either side of the patient (Fig. 8.17) and ask the patient to look at the fingers of the examiner alternatively. Saccades are also tested in this manner.

To examine vergence, the patient is first asked to look at a distant object. A pencil is now placed 30 cm from the patient and he is asked to move his fixation from the distant object to the pen-

cil. His ability to look at the pencil should be noted along with the pupillary constriction. The section on neuro-ophthalmology will describe in more detail the examination of versions, nystagmus and other neuro-ophthalmology-related examinations.

8.10.2 Head Position in Ocular Motility Testing

When there is paresis of a muscle later in life, for the sake of maintaining fusion and single vision, the head is positioned in a way that it tries to compensate for the eye movement. For example, if the right lateral rectus is weak, the head with the eye is turned to the right to compensate for the deficit in eye movement in that direction. If the right superior oblique is weak, to compensate for the resultant lack of down ward movement and intorsion, the head is flexed and tilted to the left side (Fig. 8.18).

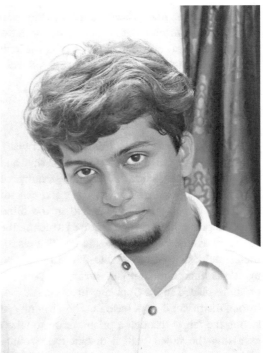

Fig. 8.18 Head position in right superior oblique palsy

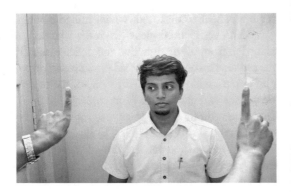

Fig. 8.17 Position of the examiner's fingers when examining for versions and saccades

Abnormal head positions can also be seen in patients with nystagmus whose nystagmus is minimal in a particular head position (**Null point**). These patients position the head to minimise nystagmus and improve vision.

8.11 Testing in Special Situations

8.11.1 Forced Duction Test and Force Generation Test

When one notes a limitation in the eye movement, it could be due to an underaction of the muscle (paresis/paralysis) or a limitation of movement of the globe by an external force. To distinguish between the two, one can do a **force duction test** (FDT) and a **force generation test** (FGT).

FDT is done to see if the globe can be moved passively by the examiner in order to rule out a mechanical restriction. To check if there is a mechanical cause for the lack of adduction in an eye, the patient is asked to make an effort to move the eye medially so that the medial rectus action if any is working. The eye is then manually rotated medially to see if the eye can be moved any further. Inability to move the eye medially suggest that there is a mechanical cause for the restriction. The cause can be either a mass in the orbit, entrapment of muscle or fibrosis of the antagonist muscle. The movement should only be a rotation and one should not push the globe into the orbit while doing this lest the leash effect (pushing the eye in, relaxes a tight fibrotic muscle) is released. If the eye is pushed in, the restriction will be missed. Doing the test correctly is important to come to the right conclusion.

To do the test, the limbus of the eye is anaesthetised with the use of repeated topical proparacaine drops. A pellet of cotton soaked in local anaesthetic can also be placed at the area of the limbus that is going to be held with the forceps. Using two fine Hoskins forceps, the limbal area at 3 and 9 o'clock positions are held. To test the medial limitation, the patient is then asked to adduct the eye. As the patient is adducting, the eye is rotated medially without pulling the eye outward or pushing it backward into the orbit. Pulling the eye outward while rotating the eye will cause the lateral rectus to stretch and prevent the eye from moving medially giving a false sense of restriction. The position of the forceps and the direction of rotation depend on the muscle being tested.

In **FGT**, one is making an assessment of the amount of muscle force present in a weak muscle. Here after anaesthetising the eye like above, Hoskins forceps is used to hold the limbal conjunctiva. To check the lateral rectus muscle action, the medial limbus is held with the patient looking straight ahead. Now the patient is asked to abduct the eye and the power of the tug assessed. In normal eyes, the power of movement is so much that the hold may even tear the conjunctiva. When learning to do the test, examine normal patients first to see what normal is, it may be a good idea not to hold too tightly at the limbus. Holding at the medial limbus also prevents corneal abrasions if the eye moves laterally. Patient should be warned about the possibility of having a sub-conjunctival haemorrhage after these tests.

8.11.2 Pupil Examination

Examination of the pupils (see Chap. 11) which is also supplied by the third nerve is necessary for any eye movement examination to figure out the aetiology. A pupil sparing third nerve is classically seen in a diabetic third nerve palsy.

8.11.3 Sensory Examination

In suspected cases of blow-out fracture, when there is a restriction of elevation or depression one should also look out for infra-orbital anaesthesia caused by the fractured inferior orbital wall bone injuring the infra-orbital nerve passing through the floor of the orbit. Crepitus of the regional soft tissue may be seen due to air getting in from the sinus due to the fracture of floor of the orbit. Fracture of any orbital wall in relation to the nose or the sinuses can cause soft tissue crepitus due to subcutaneous air.

8.11.4 Checking for Globe Retraction

Globe retraction should be looked for when examining patients with suspected Duane retraction syndrome or related pathologies. This is best done by looking at the eye position from the lateral side of the patient and seeing if the corneal plane moves backward into the orbit when the eye abducts or adducts. Since these patients have abnormal eye movements from birth, these patients are asymptomatic and may be picked up only during a routine eye examination.

8.11.5 Parks 3 Step Test

The **Parks–Bielschowsky three step test** is a method to identify the muscle causing a vertical deviation abnormality, particularly the superior oblique muscle which is the only muscle innervated by the IV nerve. First, any abnormal head posture if present is noted. The head is then straightened and the patient is asked to look at the distant target for the three-step test.

1. **Step 1**: While fixing the distant target, the position of the eyes is noted. Determine which eye is hypertropic in primary position. If there is a right hypertropia in primary position, then the depressors of the right eye (IR/SO) or the elevators of the left eye (SR/IO) are weak. If the eye position is difficult to discern, one can do a cover test to see if there is a vertical movement.
2. **Step 2**: Determine whether the hypertropia increases in the right or left gaze. The vertical recti, superior and inferior recti have their maximum action in the abducted position. In a right superior oblique palsy, moving the eye to the right removes the hypertropia and exaggerates it when the right eye is adducted.
3. **Step 3**: The patient is asked to tilt the head to the right and then left; the position of the eye

is observed. In right SO muscle palsy, on tilting the head to the right the hypertropia is exaggerated due to the unopposed action of SR on the same side, which acts to counteract the depression (along with intorsion) of the SO muscle which normally comes into play to counteract the extortion caused by the head tilt. This hypertropia decreases or disappears when head is tilted to the left side, thus confirming the diagnosis of a superior oblique paresis. Likewise, the eye movements for each of the other three elevator/depressor muscles can be worked out.

8.11.6 Prism Adaptation Test

The **prism adaptation test** (PAT) is useful in patients with long-standing esotropia. PAT may predict how the sensory mechanisms will react to the mechanical correction by surgery. There are patients who after surgical correction will have a recurrence of esotropia after surgery. This sub-group can be detected by using prisms to just over correct the esotropia (prisms put till there is a minimal inward movement on cover test) and waiting for some time. If after an hour the esotropia returns while the prisms are still on, then the prognosis is poor and additional strategies have to be employed to correct the squint. It is postulated that the optic disc is used as the suppression area in these esotropia patients and the recurrence is due to the eye trying to put back the image on to the disc in one eye.

A vertical element may be present in horizontal squints during measurements and the question then arises if the vertical component will be corrected with the correction of the horizontal component. Jampolsky has suggested that here the cover test be done with the head position in such a way that the deviating eye is in the straight ahead position. For example, in a patient with right exotropia the face is turned to the left till the deviated right eye is looking straight ahead. If the vertical deviation persists after neutralizing the horizontal deviation in this head position, then the vertical component can be significant after surgery.

8.11.7 Examination of the Unconscious and Preverbal Patients

Unconscious patients need a different strategy because they cannot follow your commands. Examination of children will be discussed in Chap. 16. In unconscious patients, one does not need the detailed information one normally looks for in the conscious patients. The examination is targeted according to the objectives and will be discussed in the section on neuro-ophthalmology examination. Moving the head passively in an unconscious patient moves the eye as part of the vestibule kinetic reflex and the eye movement can be studied to a certain extent. One needs to be careful when examining a patient with head injury who may have cervical spine injury.

8.12 Tests of Stereopsis and Fusion

In patients with squint, an idea of the fusion capabilities and the ability to have a stereoscopic vision is useful to decide on how aggressive the treatment effort should be. Patients with fusion potential and stereopsis have a much higher chance of the eye remaining aligned after a squint surgery.

The vision, time of onset of squint, symptoms, the results of the cover test, the type of squint, etc. gives us a good idea of the sensory function and adaptations in patients with squint. Trying to demonstrate them again in very case is not necessary. In addition, none of the tests available in the clinic simulates the real-life seeing. This makes the test results variable and contradictory. It is this variability that prevents clinicians using the tests described below as often as theoretical considerations would warrant. In addition, it does not add much value in the management.

The Worth Four Dot test is readily available with most vision testing systems but rarely done. The test board consists of four dots, two green, one red and one white spot placed as shown in Fig. 8.19. The patient is made to wear a red,

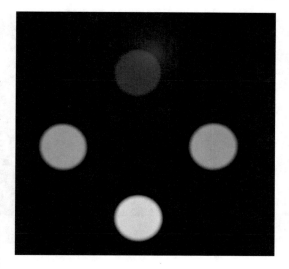

Fig. 8.19 Screen used to do Worth 4-dot test

green goggles with the red colour in front of the right eye and asked to record what he sees. This is done at the 6 m and 33 cm distance. At 6 m, the image falls on a small area of the retina as opposed to the image cast from 33 cm. A normal patient will say he can see two green spots (through the left eye), one red and one which can be red or green. If the eyes are straight and there is a suppression of the right eye, three green spots are seen; the third spot being the white spot seen through the green filter. If there is a suppression of the left eye, then two red spots will be seen through the right eye. If the suppression area is small, bringing the target (Worth Four dot) to 33 cm will make the images fall outside the suppression area and the patient will perceive more than two dots. If there is squint without suppression, then the patient will see five dots. Besides the usual red and green spots, the white dot will be seen as red by the right eye and as green by the left eye due to diplopia. Having described this test, one should also know, great variability and contradictions have been noted with this test. The fact that the red, green goggles can break fusion even in orthotropic patients, and the test itself being a psychophysical test causes problems in its interpretation.

Stereopsis can be assessed using special plates that may not be readily available in a general outpatient examination unit and so will not

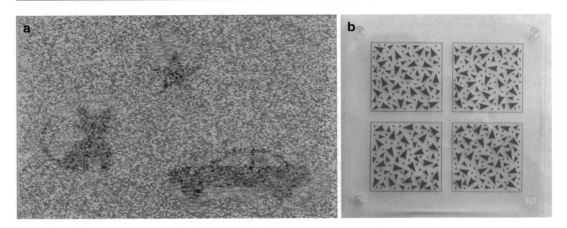

Fig 8.20 Stereo acuity testing plates (**a**) random dot stereo acuity chart and (**b**) Frisby plate

be discussed in detail. This test can be done with or without special glasses.

The **Random dot test** uses a test plate (Fig. 8.20a) and a polaroid glasses with each lens polarised at right angles to the other and kept in front of either eye of the patient. Each eye sees slightly different image (due to different polarisation) that is then fused by the brain. With the glasses and both eyes open, normal patients with stereopsis will be able to see one of the figures in the plate standing out in 3D above the level of the plate. The test comes with the instructions to do the test and identifies which figure in each set is the one that gives the stereoscopic effect. The measure of stereopsis in seconds is also given. The problem of tests with glasses is that it is an artificial testing condition and the glasses may break fusion.

Lang Stereo test and the Frisby test do not require glasses. In **Lang Stereo test,** the two random dot pattern is separated by using a grid of cylinders place on top of the random dots instead of polaroid glasses. The grid of cylinders shows one dot to the left eye and the corresponding disparate dot to the right eye. In the areas where there is a pattern that can only be seen in patients with stereopsis, the images appear to stand out. In preverbal children, the fixation of their eyes on the patterns gives the clue to the presence of stereopsis.

Frisby test are thick plastic plates with four squares in one plate (Fig. 8.20b). A central cir-

cular pattern in one of the squares is painted on the proximal part of the thick plate. All the other three squares have the circle and the background pattern painted on the distal flat side of the sheet. The thickness of the glass gives the appearance that the central pattern is elevated in the test circle and will be seen likewise by a patient with normal stereopsis.

Synoptophore or amblyoscope is a machine having two tubes which can be moved on a graduated arcuate scale to measure the angle between the tubes. Specially designed slides are kept at the distal end of the tubes into which the patients look and respond. Breaking fusion by the use of independent tubes make the testing artificial and unreliable. This machine available in specialty clinics will not be discussed here, and there is nothing that this machine can add by way of diagnosis. It is useful for measuring angle of squint, especially cyclotorsion and giving orthoptic exercises that is done by an orthoptist specialist.

Further Reading

Jampolsky A. A simplified approach to strabismus diagnosis, Symposium on strabismus. Transactions of the New Orleans Academy of Ophthalmology. St. Louis, MO: C.V. Mosby Company; 1971.

von Noorden GK, Campos EC. Binocular vision and ocular motility: theory and management of strabismus. 6th ed. St. Louis, MO: C.V. Mosby Company; 2002.

Examination of the Cornea and Ocular Surface

The **ocular surface** comprises of the conjunctiva and the anterior layers of the cornea. A healthy ocular surface is integral to keeping the cornea clear and transparent. In fact, the most important layer of the cornea in terms of its refractive power and clarity is the tear film bathing the epithelium. The tear film owes its integrity to the proper secretion of the conjunctival goblet cells, the tear glands and the meibomian glands of the lids. Besides THE secretions, the resurfacing capacity of the lids also play a role. Majority of patients seen in a general Ophthalmic clinic come with ocular surface related issues. Cornea cannot be seen in isolation without an assessment of the ocular surface too.

9.1 Applied Anatomy and Physiology

The conjunctiva extends from the muco-cutaneous junction at the lid margin (Fig. 9.1) to the limbus of the cornea. It coats the inner surface of the lid (**tarsal conjunctiva**) tightly adherent to the tarsal plate to reach the fornix. At the fornix, the conjunctiva becomes freely mobile (**forniceal conjunctiva**) with a loose areolar sub-conjunctival fibrous tissue. From the fornix the conjunctiva goes posteriorly and drapes the globe (**bulbar conjunctiva**) till the limbus. Over the globe, the conjunctiva is still loose and freely mobile. The sub-conjunctival fibrous tissue joins the tenon capsule and go as one sheath till the limbus. At the limbus, the tenons first get attached to the sclera. A millimetre further anteriorly the conjunctiva too attaches to the limbus.

The conjunctiva is a non-keratinising mucosal epithelium, 2–5 layer thick with numerous goblet cells in between that secrete mucin. The **subconjunctival fibrous tissue** or **substantia propria** is very vascular with additional lymphatic vessels, mast cells, macrophages and plasma cells. Collections of lymphoid tissue are seen in areas here called **CALT** (conjunctiva-associated lymphoid tissue). These tissues are involved in antigen processing.

The tarsal conjunctiva is supplied by the branches of the marginal arterial arcade of the lid. The forniceal conjunctiva and most of the bulbar conjunctiva up to about 3 mm from the limbus is supplied by the proximal arterial arcade present at the forniceal edge of the lid. Anterior ciliary artery which pierce the sclera 2 mm from the limbus to supply the ciliary body then runs anteriorly on the inside surface of the sclera till it reaches the limbus. At the limbus, it curves backward to supply the limbal conjunctiva as the anterior conjunctival vessels. It is due to this course that the circum-corneal vessels get congested in uveitis and keratitis. For the same reason unlike other conjunctival vessels, the blood in these vessels fills from the limbus rather than from the fornix.

The sensory nerve supply of the conjunctiva and cornea is mediated by the V_1 (ophthalmic) branch of the trigeminal nerve. The lower tarsal

© Springer Nature Singapore Pte Ltd. 2020
T. Kuriakose, *Clinical Insights and Examination Techniques in Ophthalmology*,
https://doi.org/10.1007/978-981-15-2890-3_9

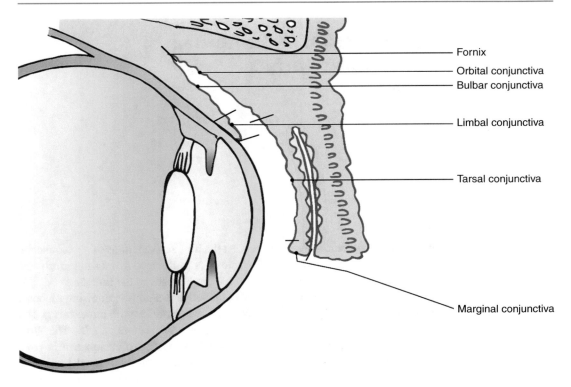

Fornix

Orbital conjunctiva

Bulbar conjunctiva

Limbal conjunctiva

Tarsal conjunctiva

Marginal conjunctiva

Fig. 9.1 Cross-section of the ocular surface and upper lid

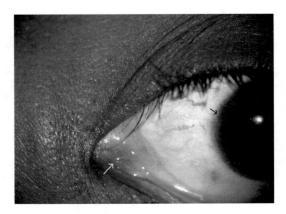

Fig. 9.2 Eye showing the caruncle medially (white arrow) and palisades of Vogt (black arrow) harbouring the limbal stem cells

conjunctiva is supplied by V_2 (maxillary) branch. The non-keratinised epithelial cells and the goblet cells of the conjunctiva are replenished by stem cells distributed all over the conjunctiva. Though the demarcation is not exact, broadly the lymphatic drainage of the lateral conjunctiva is into the pre-auricular nodes. The medial conjunctiva drains into the submandibular nodes.

The caruncle is a reddish mass of tissue seen at the medial canthus (Fig. 9.2). It is non-keratinised skin with sebaceous glands and fine hair. Associated with the caruncle at a deeper plane is a crescentic fold of reddish conjunctival tissue with fat and non-striated muscles called plica semilunaris. This represents the vestigial nictitating membrane seen in dogs and other animals.

Opening into the supero-temporal fornix are about 15 fine ducts from the main lacrimal gland that secrete the tears. Tears are also produced by multiple accessory lacrimal glands located mostly in the fornix and some under the bulbar and tarsal conjunctiva. Basal tear production is by the accessory glands. Secretomotor fibres originate in the seventh cranial nerve to finally reach the eye via the lacrimal nerve to supply the lacrimal glands.

The lacrimal glands produce the aqueous part of the tear secretion. In reality, the tear fluid is an emulsion containing an aqueous portion from the tear gland, mucin from the goblet cells and a lipid portion from the meibomian gland. The mucin coats the corneal epithelial cells making it hydrophilic and is more concentrated in the deeper layers of the tear film. The lipid portion floats on the surface of the tear film and prevents evaporation of the tears. Though the tear is described as three layered, in reality it is a continuum with no distinct layers. **The tears play a crucial role in the health of the ocular surface**. Besides the various cytokines, it also supplies the oxygen and other nutrients required for the cornea and the ocular surface. The tear lubricates the ocular surface and the blink reflex constantly resurfaces the tear film and aids its removal through the lacrimal drainage system.

The cornea is the transparent central part of the eyeball. It is a near circular disc with a vertical diameter of 10 mm and a horizontal diameter of 11 mm. Both the surfaces of the cornea is curved anteriorly. The iris can be seen clearly through the transparent cornea. Anteriorly the cornea is bounded by non-keratinised corneal epithelial cells derived from the surface ectoderm. The epithelial layer is 4–6 cell thick with the cells becoming progressively flatter as they come to the surface. The surface cells have microvilli that make it very irregular. The mucin layer of the tear film fills the spaces and coat the surface to make it smooth. The corneal epithelial cells are continually shed but are replenished by the cells migrating from the corneal limbus. Located at the corneal limbus are the corneal limbal stem cells. In pigmented race, their location can be identified by the radial rugae at the limbus called **palisades of Vogt** (Fig. 9.2). The corneal basal layer of columnar epithelium rests on its basement membrane or basal lamina.

Under the basal lamina in apposition with it is a layer of condensed tough collagen fibrils called the **Bowman's layer**. Disruption of this layer causes corneal scarring.

Deeper to the Bowman's layer is the **stroma** which constitutes 90% of the total corneal thickness. Embryologically, the stroma is derived from the mesodermal layer. It consists of tightly packed fine collagen fibrils arranged in such a way that it allows light to pass through and hence is transparent. If this structure is disrupted or water collects in between the fibrils, it loses the transparency. The stroma has keratocytes which produce the collagen and cells that mediate immune reaction. The stroma is in a constant state of dehydration. The state of corneal dehydration is maintained by the pumps on the endothelial cells that form the inner most layer of the cornea. These cells rest on the **Descemet's membrane** derived from the endothelial cells. The endothelial cells have a neuro-ectodermal origin. The posterior most part of the stroma is postulated to have a condensation of the collagen fibrils called **Dua's layer**. This layer is more important surgically. The endothelial cells derived from the neural crest cells pump water from the corneal stroma to the anterior chamber. It is a single sheet of cells mostly hexagonal in shape. The cell density in the young is about 3000 cells/mm^2. This reduces with time. The area of the cells undergoing apoptosis is filled by the remaining cells enlarging and in the process losing its hexagonal shape. An endothelial cell count below 500/mm^2 makes stromal dehydration difficult to maintain and the cornea starts to lose its transparency. The cornea is about 500 μm thick in the centre and about 1000 μm thick in the periphery.

The cornea has an aspheric surface to control spherical aberration. The anterior and posterior surface of the cornea is curved anteriorly and is responsible for about 43 of the 60 D of convergence the eye produces to focus parallel rays of light onto the retina. In reality, it is **not** the corneal epithelium but the tear film coating of the eye that bends the light rays. Tear film abnormalities can therefore significantly affect vision.

It thus becomes clear how the lid, conjunctiva, tear secretion and cornea all play an important role in the health of the ocular surface and vision.

9.2 History

Decrease in vision, photophobia, ocular discomfort mostly in the form of irritation, foreign body sensation, localised pain on the globe are the commonest complaints seen in ocular surface disorders (OSD). If there are no opacities in the cornea, decrease in vision occurs due to tear film instability. A smooth tear film is the first refracting surface of the eye. Irritation and ocular discomfort are due to the cytokines released by the inflammatory cells. Therefore, any inflammation even subclinical can cause irritation of the eye.

Itching is commonly complained of when there is an allergic component. Itching is caused by histamine and other related cytokines released in allergic conditions. It is important to distinguish between itching and irritation as patients mistake one for the other. As with other history taking, one should ask for constancy of symptoms, aggravating and relieving factors. Discomfort worse in the morning or evening can be related to OSD. Irritation worse in the morning is usually meibomianitis related and later in the evening is dry eye related. Often in conditions like mild dry eyes, one will have go by symptoms because clinical examination may not reveal any abnormality.

Use of contact lens, history of something going into the eye, past history of ocular surgery including refractive surgery, history of allergies including asthma, exanthematous fevers, blisters on the body, etc. are other useful questions to explore if one is dealing with an ocular surface disease. History of use of medications that suppress tear production like oral antihistamines, anticholinergics may give a clue to the cause of the OSD.

Three things that wake patients up in the middle of the night with pain are CL over wear, recurrent epithelial erosion and UV light exposure. Patients who come to the emergency department with severe pain in the eye on getting up should be asked if they used contact lens during the day or looked at welding or actually did welding. Patient should also be asked if he had an injury to the eye in the past (classically an injury with finger nails) after which he had some ocular discomfort and settled. This could indicate the injury that caused the primary corneal erosion. Examination of these patients may not show a stain-positive area because the epithelial defect would have closed by the time patient reaches the doctor. History therefore becomes very important. Careful examination of these patients, however, would show intraepithelial cysts within the negatively stained area and gently touching the epithelium would show the extent of the epithe-

lium that is actually loose. Care should be taken not to dislodge the epithelium and make the patient more symptomatic.

9.3 Examination

Since the tear film is integral to the health of the eye, examination of the ocular surface starts with the examination of lids and ocular adnexa (see Chap. 7). Once the position of the lashes, meibomian gland orifices and effectiveness of the blink, etc. is assessed one turns the attention to the ocular surface. With the torchlight (diffuse broad illumination) one should get a bird's eye view of the pattern of redness of the eye, if any. See if the redness is localised (**localised congestion**) to any part of the eye, e.g. medial part, inter-palpebral area, etc. Check to see if the congestion is predominantly around the cornea (**circum-corneal congestion**) or generalised congestion (**forniceal congestion**). In conjunctivitis-related congestion, the circum-corneal area will be spared comparatively.

9.3.1 Tear Film Examination

Tear film forms the anterior most layer of the ocular surface and its integrity should be assessed first. Normally, on torchlight the shine of conjunctiva and cornea should be preserved. There should be no pooling of the tears at the medial canthus.

Rest of the assessment is best done with the slit lamp. Assessment of the tear film should be done first. Normally, at the lower lid margin the tear collects in a triangular shape with the upper margin reaching 1 mm above the lid margin (Fig. 9.3). There should be very little debris collected in the tear lake. Absence of this tear collection or lots of debris in the tears suggest dry eye. A specular reflection study of the tear film should be done next by keeping the lighthouse around 60° to the eyepiece. Normally, the lipid layer would reflect multiple colours like the rainbow. If the lipid layer is absent or broken up, this reflection will be absent.

Since tear film is transparent, staining the tears with fluorescein helps in its evaluation. Before

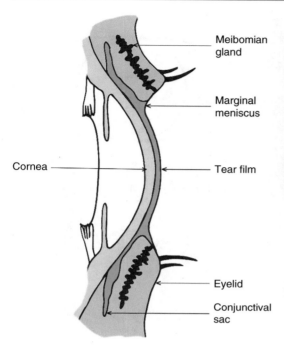

Fig. 9.3 Tear film on the ocular surface taking on a triangular shape at the lid margin

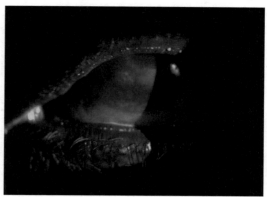

Fig. 9.4 Fluorescein staining of the tear film in a patient with few punctate staining dots on the cornea

applying the stain one should not only ask the patient if he has a contact lens on but also look for one and remove it. Soft lenses which can get stained with fluorescein is best seen if one looks for an extra ring outside the limbus that marks the edge of the soft lens. If present, it should be removed by pinching on the cornea when the contact lens will come between your fingers.

The tip of a wet fluorescein strip is touched on the edge of the lid margin so that the paper itself does not get stuck to the conjunctiva. If the conjunctiva comes in contact with the fluorescein strip, the conjunctiva could get stained in that region and may be mistaken for pathological staining. Once the tear is stained the marginal strip of tears at the lower lid is seen clearly.

Normally, the conjunctiva does not take up stain. With cobalt blue light, a thin layer of fluorescein stained tear coats the cornea with the cornea looking dark in the background (Fig. 9.4). Break-up time of the tears should be assessed next. After a blink, the patient is asked not to blink and the cornea is observed to see how long it takes for the tear film to break on the cornea

(**tear break-up time, TBUT**). Where the tear film breaks the cornea appears dark. The timing should be taken again after one more blink. A tear break-up time of less than 10 seconds is taken as abnormal. The drying spot should be at a different location each time. If the tear break-up occurs at the same spot, then it is due to a local pathology/irregularity rather than dry eyes.

The conjunctiva and the cornea should be examined for stain-positive spots on it. Less than five isolated stain-positive spots in the interpalpebral region of the cornea and conjunctiva may not be significant. More than nine spots suggest drying of the surface and unhealthy epithelium. Lissamine green and fluorescein dye is now used to assess dry eyes. Rose Bengal dye is the other dyes used. Lissamine and Rose Bengal dyes are supposed to stain unhealthy epithelial cells better than fluorescein. Figure 9.5 gives the current assessment scores for dry eyes. This used for follow up rather than to make a diagnosis.

In the clinic, one can also do a Schirmer's test to assess the amount of wetting by the tears using a Whatman 40 filter paper strip cut 5 mm in width. These strips, now available commercially is bend at the tip so that it can be hooked on the lower lid. After placing in both eyes, the eye is now gently closed for 5 min before measuring the length of wetting from the bend. The test can be done (Schirmer's test 1) before putting anaesthetic in the eye (measures some reflex secretion too) or after putting a drop (Schirmer's test 2) of anaesthetic

Ocular Staining Score

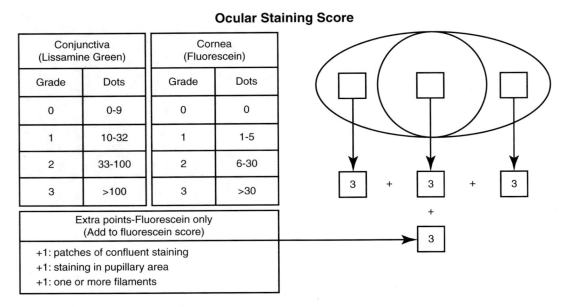

Conjunctiva (Lissamine Green)		Cornea (Fluorescein)	
Grade	Dots	Grade	Dots
0	0-9	0	0
1	10-32	1	1-5
2	33-100	2	6-30
3	>100	3	>30

Extra points-Fluorescein only
(Add to fluorescein score)

+1: patches of confluent staining
+1: staining in pupillary area
+1: one or more filaments

Fig. 9.5 Ocular staining score for dry eye

(only basal secretion measured). Schirmer's 3 test is done by keeping the paper and then stimulating the nasal mucosa to trigger reflex secretion.

Schirmer's test 1 is the most natural test to do. In Sjogren's syndrome, Schirmer's test 1 with wetting below 5 mm in 5 min gave a sensitivity and specificity of around 70%. If the cut-off for wetting is increased, it will increase the sensitivity but reduce the specificity. Likewise, for tear break-up time if the cut-off time was 10 s the sensitivity was about 70% but specificity was only 30%. If the break-up time was reduced to 5 s, it increased the specificity but reduced the sensitivity. Interestingly, a history (do not forget is a test!) of irritation of the eye or a feeling that the eye is dry had a sensitivity and specificity equal to the more elaborate clinical tests! Such is the power of history we often overlook. Combining Schirmer's and staining of the cornea increases the specificity in detecting dry eye.

9.3.2 Examination of the Conjunctiva

The conjunctiva is best examined with the slit lamp. Direct, indirect and diffuse illumination is

useful to examine the conjunctiva. Examination of the conjunctiva should start at the lid margin where the conjunctiva starts. Normally, the muco-cutaneous margin of the lid is sharp. If the keratinised cells start moving into the conjunctival region distorting the opening of the meibomian glands, one should suspect one of the more severe forms of dry eye. One might also see thick plaques of keratinised cells at the lid margin in severe dry eyes.

The lower lid tarsal conjunctiva and the lower forniceal conjunctiva are easily examined by pulling the lower lid down to expose the inner surface of the lid.

The upper lid is more difficult to see and one needs to evert the lid to see the underside of the lid (Fig. 9.6). Before everting the lid, patient should be told what you are going to do and that there could be mild discomfort. The patient is first asked to look down without closing the eye. Now hold lashes and the margin of the lid with the thumb and index finger and pull it gently downward and towards the examiner. Once this is done, using the index finger as the fulcrum, the lid is turned up to evert the lid and at the same time removing the fulcrum to give space for the lid to evert. Once everted the lid is pressed against

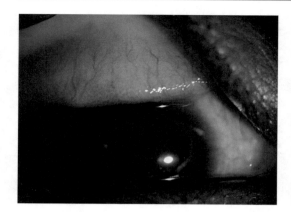

Fig. 9.6 Everted lid with papillae

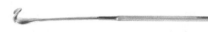

Fig. 9.7 Desmarres retractor used for double eversion of the lids

the eyeball to maintain the eversion. If everting with the finger is difficult, a thin cotton bud can be placed at the upper lid sulcus with the other hand and lid everted using that as the fulcrum for eversion. The exposed tarsal conjunctiva should be examined for papillae, follicles, scarring foreign bodies, etc. One of the places foreign bodies get lodged is the subtarsal sulcus located 2 mm from the upper lid margin. These foreign bodies will be missed if the lid is not everted. To see the upper fornix for toxic particles especially in cases of chemical injury, one needs to do a double eversion by everting the once everted upper lid using a Desmarres retractor (Fig. 9.7) or hairpin (hairpin, bend as a U) retractor. Double eversion should be done only after anaesthetising the eye with topical proparacaine drops.

Fine insect hair can sometimes get lodged in the tarsal conjunctiva and may be difficult to see even with the slit lamp. In such cases, a drop of fluorescein will show disturbance in the tear film at the site of the hair being lodged. The cornea in these patients will show vertically stained striations due to the rubbing of the hair on the cornea with each blink.

In conjunctival inflammation, one can see fine red-centred elevations on the tarsal conjunctiva called **papillae** (Fig. 9.6). This is the dilated vas-

cular system of the tarsal conjunctiva containing capillaries. If the inflammation is chronic, they become hyperplastic and form **giant papillae**, seen usually in chronic allergic conjunctivitis or contact lens wear.

Sometimes with the red-centred papillae, one sees white-centred elevations that are actually collection of lymphocytes. These are called **follicles** and should be differentiated from papillae. Follicles are seen in viral infections and other infections associated with intracellular organisms like chlamydia. One may see isolated follicles without inflammation in normal patients.

The tarsal plate may have a yellow coating in some conditions, and it represents an inflammatory membrane on it. This is seen in membranous conjunctivitis. Usually seen in children, gonorrhoea should be ruled out before other infectious and non-infectious causes are considered. Red pedunculated tissue may be seen on everting the lid. The commonest cause for this is pyogenic granuloma from a chalazion that has burst inward. Palpation of the tarsal plate will confirm the diagnosis. Papillomas and oculosporidiosis (rhinosporidiosis) are the other common differentials. In oculosporidiosis, white dots may be seen on the surface of the lesion and they bleed easily.

The tarsal plate on eversion can sometimes have yellowish white, pinhead or smaller sized elevated dots which are collections of old epithelial cells called concretions. Its presence suggest old inflammation including allergies and is usually harmless. Rarely, it can become very large and cause ocular irritation.

When examining the bulbar conjunctiva if the patient has come with a red eye, the distribution of redness must be noted first. If the congestion is localised, the first thing to check is to see if the congestion is conjunctival or scleral. In scleritis or episcleritis, the congestion is deeper. Best seen under sunlight, in scleritis one sees a deep localised pink colour with distinct conjunctival capillaries superficially. There will be tenderness over the area in scleritis. Localised conjunctival congestion will have a deeper red colour. When in doubt, put a drop of 5% phenylephrine in the eye. This will blanch the conjunctival vessels, but the redness due to the scleritis will remain. A fleshy mass under the conjunctiva with a pinkish colour points to a lymphoma.

Medial conjunctival congestion may be due to lacrimal conjunctivitis related to infection from a blocked duct. Congestion in the inter-palpebral area may be related to dryness or exposure to excessive dust or allergens. History needs to be explored again to make the diagnosis. If one sees very localised conjunctival congestion with a stain-positive centre, usually in the lower fornix, a mucous fishing syndrome should be considered.

Conjunctivitis due to infection or inflammation will show generalised congestion more so in the forniceal region. The area around the cornea will be less congested compared to the rest of the eye. On the other hand, if the circum-corneal region is very congested, inflammation of the cornea, uvea or an acute rise in pressure should be suspected. Since circum-corneal conjunctival vessels come from within the eye, inflammation within or inside the coats of the eyeball causes congestion of these vessels. Circum-corneal congestion may also be associated with generalised conjunctival congestion. Table 9.1 gives the differential diagnosis and features of red eye.

In autoimmune conjunctivitis, there is marked generalised congestion and one should stain the conjunctiva to look for areas of conjunctival ulcers that may be seen all over the surface.

Redness which is bright red restricted to a well-defined area can be **sub-conjunctival haemorrhage**. The vessels of the conjunctiva will not be seen distinctly in these cases as it will be obscured by the sub-conjunctival blood that is causing this condition. Injury, hypertension, raised blood pressure or sudden Valsalva manoeuvre can cause a break in the sub-conjunctival blood vessel and cause the bleeding. Therefore, a specific history to explore this should be taken. If the posterior border of the sub-conjunctival bleed cannot be made out, it could mean that the blood is coming from the orbit. Small sub-conjunctival haemorrhages may be seen associated with viral or pneumococcal conjunctivitis.

In patients with chronic allergic conjunctivitis, the conjunctiva may appear muddy especially in the pigmented race. The conjunctiva will have a yellowish colour in patients with jaundice. Sometimes, it is difficult to make out icterus in patients with muddy conjunctiva. The limbal area in some patients with severe allergic conjunctivitis will have multiple nodules with fine dusting on the surface that take up fluorescein stain. These are called **Horner Trantas dots**.

In some older patients, there will be a lot of redundant conjunctiva that forms folds inferiorly and even block the inferior puncta. This condition is called **conjunctivochalasis** and should be distinguished from conjunctival folds due to collection of fluid under the conjunctiva (**chemosis**) seen mostly in acute conjunctivitis and rarely in systemic fluid overload.

In chronic inflammatory conditions of the conjunctiva like ocular cicatricial pemphigoid, the conjunctiva becomes shortened and develops **symblepharon** (lid sticking to the bulbar conjunctiva due to fibrosis in the fornix). The earliest sign of symblepharon is the foreshortening of the fornix characterised by fold of conjunctiva extending from the bulbar conjunctiva to the lid.

Table 9.1 Showing the differential diagnosis of red eye

	Vision	Extent of redness	Colour	Cornea	Anterior chamber	IOP
SC haemorrhage	Normal	Well-defined margins	Bright red, conjunctival vessels hidden	Clear	Normal	Normal
Conjunctivitis	Normal	Bulbar conjunctiva	Red	Clear	Normal	Normal
Keratitis	Decreased	CCC	Deep red	Opacity	Cells and flare	Normal
Angle CG	Decreased	CCC	Deep red	Cloudy	Shallow	High
Uveitis	±	CCC	Deep red	Clear	Cells and flare	Low
Scleritis	Normal	Localised, deep	Salmon pink	Normal	Normal	Normal

SC Sub-conjunctival, *CG* Closure Glaucoma, *CCC* Circum-corneal congestion

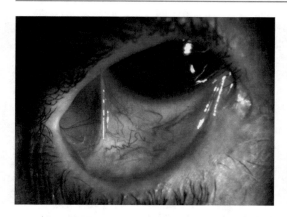

Fig. 9.8 Conjunctival folds extending from the lid to the bulbar conjunctiva indicative of conjunctival shortening due to fibrosis

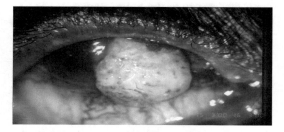

Fig. 9.9 Squamous cell carcinoma at the limbus

The fold can be demonstrated by pulling the lower lid away from the eyeball (Fig. 9.8).

In certain infection like trachoma, chronic allergies, trauma, etc., one can find scarring of tarsal conjunctiva characterised by star-shaped and linear white scar tissue replacing the normal light red tarsal mucosa. In severe scarring, the tarsal plate will bow inward causing entropion.

The conjunctiva may show mass lesions on its surface or underneath. The commonest mass seen on the conjunctiva is a nevus which needs no treatment. Melanomas (black or red coloured) and squamous cell carcinoma (vascular, irregular surfaced whitish red lesion) are other mass lesions seen on the bulbar conjunctiva usually at the limbus (Fig. 9.9). Kaposi sarcoma which appears as a bright red lesion is seen in immune-compromised patients. Sometimes, a mass lesion is seen under the conjunctiva. Lymphoma appears like fish flesh under the conjunctiva. The con-junctiva can be moved over the mass by pressing

the lid against the conjunctiva and moving it from side to side. Yellowish red mass with hair on its surface, usually seen in the lateral canthal area is suggestive of a dermolipoma.

The conjunctiva appear dry and leathery with curved folds laterally in vitamin A deficiency (xerosis). A foamy triangular patch (Bitot's spot) may also be seen near the lateral limbus along with xerosis. Bitot's spot may also be seen in patients who are currently not vitamin A deficient.

When examining a case of suspected conjunctivitis, discharge if any should be looked for. In viral conjunctivitis, the discharge is watery, with allergic aetiology the discharge is more mucoid. Stringy ropy discharge is associated with dry eyes. If the discharge is sticky, white or yellowish white a bacterial aetiology should be considered. In mucous fishing syndrome, the discharge will be stringy and yellowish white because of the constant trauma. The discharge can be bloody if there is conjunctival ulceration. If some foreign body is being put in the eye to induce irritation, bits of that will also be there in the discharge.

In Munchausen's syndrome, the discharge can have bizarre things like hair, blood, etc. and should be kept in mind when no other sinister pathology can be made out. In a condition call 'Munchausen's by proxy' babies may have these odd discharges that is induced by the carer.

9.3.3 Pre-Auricular Node Examination

Examination of the conjunctiva especially if an infection is suspected is not complete without examining the pre-auricular nodes. To examine the pre-auricular node, one should gently move the middle three fingers of the examiner's hand forward and backward in front of the tragus, over the parotid region. Normally, there should be no tenderness over the area and lymph nodes should not be palpable. When palpating with both hands simultaneously, one can compare the two sides. Tenderness over the palpated area in the absence of a palpable node is a sign of soft small inflamed node beneath it. Submandibular nodes, the other group of nodes the conjunctiva drains into, can enlarge due to a variety of reasons including oral pathology and its enlargement is not specific for conjunctival infection. Organisms that cause intracellular infections like virus, chlamydia and bacteria like gonococcus cause pre-auricular node enlargement. If the pre-auricular node is enlarged and tender, especially in a case of kerato-conjunctivitis, one of the above organisms should be suspected to be the cause.

9.3.4 Examination of the Limbus

Limbus is the junction of conjunctiva and the cornea and is an important surgical landmark. It is continuous with the corneal epithelial cells anteriorly and with the bulbar conjunctiva posteriorly. The limbal area merits a focused inspection because of the multiple pathologies seen there in ocular surface diseases. It sometimes offers the only evidence of the type of surgery done on the eye in the past. The limbus contains the corneal stem cells that continuously replenishes the corneal epithelial cells. Limbal stem cell disease affects ocular surface integrity. Examination of the limbus is best done with the slit lamp.

In normal patients, the limbus is smooth with a small depression called sulcus sclerae that mark the junction of the sclera and cornea. On the surface are small pigmented radial lines called palisades of Vogt that house the limbal stem cells (Fig. 9.2). This is best seen in the upper and lower unexposed limbus. The conjunctival vessels stop at limbus with a few loops of vessels going 1 mm into the cornea. Beyond this the cornea is avascular.

The limbus should be first examined for any surface irregularity. One of the common lesions seen is a small whitish yellow lesion about 1 mm or more in size at the nasal conjunctival limbus. This is **pinguecula** which is a collection of hyperplastic sub-conjunctival fibrous tissue. Other common elevated lesions at the limbus could be a foreign body or a limbal neoplasm. A foreign body has well-defined edges and may show mild congestion around it but no increase in vascularity. A neoplasm on the other hand is highly vascular with a cauliflower-like surface (Fig. 9.9). Unlike neo-

plasm a foreign body can be dislodged easily with a 24-gauge needle inserted under its edge after instilling topical anaesthesia. The limbus is a common site of neoplasm due to the presence of replicating cells (stem cells and transient amplifying cells). In children, one may see a raised yellowish white circular lesion 2 mm or more at the limbus. The lesion may have fine hairs on it and is a limbal dermoid. The depth of the lesion should be assessed before planning excision.

Sometimes, multiple elevations like papillae are seen in the superior limbus in allergic conjunctivitis. The top of these papillae may be yellow centred due to collection of dead epithelial cells and eosinophils and stain with fluorescein. They are called **Horner Trantas dots**. Multiple depressions seen at the limbus (areas of old follicles) in treated old cases of trachoma is called **Herbert's pits** and do not need any further treatment.

Areas of localised inflammation with redness may be seen at the limbus on examination. These patients should be stained. Multiple or isolated small (1–2 mm) areas of congestion with ulcers (staining positive with fluorescein) is seen in this immune-related condition called **Phlyctenular keratoconjunctivitis**. The ulcers may progress into the cornea.

The superior limbus may be congested in a poorly understood condition called **superior limbic kerato-conjunctivitis**. In some autoimmune keratitis, the limbal area gets inflamed before the cornea becomes obviously involved.

One of the important examination of the limbal area is examination of the limbal stem cells. If the palisades of Vogt are well seen, it is a sign of healthy limbal cells. If the demarcation of the limbus (maintained by the healthy stem cells) is absent and conjunctival vessels grow over to the clear side of the cornea, it is a sign of unhealthy limbal stem cells. Vessels growing over the cornea with or without a preceding area of inflammatory cells is called **pannus**. Here fine vessels along with conjunctival epithelium grow onto the cornea. In fact before the vessels grow, the conjunctival epithelium grows which is not as clear as the corneal epithelium. Conjunctival epithelium has **goblet cells** in it. When stained with fluorescein; speckled staining appears, as the abnormal conjunctival epithelial cells do not have tight junction as the corneal epithelium. Limbal scars, surgical or secondary to limbal injury like chemical injury or cryo-therapy suggest limbal stem cell insult.

Pterygium is a triangular fibrovascular tissue covered with conjunctiva that grows from the nasal conjunctiva and limbus on to the cornea (Fig. 9.10). Here the UV rays from sun hitting the more exposed temporal cornea gets focused on the nasal limbus causing alterations in the subconjunctival fibroblast and destroying the limbal stem cells. With the barrier function of the nasal stem cells gone altered fibroblasts multiply and grow on to the cornea. If the limbal stem cells are preserved, only a **pinguecula** forms on the conjunctival side of the limbus.

Since limbus is the site of entry for many, an ocular surgeries examination of this area gives clue to past surgeries. A boggy elevated conjunctiva especially if associated with a peripheral iris hole suggest a previous trabeculectomy. Sometimes, a suture at the limbus may be the cause of the ocular irritation the patient has or the nidus of infection for a peripheral corneal ulcer.

9.3.5 Examination of the Cornea

A torchlight examination of the cornea along with the anterior ocular surface gives us the big

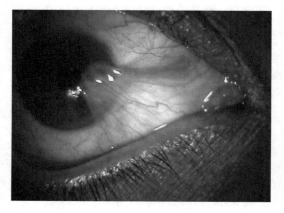

Fig. 9.10 Pterygium on the medial side of the right cornea

picture. An assessment of the corneal size and shape should be made. Small corneas less than 10 mm diameter should raise the suspicion of a microphthalmos or microcornea. Large corneas above 11 mm should raise the suspicion of raised intraocular pressure (specifically in children), megalocornea or corneal thinning. A cornea that looks pointed when patient looks down is suggestive of advanced keratoconus (**Munson's sign**).

Since cornea is a transparent structure, slit lamp finds its greatest use in the examination of the cornea. Due to the glare from the mirror-like surface of the cornea, examination with bright focal illumination gives the least information. Diffuse illumination, slit illumination, indirect illumination, sclerotic scatter and retro-illumination methods of slit lamp examination (see Chap. 6) gives the maximum information about the cornea. To study the endothelium, one can use specular reflection. The more subtle lesions are best seen by indirect illumination, sclerotic scatter and retro-illumination. **Dynamic slit lamp examination,** i.e. observing the cornea while shifting the illumination also highlights lesions on the cornea.

In cases where there is corneal or anterior segment inflammation, the patient may be photophobic and not very cooperative due to lid spasm. This reflex is mediated by the trigeminal nerve rather than the optic nerve. A drop of topical anaesthetic before the examination relieves the spasm and eases the examination.

After examining the tear film, attention should be directed at the epithelium. The epithelium must be smooth without any pigmentations. Diffuse illumination may show fine punctuate lesions on the cornea. Punctate lesions can be seen better if the angle of illumination is kept the widest possible. These lesions could be secondary to a variety of reasons. Dry eye, drug toxicity, vitamin deficiency, conjunctivalisation of the cornea, healed epithelial erosion are some of the reasons. Larger lesions with some sub-epithelial infiltrations can be seen in post-viral conjunctivitis, microsporidial keratitis, etc. If one finds vortex patterned radial lines, pigmented or otherwise, it suggests rapid turnover of epithelial cells (Fig. 9.11) due to a primary pathology. Vortex

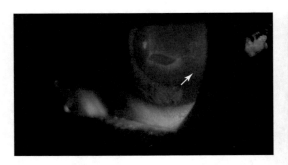

Fig. 9.11 Radial pigmented lines (white arrow) seen in conditions causing rapid epithelial turn over

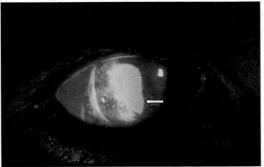

Fig. 9.12 Medial part of the left cornea taking up fluorescein stain (white arrow)

keratopathy seen in Fabry's disease and intake of drugs like Indomethacin, Chlorpromazine and Hydroxychloroquine (HCQ) are other rare possibilities here.

The corneal epithelial layer may show fine wavy lines like a fingerprint with or without fine nebulous opacities of different geographical shapes. This could be suggestive of an epithelial dystrophy called **map dot fingerprint dystrophy**. The level of the lesion is checked by directing a thin slit beam on the lesion and seeing where the lesion cuts the slit.

Corneal opacities that can just be seen with difficulty, with the iris details seen clearly is called **nebulous opacity**. More obvious opacities were the iris can be seen through but its details are not clear is called **macular opacity**. White opacities where the iris cannot be seen through at all is called **leucomatous opacity**.

The corneal epithelium may show filaments attached to its surface (**filamentary keratitis**). These mucoid strands with epithelial cells are seen in dry eyes especially after bandaging the eye. The underlying reason for bandaging should not be thought of as the culprit.

Epithelial defects may be difficult to make out if one does not look for it. Staining using a drop of fluorescein helps delineate the epithelial defect. The area without the epithelium takes up the stain and can be seen distinctly from the rest of the cornea (Fig. 9.12). Staining also helps define areas of corneal epithelial irregularities and unhealthy areas better. In patients with healed corneal ulcers, there may be a slight depression in the area of the healed ulcer in which the stained tears collect. This **pooling** of dye may appear as

a stain-positive area. One needs to flush the eye with artificial tears to remove the dye to see if the area continues to stain.

Degenerative changes are seen in the superficial layers of the cornea and may denote other underlying causes. A horizontal white band seen across cornea in the inter-palpebral region is called **band keratopathy**. Early band keratopathy is better seen using the sclerotic scatter illumination and will be seen as fine dusting on the corneal epithelium. Here, in the epithelial and sub-epithelial layers are fine deposits of calcium salts. Vacuolated clearing is seen in between. Chronic uveitis, systemic hypercalcaemia, long-standing presence of silicone oil in the eye, genetic predisposition and exposure to sun and dust are some of the reasons for this change and should be looked for.

The epithelial surface may show single or multiple elevated yellowish or white nodules or scar tissue that is seen predominantly in the inter-palpebral area. Most of these changes are seen in patients who are out in the sun in dusty environments and who may have injured their eye inadvertently in the past. In **climatic droplet keratopathy,** one sees oil droplet like deposits in the epithelial layers and is again best seen with sclerotic scatter or retro-illumination. Whiter and larger lesions are called **Salzmann's nodular degeneration**. As long as the condition is recognised and aetiology confirmed from history, the exact naming is not important.

If conjunctivalisation of the cornea is suspected staining will show fine stain-positive spots in the area covered by conjunctiva due to lack of tight junction in the epithelium. Fine spots much more closely packed can also be seen when there is corneal toxicity or some form of punctate keratopathy.

Cornea is not normally vascularised beyond 1 mm from the limbus. If corneal vascularisation is noted beyond this limit, its level, depth and extent should be noted. Superficial vessels accompanying the conjunctiva and growing onto the cornea is called pannus. These vessels do not penetrate the corneal stroma and is due to ocular surface disorders like allergies, stem cell deficiency, dry eye, etc. These vessels arise from the conjunctival vessels supplying the posterior bulbar conjunctiva.

Deep corneal vessels, on the other hand, arise from the anterior ciliary artery which come to the cornea from inside the eye. New vessels from this go directly into the stroma of the cornea. The stimuli for these vessels to develop is corneal inflammation and oedema. Deep corneal vessels appear less distinct and cannot be seen to cross the limbus. These vessels can affect the graft survival after keratoplasty.

9.3.5.1 Corneal Staining

Corneal staining is done by wetting dry strips impregnated with dye like fluorescein, lissamine green or Rose Bengal. Liquid dye is now avoided because they can be media for bacterial growth. The dye should not be too concentrated or too dilute as it could give misleading results. If local anaesthetic is being planned, then a drop of the anaesthetic can be instilled before instilling the dye to prevent the sting due to the dye. Wetting the dye strip with the topical anaesthetic can affect the staining characteristics.

Corneal staining patterns in patients with gritty sensation of the eye can give a clue to the diagnosis. Punctate staining in the inter-palpebral area suggest dry eye-related exposure. If the stain-positive area is at the lower lid margin, it may be related to drug toxicity or nocturnal exposure. The constant contact of the drug in the tear lake with the lower cornea is the reason for this. Punctate staining at the upper cornea is seen in allergic conjunctivitis due to contact with the tarsal papillae. In superior limbic keratitis too, one can get staining in the upper part of the con-

junctiva. Areas of epithelial defect will be delineated well and better seen with fluorescein stain. If the cornea shows vertical lines on it, it means there is a foreign body (FB) in the tarsal conjunctiva rubbing the cornea. If the FB is not obvious on the tarsal conjunctiva, then one should look for fine caterpillar hair sticking out and rubbing the cornea. Fluorescein stain can help localising the area of penetration if there is corneal injury. Diffuse punctate staining of the entire cornea can be seen with toxicity to drug preservatives in eye drops, vitamin B deficiency, severe dry eye, etc.

9.3.5.2 Corneal Epithelia Iron Lines

Corneal epithelial layers may show dark brown iron lines in many situations. In many of these situations, the association do not have any diagnostic significance and are features that have been noted with the condition. **Hudson–Stahli line** is an irregular wavy line running across the lower third of the cornea and is seen in older people who have spent long hours in dusty outside environment. Small brown rings with possible depression in the centre suggest **old iron FB** that have been dislodged or removed from the cornea. Iron rings/lines are seen in areas of cornea where there is a change in surface angle of the cornea, like in front of a pterygium, filtering bleb, etc. Of particular diagnostic use is the **Fleischer ring** seen at the base of a keratoconus cone. This ring is seen even before the thinning and irregular high astigmatism is obvious clinically. These iron lines are best seen with the cobalt blue filter where they are seen as black lines against a blue background.

9.3.5.3 Corneal Stromal Examination

The normal corneal stroma has a fine granular appearance on the slit lamp cross-section and is clear. Once opacities are seen in the stroma by the diffuse or other appropriate illumination the slit light is used to assess the depth and any finer features of the lesion. The intensity of the opacity, its distribution, the margins, shape, the area in between the opacity, involvement of the fellow eye should all be noted for making a diagnosis. A nebulous opacity may mean a previous mild corneal insult due to trauma, infection, etc. A leucomatous opacity suggest a more severe insult. Multiple opacities of a similar nature in both eyes suggest a dystrophy. An opacity with spiky edges like a crystal is suggestive of a **crystalline keratopathy**. If the area between opacities is not clear, then the disease may be more generalised or there is an associated corneal oedema. In some corneal dystrophy, the space between opacities may be clear, e.g. **granular dystrophy**. Some corneal dystrophies affect both the epithelium and superficial stroma. Some characteristics of the corneal lesion can only be made out on retro-illumination. The Y shaped pattern of amyloid deposits seen in **lattice dystrophy**, assessment of the clarity of the areas between the opacities and the density of the opacity itself are all better appreciated on retro-illumination.

When corneal opacity is associated with swelling of the cornea in the area of opacity, it is not due to scar tissue. Water logging in the corneal stroma causes the opacity here. Stromal oedema is made out by the flattening of the posterior corneal curvature and associated Descemet's folds. If there is no epithelial defect, corneal epithelial oedema may be seen as fine bubbles on indirect illumination. This is classically seen in **disciform keratitis** caused by a viral endotheliitis that causes an endothelial pump failure. The eye may be white in this condition and should not be mistaken for an old healed suppurative keratitis.

In the superficial stroma, concentric to the limbus, one may observe a whitish discolouration of the superficial stroma. This is a normal degenerative change due to deposit of lipid material and is called **arcus senilis**. The arcus senilis has a clear area of cornea between the corneal limbus and arcus. If this condition occurs in patients less than 40 years of age, it is called **arcus juvenilis** and one needs to rule out hyperlipidaemia. A similar concentric circle of deposit is seen deep in the corneal stroma just above the Descemet's membrane in Wilson's disease. Called KF (**Keyser Fleischer**) ring, here copper gets deposited without a gap between the limbus and the ring. The deposit starts in the upper and lower cornea first and is also the last areas from where it will disappear on treatment. Presence of bilateral KF ring is near 100% specific (pathogno-

monic) for Wilson's disease. If patients have an associated arcus senilis that hinders the view of the pre-Descemet's area from the front, then one can use a gonioscope to see the Descemet's area from below to look for the deposit. Patients with Wilson's disease may also have similar deposits on the anterior surface of the lens in a flower petal pattern called sunflower cataract.

In patients who have had blood in the anterior chamber (hyphaema) and raised pressures, the RBCs can enter the corneal stroma and stain it. This **corneal blood staining** starts in the centre of the cornea and spread outward. It disappears from the periphery when the insult is removed. In **Chalcosis** (copper foreign body in the eye), there can be diffuse deposition of copper on all basement membranes of the eye including the Descemet's membrane in that eye.

When examining the corneal stroma with the slit beam, one should also note the curvature of the cornea by looking at the anterior and posterior edges of a broad beam of slit. After seeing many normal corneas in cross-section with the slit illumination, one gets a visual impression of the normal corneal curvatures.

The cornea will appear flat with some corneal folds and stromal opacity in a bilateral condition called **cornea plana**. The central or paracentral areas of the cornea will look steeper with thinning of the corneal stroma in that region is **keratoconus**. In these patients, one should look for a vertical fibrillar alteration in the corneal stroma called Vogt's striae. In patients with suspected keratoconus, one should also look at the tarsal conjunctiva for papillae suggestive of an allergic conjunctivitis that can worsen the condition. As opposed to localised ectasia, the whole cornea can be very thin and bulging forward in **keratoglobus**.

Both anterior and posterior surfaces of the cornea are near parallel to each other normally. If there is a sudden change in curvature of either of the surface, a cause has to be looked for. Localised thinning of the cornea can occur near the limbus of the cornea due to stromal thinning secondary to marginal ulcers like **Mooren's ulcer**. Degenerative changes like **Terrien's marginal degeneration** cause thinning of the cornea usually near the upper limbus with intact epithelium.

There may be fine vessels in the depression with some yellow deposits superficially. This thinning can change the corneal curvature to affect vision.

The corneal nerves appearing as white threads can be seen coming into the stroma at the limbus. This branches and progressively become thinner to disappear in the mid periphery. These nerves can be seen coming to the centre of the cornea in conditions like keratoconus, neurofibromatosis and multiple endocrine neoplasia (MEN). In some corneal infections, especially those caused by Acanthamoeba, one may see infiltrations around the corneal nerves.

9.3.5.4 Examination of the Corneal Endothelium

Corneal endothelial dysfunction causes oedema of the cornea with eventual loss of transparency. Early signs of corneal endothelial function loss may only be an increase in the corneal thickness compared to the other eye. Even before the signs appear, patients with endothelial dysfunction may complain of early morning blurring of vision which clears after the eye gets dehydrated when exposed to the atmosphere. The evaporation caused by the open eye and better oxygenation of the cornea removes the excess fluid collected overnight. Corneal oedema causes flattening of the posterior corneal curvature as that part of the cornea is less rigid and moves backward. The backward movement of the endothelial surface is associated with a reduced surface area causing it to produce folds. These posterior folds are best made out on indirect illumination or retro-illumination. Epithelial oedema if present too is best seen with indirect or retro-illumination. They appear as fine droplets on the corneal surface. To observe the endothelium clinically, one should do the specular reflection described in Chap. 6. Low endothelial density, loss of the hexagonal shape of the cells and wart-like projections on the endothelium are all suggestive of poor endothelial function. In Fuchs endothelial dystrophy, there are small warty lesions on the endothelium that project into the anterior chamber called **corneal guttata**. In these patients, slit lamp examination with a thick slit will show cop-

per beaten appearance of the endothelial surface with pigment deposition.

If one sees patients suspected with endothelial dysfunction and an area of localised corneal oedema inferiorly, one should suspect a corneal foreign body in the angle causing trauma to the endothelium. A gonioscopy should be done in these cases.

When cornea is examined with a thin slit light, the endothelial layer of the cornea should also be examined. White blood cells due to inflammation in the anterior chamber gets deposited on the endothelial surface and is called keratic precipitates (KP). In granulomatous uveitis, there will be a collection of cells forming one KP and is called mutton fat KP. In cases of suspected disciform keratitis with viral endotheliitis, one should look for KPs on the endothelium underlying the oedema. In suspected corneal graft rejections, one should look for KPs arranged in a row (rejection line) called **Khodadoust line**. On the endothelium, one should look for pigment dusting more concentrated in the vertical meridian like a cigar (seen in pigmentary glaucoma).

Breaks in endothelium should be looked for in congenital glaucoma, non-resolving corneal oedema after surgery, trauma, etc. Haab's striae are breaks seen in the endothelium in cases of congenital glaucoma. Retro-illumination is the best way to look for endothelial breaks. Breaks will appear like a rail track on retro-illumination.

9.4 Examination of Corneal Ulcer

Corneal ulcer is a serious disease of the cornea and an emergency. Corneal ulcer should be examined with an idea to make a diagnosis, prognosticate and to follow response to treatment. The initial assessment of the ulcer should be like any surgical ulcer. Site, size, shape, base of the ulcer, surrounding areas, drainage nodes, etc., should be looked at. Central ulcers are usually infective, e.g. bacterial or fungal. The ulcers near the limbus are more likely to be toxic or autoimmune in nature. Viral ulcers though seen more towards the centre can be seen near the limbus too.

Size of the ulcer should be noted to monitor progression. There are two aspects to size of the ulcer. First is the size of the epithelial defect delineated better by staining the ulcer with fluorescein. The next is the size of the infiltrate. The extent of both should be recorded. Large ulcers and infiltrates are seen in fungal and bacterial ulcers. To measure the ulcer diameter, one needs to keep the microscope and the lighthouse co-axial. Angulation of one can make the measurements variable. The height of the slit beam is adjusted till the beam is equal to the extent of the lesion. The height of the beam is now read off from the scale. To measure the size in any other axis, the lamp housing is rotated so that the slit beam also rotates. At the required axis, measurements can be taken.

The shape of the ulcer can give a clue to the etiological diagnosis. Ulcer with a dendritic shape is suggestive of a viral aetiology (Fig. 9.13). Ulcer with long feathery margins can be fungal (Fig. 9.14). However, acute ulcers with fine small feathery margin are more likely to be due to pseudomonas. White ulcers looking like a comet may be due to pneumococcus (Fig. 9.15). If this is associated with a blocked nasolacrimal duct, the diagnosis is even more certain. Ulcers with margins like a string of pearls is suggestive of a nocardial ulcer (Fig. 9.16).

Attention should now be directed at the floor of the ulcer. If the ulcer has a mucoid base, it may be a bacterial ulcer or there is corneal melt. A dry

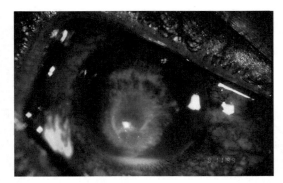

Fig. 9.14 Feathery margins seen in fungal ulcers

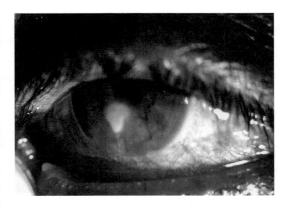

Fig. 9.15 Pneumococcal ulcer with a leading edge like a comet

surface is more likely to be seen in a fungal rather than a bacterial ulcer. Black pigment on the floor of the ulcer is pathognomonic of a fungal ulcer (Fig. 9.17). Iris prolapse is a differential diagnosis and one should rule out a corneal perforation before calling it a fungal ulcer. The base of the ulcer may be elevated in a fungal ulcer (Fig. 9.18). Epithelial defects without much infiltration in the underlying stroma can be viral or early Acanthamoeba ulcers. Neurotrophic ulcers (due to fifth nerve palsy) can be recalcitrant and difficult to heal in spite of having no infection (Fig. 9.19).

Examining the area surrounding an ulcer may show a ring infiltrate. This may be an immune ring or infective. Rings around the ulcer have been seen in fungal, bacterial, viral and acanthamoebic ulcers. Ulcers older than a month with a persisting ring around the ulcer is very sugges-

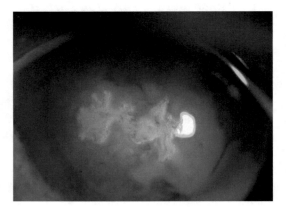

Fig. 9.13 Viral ulcer stained with fluorescein showing dendritic pattern

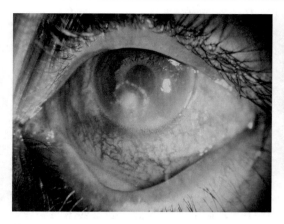

Fig. 9.16 Nocardia ulcer showing a string of pearls appearance

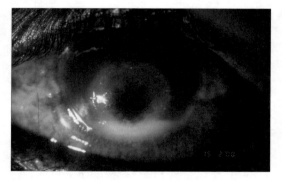

Fig. 9.17 Fungal ulcer showing pigmentation at the base of the ulcer

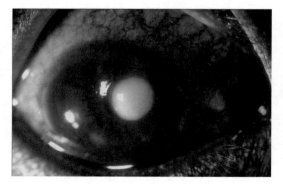

Fig. 9.18 Elevated base due to a fungal colony in fungal keratitis

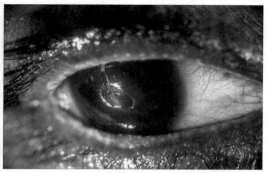

Fig. 9.19 Persistent epithelial defect in a patient with corneal anaesthesia and dry eye

The depth of the ulcer is difficult to make out due to overlying infiltrates. A look through the edges of the ulcer can give a fairly good idea of the depth of the ulcer. Small perforation of the ulcer cannot be made out easily due to infiltrates. Radial folds seen in the deeper layers of the cornea or a sudden decrease in the hypopyon may be pointers of a silent perforation.

Satellite lesions (small lesions away from the main ulcer) has been attributed to fungal ulcer but is seen with equal frequency in ulcers of other aetiology too.

Peripheral corneal ulcers with localised conjunctival congestion is usually due to an autoimmune cause; however, a focal reason like a foreign body or suture in that clock hour should be looked for.

Examination for corneal sensation (see Chap. 15) may reveal significantly reduced sensation even in small viral ulcers and should be examined before instilling any topical anaesthetic drops. Sensation between the two eyes should be compared. In suppurative large corneal ulcers of any aetiology, the corneal sensation is poor due to destruction of the corneal nerves and checking the corneal sensation does not have any diagnostic value. Corneal anaesthesia should be ruled out in any case of non-healing epithelial defect.

Pre-auricular lymph nodes should be palpated. They are not enlarged in any corneal ulcer except that of viral aetiology.

Factors like poor lid closure, underlying dry eye, inturned lashes rubbing on the cornea, sub-

tive of an Acanthamoeba aetiology. Old corneal opacities in the same or fellow cornea points towards a viral aetiology.

tarsal FB, blocked nasolacrimal ducts, ocular co-morbidity like endothelial dysfunction, nutritional status, diabetes are other findings that one need to look for when evaluating a patient with corneal ulcers.

Raised intraocular pressure has been mentioned as reason for non-healing ulcer. Though the causal relationship is not clear, IOP monitoring can be done by digital tonometry (see Chap. 13) if there is no access to a Tonopen that can be used outside the area of the ulcer.

9.4.1 Examination of patients with corneal injury

In patients with suspected penetrating corneal injury the depth of the penetration may be difficult to assess especially because the whole injury track may not be in one slit plane. To assess this, one should do a dynamic slit lamp examination to compute and reconstruct in one's mind the injury tract, to see the extent. Full thickness corneal injury wounds may self-seal due to the valve-like action of the corneal stroma if the wound in bevelled. If a wound leak is suspected, it can be confirmed by doing a **Seidel test** where a wet fluorescein strip is touched on the area of leak. Concentrated fluorescein appears dark, but as it gets diluted by the aqueous from the wound, that area alone becomes green and then yellowish green. If there is a good leak, then a rivulet of dye flow can be seen.

Corneal surgeries: Examination of the cornea is also done after corneal surgeries and follow the principles of examination mentioned before. The things to specially look for after keratoplasty is wound apposition, wound leaks, suture integrity and tightness of sutures in the immediate post-op period. In the late stages, one should look for signs of graft rejection in all the layers of the cornea characterised by signs of inflammation and loss of corneal clarity. Examination of the anterior chamber is also a must.

Following photorefractive corneal surgery, all one may see is a mild corneal haze or the edge line of the flap. After LASIK, one may see few interface opacities between the corneal flap and the stoma. Rarely, some surface wrinkling may be seen.

9.5 Contact Lens Fitting Examination Principles

Contact lenses are lenses that lie in contact with the eye. In fact, it is really floating on the tear film rather than resting on the corneal tissue. The power of the contact lens along with the power of the tear lens (formed between the surfaces of the contact lens and the cornea) corrects the refractive error of the patient. This is more true in rigid gas permeable lens users. The tear lens is not effective in soft lens users because it moulds according to the curvature of the lens. In contact lens fitting, the idea is that one chooses a stable lens that floats on the tears and move enough so that there is tear exchange under the lens for nutrients to pass.

The soft lens is an easy lens to fit. Since the soft lens extends just outside the limbus, the curvature (base curve) selected for the trial soft lens should be 1 mm more than the average central corneal curvature of the patient. This makes the lens flat enough to go from one limbus to the other. The power of the trial lens should be the closest possible to the patient's spherical power. After insertion of the trail lens, one needs to wait for the tearing to settle in about 20 min. The eye is checked under slit lamp for movement of the lens. On blinking, there should be a 1 mm movement of the lens. The lens should not be pressing against the sclera and if it does, it is suggestive of a tight fit. During examination, the lens should be pushed up with the lower lid (**push up test**) to see if it comes back to position. If it does, then that lens has the base curve appropriate for the patient. If the lens appears tight, a flatter lens should be tried. Once the fit is right an over-refraction and acceptance with the contact lens on, is done. This power is added to the power of the trial lens to get the final contact lens power. For example, if the power if the trial lens is −2 D and over-refraction shows −1 D. The patient needs a lens of the same base curve as the fitted lens and a power of −3 D. No fluorescein dye is used for this assessment as the soft contact lens material takes up the stain.

Rigid gas permeable lenses are more difficult to fit and less comfortable for the patient. Here the first trial lens for the fit is chosen based on the flatter corneal curvature of the cornea. **On K fit** means a lens corresponding to the flatter radius of curvature is chosen. After inserting the lens, one has to wait for 30 min or more before assessing the patient. If there is excessive discomfort, a drop of paracaine eases the pain. Once the watering has settled a drop of fluorescein is put into the eye and with the cobalt blue light the tear lake under the lens is examined. When the fit is correct, there may or may not be a mild central corneal touch with very little fluorescein underneath it. Then there is an area of dye pooling around in the mid periphery of the lens following which there may be a mild touch on the cornea more peripherally (Fig. 9.20). In the periphery of the lens, there should be enough of a lift to see the dye well. With each blink the lens should move

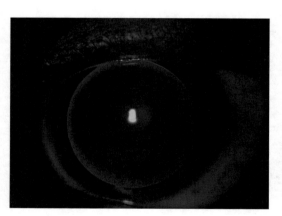

Fig. 9.20 Ideal rigid contact lens fitting pattern with fluorescein

well and the lens should settle in the centre of the cornea within a second. The lens should not ride either too high or too low. If it rides too high, it means the lens is too flat and is getting caught by the lid. If the lens is too steep, the central area of the lens will have a large pool of dye and there will be a corneal touch in the periphery of the contact lens with no dye seen there. The movement of the lens will be poor. Depending on the dye collection and the movement of the lens, flatter or steeper lens is chosen. Once a good fit is achieved, like soft lens, an over-refraction is done to see the power required to get the best vision. This power is now added to the trial lens fitted to get the final power of the lens.

To select the power of the rigid gas permeable heard contact lens, the spectacle correction is done in the negative cylinder form and then only the spherical component is used. The theory is that the negative cylindrical lens power is neutralised by the tear lens.

With soft lens the spherical equivalent is used. Normally, soft lens is not given if the astigmatism is more than 1 D.

When evaluating patients on contact lens, one should look for the tear secretion of the patient and see if the lens fit is ideal. Allergy to the lens or other irritants should be checked for by looking for papillae on the upper tarsal conjunctiva. Corneal scarring and vascularisation suggest contact lens over wear and should be looked for with slit lamp.

A digital anterior segment photograph is the best way to record ocular surface and corneal findings. The colour-coded drawings described is time-consuming and less accurate than the digital slit lamp photographs which is now widely available. Lesions can be measured with the slit lamp by keeping the lamp housing and the microscope coaxial and it is noted down.

Examination of Sclera

10

In this age of sub-specialization one does not normally hear about a scleral specialist! Covering about 80% of the globe surface, the sclera one would have thought would have caused more trouble than it is credited for. On the whole, the sclera appears like an inactive tissue with no major function except to protect the delicate internal layers. Examination of the sclera is not emphasised normally. For this reason diseases of the sclera especially that occurring posteriorly is missed commonly.

10.1 Applied Anatomy

The sclera is the thick fibrous sheet that covers most of the globe. It is white in colour normally. In children below 5 years it may have a bluish hue due to the underlying choroid that is seen through the thinner sclera of children.

The sclera can be divided into three layers for convenience. The outer most layer is the episclera that is attached to the sclera proper and consists of loose fibrous tissue that merges with the tenons superficially. This layer is more prominent anterior to the muscle insertion. It is supplied by the anterior ciliary arteries that forms a deep plexus and is normally not seen under the conjunctival vessels.

The middle layer is the actual scleral stroma. It has a dense fibrous tissue made of collagen that is packed irregularly in whorls and loops.

The haphazard arrangement makes it opaque unlike the cornea. The stoma has fibroblast and a few melanocytes. The scleral stroma is 1 mm thick posteriorly and gradually becomes thinner anteriorly. At the insertion of the rectus muscles it is the thinnest at 0.3 mm. It becomes thicker anteriorly and is about 0.8 mm at the limbus. The trabecular meshwork lies in the sclera at the limbus. At the limbus the sclera fuses with the cornea.

The innermost layer of the sclera is the lamina fusca. This is a membranous layer composed of fine avascular lamellae. It has brownish tinge due to melanocytes and connects to the underlying choroid in certain areas with fine collagen fibres. Between these connections is a potential space called suprachoroidal or perichoroidal space. Anteriorly there are only about four radial connections whereas posteriorly there are many more. It is for this reason that the suprachoroidal effusion form elevated mounds anteriorly with the mounds dipping down at the four or five sites of attachment of choroid to the sclera.

The sclera has a mesh-like opening posteriorly to allow the optic nerve and vessels to pass through. Just outside the optic nerve entry are multiple openings to let the short and long posterior arteries and nerves to pass through. 4 mm posterior to the equator are 4–5 openings in the sclera for the vortex veins to exit. Further anteriorly in front of the insertion of the rectii are the seven openings for the entry of the anterior cili-

© Springer Nature Singapore Pte Ltd. 2020
T. Kuriakose, *Clinical Insights and Examination Techniques in Ophthalmology*,
https://doi.org/10.1007/978-981-15-2890-3_10

ary arteries. Intraocular tumours can come out of the eye through these openings.

The four recti are inserted 5.5–7.5 mm behind the limbus and can be seen clinically especially if the muscles are inflamed. Scleral inflammation can cause eye pain when the eyes move due to the pull of the muscle tendon on the inflamed sclera.

The sclera is relatively avascular and is supplied by the long, short and anterior ciliary arteries. When congested, these deep vessels appear indistinct and pink.

The scleral nerve supply is from the short and long ciliary nerves that pass through the sclera. It is for this reason that scleral inflammation can be painful. Scleritis may also cause sectoral corneal anaesthesia due to the involvement of the long ciliary nerves which supply the cornea.

Normal sclera appears white in young adults. In young children the sclera appear blue due to the choroid showing through the thin sclera. In older people sclera may have a yellowish colour due to fat deposition. In people around the age of 80 years, at the insertion of the recti, especially the lateral rectus, one may see a translucent vertically oval plaque called *hyaline scleral plaques* (Fig. 10.1).

In the area around the entry of the anterior ciliary vessels in front of the rectus muscle insertion the sclera may be pigmented due to migration of pigments from inside the eye. This is more commonly seen in pigmented race and does not signify an underlying melanoma unless it is

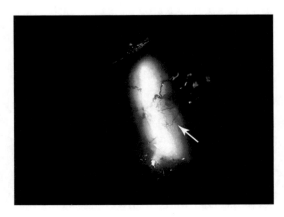

Fig. 10.1 Hyaline scleral plaques just anterior to the lateral rectus insertion (white arrow)

extensive with dilated vessels. The sclera, the size of the anterior ciliary artery, the pigmentation around it, insertion of the rectus muscle, etc. should be noted in all patients so that the normal and its variations can be understood.

10.2 History

Pain in the eye is one of the commoner symptoms with which patients with scleral problems present. In any patient with eye pain the possibility of a scleritis should be kept in mind. The pain can be very severe, waking up the patient at night. One can also get a dull boring pain or mild intermittent shooting pain that lasts a few seconds. Dry eye also can cause intermittent shooting pain in the eye. Sometimes scleritis can occur without pain. If a scleritis patch is near a muscle insertion, the patient will complain of pain while moving the eye.

History of redness of the eyes is the other common presentation. The redness can be localised or general. There will be no history of discharge. Watering can be present. A past history of similar redness of eyes should be asked. Redness of the eye is not a must, especially for posterior scleritis.

If there is underlying uveitis, patient may complain of photophobia. The patient may have uveitis as part of the primary diseases causing a scleritis.

Decreased vision can be a presentation of posterior scleritis and there is usually pain associated with it. If the scleral inflammation spreads to the cornea, it can affect the vision.

Some patients present with black discolouration in the white of the eye. Patient should be asked how it was noticed to give an idea of the duration. Some patches may have been noted while retracting the upper or lower lid and may have been there for a long time. Long-standing lesions are congenital pigmentation of the sclera or nevai. A staphyloma following past injury, rhinosporidial infection, scleral melt due to scleritis, etc. can also cause black discolouration due to the uveal tissue bulging out through the thin or deficient sclera.

Patient should be asked about a recent history of pain and blisters around the eye to rule out an attack of herpes zoster ophthalmicus as it too can cause scleral inflammation.

Like the work up of a uveitis patient, a good systemic history is important for these patients too. Patients should be asked about joint pains, haemoptysis, history of exposure to venereal diseases, etc. Autoimmune diseases like rheumatoid arthritis, Wegner's granulomatosis, etc. can also cause scleritis. The latter is particularly notorious for causing scleritis, and a high index of suspicion should be present when dealing with a case of suspected scleritis. History of any present or past treatments should be taken to get an idea of any underlying diseases.

Finally, patient should be asked about a history of trauma or eye surgeries in the past as these can cause scleral inflammations.

10.3 Examination

Before examining the sclera one should stand back and see the patient as a whole, the joints, the posture, etc. to look out for any evidence of autoimmune diseases. It may be even worth asking the patient to put out his hands to look at the joints.

In patients with eye pain, proptosis or prominence of one eye should be looked for. If this is not consciously looked for, it can be missed. Even if the prominence is not obvious, it is worth looking for proptosis from behind the patient as it is good method to pick up asymmetric proptosis. Here one stands behind the seated patient and looks from above along the plane of the forehead to see which eye is more prominent (see Chap. 7). Standing behind the patient, the head of the patient is tilted back about 20° with the palm of the examiner's hands kept on either side of the face. The index fingers of each hand is used to raise the upper lid and patient asked to look straight. The examiner now moves his head back till the patient's eyes cannot be seen. Now the examiner brings his head forward looking over the patient's forehead till he sees the cornea of the patient. If the apex of both the corneas are seen at the same time, then both eyes are at the same level. If one

cornea is seen earlier, it means that eye is more proptosed compared to the other.

When looking at the face, one should look for areas of increased pigmentation on the face if nevus of Ota is suspected.

The eyes are first examined with torchlight and then sunlight if possible. This gives an overview of the position of the lesions and their colours. The classical salmon pink colour of scleritis patch is seen best with sunlight. Since the sclera lies under the conjunctiva the conjunctival colour may mask the scleral colours, scleral colours are best assessed in the sunlight. The conjunctiva can be moved over the sclera by pressing the lid against the conjunctiva with a finger and moving it to figure out which tissue has the colour. In suspected cases of posterior scleritis the only evidence of inflammation will be redness in the forniceal region. To examine the upper sclera, the patient should be asked to look down as much as possible to expose the posterior sclera. Likewise, all quadrants of the eye is examined.

When examining the redness of the eye one should make an effort to see which of the three tissues, namely conjunctiva, episcleral or sclera, is primarily at fault. In conjunctivitis the sclera will not be affected and the white sclera will be seen well. In episcleritis since slightly deeper vessels are involved, the scleral white is not that clearly seen. However the vessels are still superficial enough to be blanched by 5% phenylephrine drops applied topically. The classical teaching is that in patients with suspected scleritis/episcleritis if the congestion disappears with 5% phenylephrine one is dealing with episcleritis. This is seldom used in clinics as the demarcation is not clear cut and the presence of other signs and symptoms is enough to differentiate the two if needed. In scleritis, there will be a salmon pink colour and the redness will persist with phenylephrine. The sclera will appear boggy without any conjunctival chemosis (Fig. 10.2). The sclera will be tender to palpate in the area of scleritis.

The sclera can be palpated using the lid, by moving the lid over the sclera. Tenderness on palpation over the red patch is suggestive of scleritis. In episcleritis there is a little tenderness. In poste-

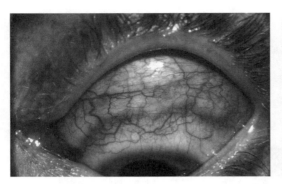

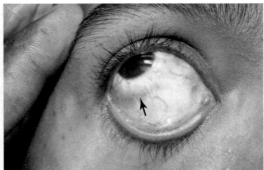

Fig. 10.2 Localised congestion and swelling of the sclera in the superior forniceal region due to scleritis. Elevation was restricted in the patient due to pain on supraduction

Fig. 10.3 Blue sclera due to scleral thinning (black arrow) seen in a patient with old recurrent scleritis

rior scleritis pressing on the globe over the closed lid in some directions will elicit pain. If on palpation the sclera feels boggy, then there is severe inflammation and some scleral melt.

In suspected cases of scleral inflammation or infection, besides history, the limbal area should be examined for evidence of previous surgeries and sutures remnants. The area of the sclera around the insertion of the rectus muscle should be inspected to see if there is evidence of a scleral buckling surgery. Previous surgery and sutures can be a trigger factor for scleral inflammation. Nocardial infection of the sclera can be seen after surgery. One may see pus coming from the sclera in these cases. In some cases of non-infectious necrotising scleritis too there can be yellow pointing nodules with pus-like material coming from it and should not be mistaken for an infection.

Evidence of localised bluish area on the sclera is suggestive of old attacks of scleritis causing scleral melt and the choroid being seen through (Fig. 10.3).

When patients come with complaint of seeing a black patch on the sclera, the first thing to do is to ensure it is in the scleral plane and not on the conjunctiva by using the slit illumination of the slit lamp. One can also move the conjunctiva over the sclera. If it is in the scleral plane, make sure it is not the normal pigmentation around the anterior

ciliary artery. If the anterior ciliary artery is grossly dilated compared to the others (*sentinel artery*) and the pigmentation is more than normal, a possible melanoma in the eye should be suspected.

One may see a black elevated area in the sclera with a thin sliver of scleral tissue on it and is called **staphyloma**. Depending on the location of the staphyloma it has been named as ciliary staphyloma, intercalary staphyloma, etc. Posterior staphyloma cannot be seen clinically. Patients may give a history of trauma or surgery in the past. The intraocular pressure should be checked in these patients. In some patients, the staphyloma is due to raised intraocular pressure pushing the uveal tissue through a previously weak sclera. Rhinosporidiosis can be a cause of staphyloma and these patients should be asked if they had some reddish mass in the eye in the past which may or may not have been removed.

Diffuse blue sclera in anybody over 5 years is suggestive of a problem with the collagen synthesis. In conditions like osteogenesis imperfecta and Ehlers-Danlos syndrome, the choroid is seen through the thin sclera giving the blue discolouration.

Nodules on the surface of the sclera suggest nodular scleritis which may not have any clinical significance in itself. One should examine the surface of these nodules to look for any foreign bodies like caterpillar hairs that may be responsible for the inflammation. Yellowish nodules

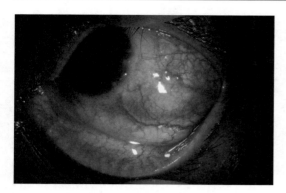

Fig. 10.4 Localised area of scleritis temporally with an area of corneal inflammation (white area) adjacent to the limbus

need not always suggest an infective origin. It just means necrotic sclera and can be seen with autoimmune necrotising scleritis. Nocardia is a common cause of infective scleritis seen after surgery to the eye.

Examination of the cornea and uveal tissue is important in cases of scleral disease. Old scleritis adjacent to the cornea can leave a tongue-shaped opacity on the cornea as a result of the corneal inflammation. In acute cases there may be segmental corneal oedema if the scleritis is adjacent to limbus (Fig. 10.4). In scleritis away from the limbus, one may find a corneal hypoesthesia in the quadrant where the scleritis is, due to involvement of the posterior ciliary nerves that traverse the area.

Since the sclera is apposed to the uveal tissue, there may be some anterior uveitis evident clinically in patients with scleritis. The presence of uveitis helps one differentiate scleritis from episcleritis and conjunctivitis.

In patients with trabeculitis with scleritis, the intraocular pressure may be elevated and so need to be monitored.

In patients who come with trauma and suspected globe (scleral) rupture, one has to go by indirect evidences. If the eye is very soft, a globe rupture should be suspected. If the anterior chamber is very deep again, it suggests that the content of the globe has escaped from the eye making the eye soft and iris and lens go backward. If fundus examination shows vitreous haemorrhage along with a low IOP again a posterior globe rupture should be suspected. Many of these patients will have sub-conjunctival haemorrhage and a boggy conjunctiva.

Examination of the eye movement can give useful information in patients with scleral disease. In scleritis the patient may not be able to move the eye to the extreme gaze due to pain on ductions. In globe rupture the eye movements will be restricted due to the collapse of the globe.

In patients who complaint of eye pain and decreased vision, the posterior segment examination will show elevation of the posterior pole with or without some retinal oedema due to the inflamed sclera covering the area. If the inflamed sclera compresses the optic nerve, then one may get disc oedema associated with some soft exudates. In these patients the ultrasound will show fluid in the sub-tenon's space with a 'T' sign.

Red free light has been used to highlight/delineate the area of redness in scleritis. The reddish area including the blood vessels will appear black against the sclera.

Examination of Iris and Pupil

Examination of the 'pupil' as such makes no sense because the pupil is actually a gap in the continuity of the iris. Pupil examination is actually the examination of the iris and its function!

The iris is the equivalent of the diaphragm of the camera in the eye. Its major functions are the control of light going into the eye, reduce aberrations by allowing only the paraxial rays to focus on the retina and finally increase the depth of focus of the eye.

11.1 Applied Anatomy

Iris is like a curtain that is in between the lens and the cornea and hangs from the anterior surface of the ciliary body. It divides the space into anterior and posterior chambers. The iris extends from the ciliary margin at ciliary body to the pupillary border. The iris is thinnest at the ciliary border and thickest 2 mm from the pupillary border along the collarette (Fig. 11.1). The bowing out of the thinner peripheral iris cause angle closure if there is a block in aqueous flow from posterior to anterior chamber.

The iris has an anterior stromal layer derived from the mesenchyma and a posterior epithelial layer derived from the neural ectoderm.

The stromal layer is made of vascular connective tissue containing melanocytes, fibroblasts, smooth muscles, collagen fibres, blood vessels, nerve fibres, etc. Since the anterior surface has no epithelial cell covering the stroma, it is in direct contact with the aqueous in the anterior chamber. The vessels of the iris have no tight junctions. Lymphocytes, macrophages and mast cells are also seen in the iris stroma. The stromal tissue along with the collagen fibres are arranged radially in most parts of the iris. In between tissue are depressions called crypts. 2 mm from the pupillary margin the connective tissue forms a circular ridge called the *collarette* (Fig. 11.2). This divides the iris into an outer ciliary zone and an inner pupillary zone. Deep in the stroma at the collarette and extending into pupillary zone is the sphincter pupillae muscle. This smooth muscle is supplied by parasympathetic nerves in the third cranial nerve (CN) and constricts the pupil. The colour of the iris depends on the amount of melanin in the iris.

Just anterior to the epithelial layer of the iris, in the ciliary area lies the dilator pupillae muscle. This is supplied by the sympathetic fibres in the third CN and dilates the pupil (Fig. 11.1).

The posterior epithelial layer in turn has two layers of cells facing each other. A potential space therefore exists between the two layers, making formation of cysts easy. The anterior layer gives rise to the dilator pupillae and is in close contact with it and the stroma. It has very little melanin granules and is continuous with the posterior layer at the pupillary border. The junction of the two layers lies just within the anterior surface of the iris and forms the *pupillary ruff*.

© Springer Nature Singapore Pte Ltd. 2020
T. Kuriakose, *Clinical Insights and Examination Techniques in Ophthalmology*,
https://doi.org/10.1007/978-981-15-2890-3_11

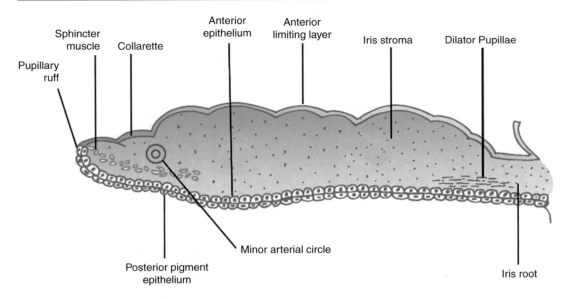

Fig. 11.1 Cross section of the iris

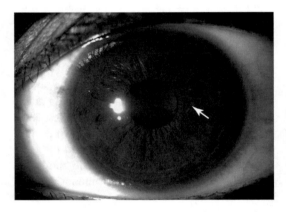

Fig. 11.2 Normal iris showing the pupillary zone and the ciliary zone delineated by the collarette (arrow)

The posterior layer is heavily pigmented with a lot of melanin pigments.

The iris is supplied by vessels arising from the major arterial circle in the ciliary body. This in turn receives blood supply from the long posterior and anterior ciliary arteries. The nerve supply of the iris and that which sub-serves the pupillary reflex is complex. This is described in more detail in the section on neuro-ophthalmology. The sympathetic nerve supplies the dilator muscles. Parasympathetic nerve fibres coming via the ciliary ganglion form the efferent pathway for the light reflex causing constriction of the pupil mediated by the constrictor pupillae muscle. Sensory supply of the iris come from the naso-ciliary branch of the fifth CN.

11.2 Normal Pupil

The normal pupil is round. It is almost central with respect to the cornea and is shifted slightly to the nasal side. It measures 2–4 mm in size in normal adults. In infants and in people over 75 years of age the pupil is smaller. The pupil in both eyes are usually of equal size though a small amount of inequality (*anisocoria*) of less than 0.4 mm may be normal. In physiological aniso-coria the pupil maintain the difference in all conditions of lighting and constrict and dilate equally.

The pupil is well seen in the Caucasian population because of contrast between the black pupil and the light coloured iris. In the pigmented race the iris is brown and it is difficult to make out the pupil from a distance without good lighting. In hypopigmented iris the blood vessels may be seen with the slit lamp and should not be mistaken for new vessels. New vessels will not follow the radial pattern of the normal iris vessels. Sometimes one can see fine strands attached to the collarette area moving in the anterior chamber. These are remnants or persistence of the pupillary membrane which forms during the developmental stage. These strands can cross the pupil and be attached to the collarette on the opposite side of the pupil. These fibres can break during pupillary dilatation and cause spontaneous hyphaema.

The commonest pupil reaction to light is an initial brisk contract followed by a slow minimal dilatation and again a mild contraction. In some patients both the constriction and dilatation are slow. Other rarer patterns of pupillary constriction like a slow contraction, quick dilatation and quick contraction have also been described in the normal population. In normal people without any pathology of the second and third CNs, both eyes react equally when light is shown in one eye. Therefore even if one eye is blind, if the third CN is intact, light shown in the good eye will cause an equal constriction of the pupil in both eyes. It takes about 2–3 s for the pupil to steady after shining the light. When examining for relative afferent pupillary defect (RAPD) this is the reason why one waits for 2–3 s after shining the light in one eye before moving the light to the fellow eye. If moved too quickly, one would catch the dilatation phase of the fellow eye's consensual reflex and mistake it for a relative afferent pupillary defect.

Besides light, pupil also constrict if eye shifts gaze to a nearby object like the tip of one's nose. This is part of the *near reflex* where in there is triad of convergence of both eyes, constriction of the pupil and contraction of the ciliary muscles to facilitate accommodation when we look at a near object.

11.3 History

Usually examination of iris and pupil is done as part of the general examination of the eye. If a patient has come with a specific complaint related to the pupil like the pupil being unequal in size, or patient perceives excessive brightness or dimness of light in one or both eyes, etc. one should take the history of using any new medications including topical medications. Splashing of medicine into the eye or even some makeup material may affect the pupil size. History of ocular trauma causing traumatic mydriasis or ocular

inflammation evidenced by redness of eye should also be asked for.

11.4 Examination of the Iris

As alluded to earlier, examination of the iris is closely related to the pupils as the latter is a defect in the iris. Though iris details are better seen with a slit lamp a good focused torchlight with preferably yellow colour light is the main stay for pupil examination. White light causes glare and photophobia making the patient blink reflexively when light is shown. A transparent millimetre scale is useful to measure the pupil size when needed. One should be aware that the pupil size is magnified due to the corneal curvature, a 3.5 mm real-life pupil will be measured as about 4 mm from outside of the eye. The first thing to notice in the pupil is to see if it is round, central and equal in both eyes. The iris in both eyes should be of the same colour. Any colour difference between the two eyes should be noted (*heterochromia iridum*). The iris in each eye should also be uniformly coloured. If there are sectoral differences (*heterochromia iridis*), it should be noted. Just to name one of the causes, congenital Horner's syndrome could be a cause for heterochromia iridum and a nevus could be the cause for heterochromia iridis.

The pupil may not be round in some patients. A teardrop like pupil with a defect inferiorly is usually due to a developmental problem of the iris like a coloboma (Fig. 11.3). A surgical exci-

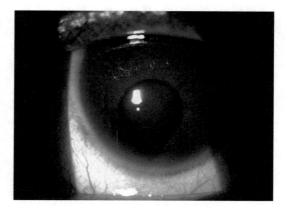

Fig. 11.3 Coloboma of the iris in the infero-medial quadrant

sion of the iris in that area is also a possibility. In coloboma the iris collarette touches the pupillary ruff. In surgical excision these two stop abruptly. In coloboma there may be associated coloboma of the lens and choroid.

The pupil margin may be peaked in areas. Fibrous or neoplastic tissue in the peripheral iris may be the cause in unoperated eyes. In operated eyes the causes would include a strand of vitreous going from the posterior chamber to the wound, internal iris prolapse, sphincter rupture, reverse iris tuck by an intraocular lens, capsule at the pupillary margin, sphincterotomy, etc. Unless the cause is specifically looked for it is easy to miss it.

There should be only one opening (pupil) in the iris. More than one opening is called *polycoria*. This is usually due to a developmental defect. Conditions like essential iris atrophy can develop defects in the iris. Additional openings in the iris may also be seen secondary to surgical intervention or trauma. A hole may be seen in the peripheral iris following a YAG laser iridotomy or a surgical peripheral iridectomy. Unless one looks for it, it is easy to miss a peripheral laser iridotomy or a hole formed by a projectile foreign body. In the pigmented eyes, on retro-illumination if one sees a red glow in the periphery it is suggestive of through-and-through defect in the iris. However in Caucasian eyes the inherent poor pigmentation of the iris can give transillumination without an actual iris defect. Here one should see the ciliary body or lens through the suspected iris defect to confirm a full thickness hole. Dis-insertion of the iris root (iridodialysis) is seen as a gap in the iris at the ciliary body area. The flat side of a 'D'-shaped pupil seen in many of these cases will point to the location of the iridodialysis (Fig. 11.4).

The colour of the pupil in normal young people is a greenish dark grey. Development of cataract with age makes it start looking more whitish grey. White-coloured pupil in younger people needs to be investigated. Cataracts, persistent hyperplasic primary vitreous, retinoblastoma, retinopathy of prematurity, etc. are some of the more commoner causes for this condition called cat's eye pupil. A jet black pupil is seen in aphakia (absence of lens from the patellar fossa of the

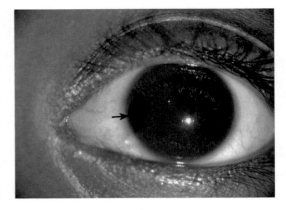

Fig. 11.4 Eye with iridodialysis in the medial aspect (black arrow)

anterior vitreous face) or pseudophakia (artificial lens in the eye).

Iridodonesis is a tremulousness of the iris and is normally absent. The iris shake or iridodonesis occurs due to two main reasons. One is the lack of support from the lens zonular diaphragm which lie in apposition to the iris. The second reason is ophthalmodonesis were the jelly-like vitreous body hits against the iris in the absence of the lens and moves it. The latter seems to be the predominant reason for the iris tremulousness because iridodonesis is only rarely present in pseudophakia where the IOL (intraocular lens) is far away from the iris. The IOL also prevents the vitreous body coming and hitting the iris. Iridodonesis is best seen in aphakia after an intracapsular cataract extraction. The sign of iridodonesis is best made out soon after a blink or when the eye makes short jerky movement. It can be seen under the slit lamp soon after the eye makes spontaneous movements. The torchlight or slit lamp light should be shown from the temporal side to see the shake better.

The iris should be examined un-dilated first. The details of the iris is best seen with the slit lamp. The radial iris pattern with crypts is seen clearly with the slit lamp. Iris pattern, discolouration, swelling, nodules, new vessels, defects, etc. should be noted with the slit lamp. The pattern of pupillary contraction, e.g. vermiform movements, can also be made out better with the slit lamp.

If the iris pattern becomes indistinct or muddy, it suggests previous inflammation of the iris like uveitis. Segmental areas of atrophy (whitish discolouration) seen on the iris suggest previous trauma or viral infection (herpetic). Hyperpigmented lesions could be nevus or melanoma. Table 11.1 shows the features of each.

Localised elevations of the iris suggest a cyst of the iris or a mass behind the iris. Pupillary dilatation may reveal the true nature of the swelling. If that fails, ultrasound (UBM—ultrasound biomicroscopy) has to be done.

Nodules on the surface of the iris is abnormal (Fig. 11.5). The colour of the nodules for the same condition depends on the iris colour and pigmentation. In phacomatosis, e.g. neurofibromatosis, fine small or larger nodules (*Lisch nodules*) are seen scattered all around the iris. The number of nodules can be very variable. In Down's syndrome the nodules (*Brushfield nodules*) are seen located all around near the iris root. This may also be seen in normal children. In uveitis, nodules may appear on the iris surface (*Bussaca's nodules*) and at the pupillary borders (*Koeppe's nodules*). In uveitis there will be associated cells and flare in the anterior chamber. These nodules resolve with treatment. Infections, especially fungus infections, can have fungal colonies growing on the iris in the infected eye.

Stromal vessels of the iris is not normally seen. In some lightly coloured iris (e.g. blue iris) radial vessels may be normally seen. Any vessel on the iris should be looked at in detail. New vessels should be suspected if there are non-radial and arborizing vessels over the iris. New vessels due to ischemic retina in diabetes usually starts at the pupillary border or the ciliary border (iris root) due to passage of larger amounts of vascular endothelial factors that come from the posterior segment into the anterior segment via the pupil and gets out of the eye via the trabecular meshwork. Distortion of the pupillary border, migration of the posterior epithelial layer of the iris (Fig. 11.6) anteriorly (*ectropion uveae*), peripheral anterior synechiae (PAS), etc. are all suggestive of new vessel formation on the iris.

Table 11.1 Difference between iris nevus and melanoma

Character	Iris nevus	Iris melanoma
Size and extent of lesion	Small well circumscribed. <3 mm	Circumscribed or diffuse
Thickness of lesion	Flat or minimally elevated. <0.5 mm elevation	Elevated and fleshy
New vessels on and surrounding the lesion	No new vessels	New vessels may be seen feeding the tumour
Intraocular pressure	Normal	May be high
Trabecular meshwork	No pigmentation	Unilateral increase in pigments

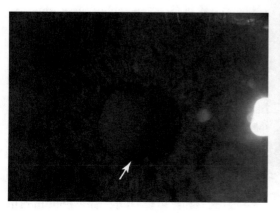

Fig. 11.5 Iris nodules (white arrow) due to uveitis

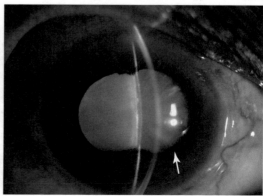

Fig. 11.6 Ectropion uveae (white arrow) due to contracting neovascular membrane pulling the posterior pigment layer of iris anteriorly

Slit lamp examination can reveal sluggish low-amplitude pupillary reactions that can be missed by torchlight examination. Here a thin beam of light is shown into the pupillary area by switching on the slit lamp light and the pupils observed.

11.5   Insights into Examination of the Pupil

The long and complex afferent and efferent pathway of the nerve fibres sub-serving pupillary reflex both within and outside skull make it amenable to be affected by multiple neurological problems. Pupil reaction is an objective test of visual function without the need for patient cooperation. It is these characteristics that make the examination of the pupil important and useful. Pupillary abnormalities can also be due to causes within the eye.

In coloured patients it is difficult to make out the pupillary margins due to lack of contrast between the greyish black pupil and dark brown iris. To see the pupil well it may be useful to ask the patient or clinical assistant to shine a torch from below the nose so that scattered light illuminates the iris without inducing a pupillary reaction (Fig. 11.7). The patient should be asked to look at the distance when the pupils are inspected. Difference in the size of the pupil between the eyes (*anisocoria*) if any should be the first thing noted. If different, the next thing is to figure out which is the abnormal pupil. For this, the pupils should be re-examined in bright light and very dim light. If the anisocoria increases in bright light, then the larger pupil is the pathological. If anisocoria is more in dim light, then the smaller pupil is the pathological one. Often one does not have to do this test because there are other related symptoms and signs that will give a clue to the abnormal pupil and needs to be looked for. Presence of ptosis associated with pupillary abnormality gives a clue. If there is ptosis with constriction of pupil, it is likely to be *Horner's syndrome*, ptosis associated with dilated pupil in the same eye suggest third nerve paresis. If aniso-

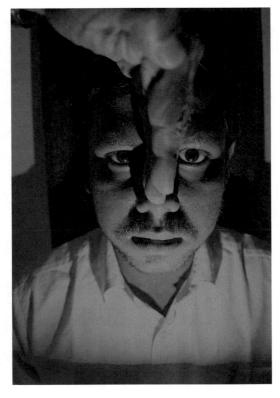

Fig. 11.7 A torch shown from below at the level of the chest to illuminate and view the pupils in darkly pigmented eyes

coria does not change with illumination, then a local cause should be suspected (drug induced, trauma, Holmes-Adie pupil, etc.).

In the extremes of age (infancy and old age) the pupils are very small and examination of pupillary reaction can be difficult. This should not be mistaken for any pathological conditions.

Once the size of the pupil is assessed and measured if needed, one should look for the pupillary reaction. Pupils react to light and near viewing as part of the accommodative reflex. Examination of the pupillary reaction is best done in a very dimly lit or dark room with the patient looking at the distant target, a dimly lit red light. This relaxes the accommodation causing maximal pupillary dilatation, any constriction now is made out more easily. Once the patient looks at the distance, a focused torchlight is shown into each eye, one eye after the other to see if the pupil constricts to

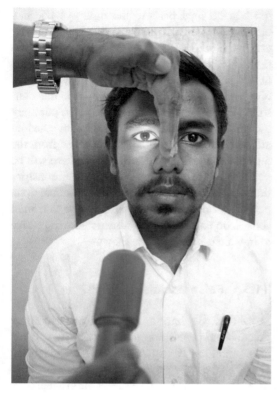

Fig. 11.8 A method of restricting light falling into the fellow eye when examining the pupillary reaction

light shown directly into the eye. This is the direct pupillary reaction. Along with contraction, the speed of contraction should also be noted; a brisk contraction of the iris with the pupil reaching 3 mm or less in diameter suggests a normal pupillary reaction. If the light of the torch is scattered, one should place the palm of the hand between the nose to prevent light reaching the opposite eye (Fig. 11.8). If direct reaction is absent or very sluggish in an eye, there are two possibilities. Either the afferent pathway (Retina, optic nerve, chiasma, optic tracts, etc.) has a pathology or the efferent pathway (third CN, iris tissue) has an issue.

Rarely lesions affecting the tectum of the midbrain can compress the pupillary reflex fibres crossing the periaqueductal area and abolishes the light reaction in both eyes. This may be associated with preserved vision and loss of upward gaze (Parinaud syndrome).

When the retina or optic nerve is significantly damaged, the direct pupillary reaction if present will be very sluggish and incomplete. Sometimes there is an initial sluggish contraction followed by significant dilatation (*escape phenomenon*). This is due to the fact that the weak signals are made even weaker by sustained light which bleaches the retinal pigments.

In lesions of the optic tract it has been suggested that focussed light shown from the unaffected half of the field gives a better pupillary reaction (Wernicke's pupil) compared to the opposite field. The test is not really worth doing because it is very difficult to elicit this sign due to light scatter within the eye. There is no point trying to elicit it and imagining a Wernicke's pupil after the field test shows a homonymous hemianopia! **There is no virtue in eliciting a sign which has no role in changing your post-test probability.**

It is also useful to remember at this stage that pupillary reaction is also sub-served by light-sensitive ganglion cells that transmit directly to the Edinger Westphal nucleus to sub-serve pupillary reaction. Such patients with intact ganglion cells and no vision at all (due to photoreceptor pathology) may still show a weak pupillary reaction.

If direct reaction is present in both eyes, then checking for consensual reflex (checking for pupillary reaction in the fellow eye when light is shown in one eye) does not give any additional information. If however one eye pupil is not reacting, then while shining the light into the non-reacting pupil, the fellow eye can be observed for consensual reaction and if present then the efferent system is at fault in the non-reacting pupil and not the afferent system. On the other hand, if consensual is also absent, then the afferent pathway including the optic nerve and the retina could be at fault. It is not a must to do consensual reaction after the direct reaction because the information got from consensual pupillary examination can be deduced when checking for a relative afferent pupillary defect (RAPD). In pigmented eyes the lack of contrast makes checking consensual reaction with an additional torch a laborious task.

RAPD can sometimes be the only sign of optic nerve/afferent pathway pathology. To check for RAPD, again patient should be looking at the distance in a dim room. The walls of the ever-shrinking consultation rooms often hinders distance viewing. A better instruction would be to ask the patient to look at the ceiling. This will give a more consistent distance viewing. Focussed light is now shown into one eye from below the pupillary border and patient's pupillary reaction and size is noted. After the pupil has stabilised (in about 2–3 s), the light is **quickly** swung to the fellow eye by moving the torch below the nose to the opposite side and light shown from below pupillary level. Besides the ease of doing the test an additional advantage of shining the light from below is that the same part of the retina (upper retina) is illuminated in both eyes. When the patient is looking up, the examiner standing in front of the patient will not hinder the patient's view.

In normal people as soon as the torch is moved quickly to the fellow eye there is a small additional constriction of the pupil or it remains the same. If there is any dilatation instead, there is an afferent pupillary defect in the eye that had the light directed on it. This means that the afferent pathway of the eye which dilates when light is shown in it, is affected compared to the fellow eye. Though obvious it should be reiterated that if both eyes are equally affected by disease there will be no RAPD. Having said that diseases like primary glaucoma which is bilateral, often have asymmetrical damage of the ganglion cells and optic nerve in the early stages and an RAPD is very sensitive in picking up this asymmetry suggesting optic nerve damage.

If for some reason one eye had to be dilated pharmacologically or the pupil of one eye is non-reactive due to past trauma, it is still possible to elicit an RAPD. Here the pupillary reaction of one eye alone is used to assess the afferent function pathway of both eyes. If suppose the right eye is the non-reacting pupil and also has an RAPD. When light is shown in the right eye there will be no constriction. Now when light is shifted to the left eye the left eye will constrict significantly. Then on

moving the light back to the right eye one can observe a consensual pupillary dilatation in the left eye. Even without looking for consensual dilatation (difficult to do in coloured eyes) when the light is shifted back to the left eye if the pupil size observed was significantly more than the constricted state one can assume there was a pupillary escape. If, on the other hand, the left eye had an afferent defect, when the light is moved from the dilated and fixed right eye to the left there will be pupillary dilatation instead of a further constriction in the left eye. If both eyes have normal optic nerve function, pupil in the left eye after the initial constriction size will stay constricted irrespective of in which eye the light is shown.

11.5.1 False Localising RAPD

In patients who have a cataract in one eye and a pseudophakic 6/6 vision in the other eye, it is not uncommon to get an RAPD in the pseudophakic eye when the optic nerve of both eyes are functioning normally. This RAPD is due to the brighter light that goes into the cataractous eye as a result of the scattering by the lens opacities. Reverse RAPD and paradoxical RAPD have been terms used for this phenomenon which is really not what it is. There is nothing that is reversed or paradoxical here.

11.5.2 Pupillary Reaction for Near

After examining the pupil for light reaction one should look at the pupillary reaction of near. As part of the near reflex, along with convergence and accommodation the pupil also constricts. This is more fully discussed in the section on neuro-ophthalmology (see Chap. 15). Here patient is asked to look at a distance and then suddenly asked to look at a near object. Normally the pupil constricts. If light reaction is present, then pupillary reaction for near need not be checked as there is no clinical condition where the light reaction is present and convergence pupillary reaction is absent.

11.5.3 Dilatation of Pupil

After the pupil and iris examination the pupil should be dilated. Pupil and iris examination is never complete without dilating the pupil with short-acting mydriatic. A combination of Tropicamide 1% and Phenylephrine 1% can be used for adults. The former relaxes the sphincter pupillae muscle and the latter activates the dilator pupillae muscles and make the dilatation process more effective. This combination of drugs should not be used if cycloplegia is the objective. If the patient is a hypertensive or has myocardial ischaemia, in an effort to prevent systemic absorption, the lacrimal punctum and canaliculi can be occluded by pressing the thumb and index finger on the medial side of the nose on either side for a minute.

The speed and amount of dilatation should be assessed. Normal patients with pigmented iris dilate fully in about 20 min if one uses a combination of Tropicamide and Phenylephrine. Lightly coloured iris dilates even faster. Pupil diameter on full dilation is about 8 mm. Patients who have had intraocular surgery or have had uveitis may have poor dilatation because of inflammatory tissue in the iris stoma. Diabetes,

use of chronic pilocarpine drops in the eye, floppy iris, pseudo-exfoliation, advanced age, etc. are other reasons for poor pupillary dilatation. On dilatation if iris is stuck to the lens in areas, it is posterior synechiae due to inflammation of the iris. Patches of pigments stuck to the lens also suggest old inflammation. If iris is stuck in multiple areas, the pupil can have a flower pattern called *festooned pupil* (Fig. 11.9). Following dilatation if one notices a cataractous spot under the area of a suspected iris hole, an intraocular foreign body should be suspected.

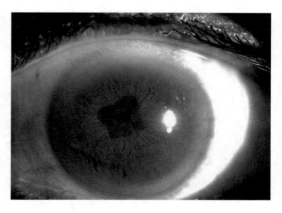

Fig. 11.9 Festooned non-dilating pupil

Examination of Lens

12

It was said in the past that the bread and butter of an Ophthalmologist is refraction and cataract surgery, respectively. This was of course in the days when an ophthalmologist true to his name looked after all the diseases of the eye!

Examination of the lens with a slit lamp is a must. However the periphery of the lens and its support cannot be seen directly and need indirect methods to assess their integrity. The examination of the lens is more than looking for a cataract to operate.

12.1 Applied Anatomy

The human lens is a transparent biconvex tissue much like a regular glass or plastic lens, placed between the iris and the vitreous body. It separates the anterior segment from the posterior segment and rests on a fossa (*patellar fossa*) on the anterior vitreous face. Though the cornea is the main refracting surface of the eye (giving about 40 dioptres (D) of the 60 dioptre produced by the eye) its power cannot be changed with changing distances of viewing. The lens evolved to meet this requirement. The human lens becomes more convex as objects come closer so that the divergent rays from near are converged more to keep the image focussed on the retina. At distance the human lens gives about +20 D. For near, in children it can give an additional 10–15 D. This converging power decreases with age and by 40 years reach a state where near vision becomes blurred. This condition is called presbyopia.

The central apical part of the convexity of the lens anteriorly and posteriorly is called the pole of the lens. The ring of tissue where the anterior and posterior convex surfaces of the lens meet is called the equator. The equatorial diameter of the lens increases from about 6 mm in an infant to about 10 mm in an adult and increases further to about 12 mm as one touches 80 years. The antero-posterior thickness (anterior pole to posterior pole) increases from about 3 mm at birth to about 5 mm in an adult. Compared to this the artificial intraocular lens (IOL) is only 1 mm thick.

Outside the equator of the lens all around is the ciliary body. The lens is held in its place by fine fibrils (zonular fibres) that start from the basal laminae of the ciliary epithelium in the pars plicata and anterior part of the pars plana. They get inserted in the anterior and posterior surface of the lens near the equator by merging with the lens capsule (Fig. 12.1). When the ciliary body is **not** contracted (state of rest) it goes further away from the lens equator making the zonular fibres taught. The resulting pull on the capsule flattens its curvature, reducing the power of the lens. Contraction of the circular ciliary muscles makes the Zonules lax and relaxes the stretch on the capsule. This increases the curvature of the lens capsule causing the lens to accommodate. The lens become more globular (increasing the curvature of the lens) due to the inherent elasticity of lens protein. The increasing curvature of lens increases the power of the lens.

With increasing age more lens fibres form and older fibres get packed into the centre making the

© Springer Nature Singapore Pte Ltd. 2020
T. Kuriakose, *Clinical Insights and Examination Techniques in Ophthalmology*,
https://doi.org/10.1007/978-981-15-2890-3_12

Fig. 12.1 Anatomy of
the lens

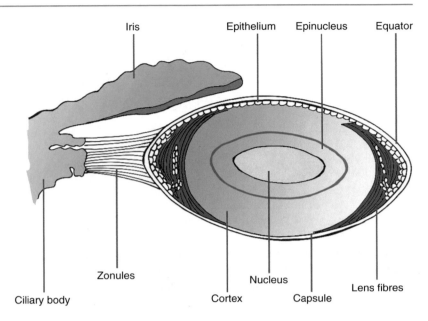

lens more rigid and reducing its capacity to change shape. This increasing rigidity may be one of the most important factors to reduce the accommodative power of the lens with increasing age. The zonular fibres keep the lens central and prevents the lens moving forward or backward.

The lens capsule is a collagenous cover of the lens and is a product of the lens epithelium just inside it. The lens is more curved posteriorly than anteriorly. The thinnest part of the lens capsule (about 2–4 microns) is at the posterior pole and is 1/10th the thickness of the human hair. Only an ophthalmic surgeon works with structures so fine during surgery!

The lens epithelial cells derived from the surface ectoderm lies just inside the lens capsule. The cells at the equator continuously multiply throughout life creating new cells that elongate to form lens fibres as they move centripetally. The newer fibres push the older fibres into the centre of the lens. In an adult the posterior capsule has no cells. The anterior capsule has a sheet of nondividing cells.

The transparent lens fibres are seen more centrally inside the capsule. The central fibres get tightly packed with age and becomes hard. This is called the nucleus of the lens. The peripheral fibres are soft and is called the cortex. In between there is an area called epinucleus were the fibres

are not as tightly packed as nucleus and behaves differently from the cortex during surgery. The lens fibres from the equator meets at two Y shape sutures in the centre of the lens. The posterior suture is an inverted Y and both can be visualised with the slit beam cross-sections of the lens.

The lens had no nerve or blood supply. It gets it nourishment from the vitreous and the aqueous.

12.2   History

The most common complaint in a patient with a lens pathology is decrease in vision as opacities in the lens either blocks the light entering the eye or changes the refraction. Depending on the pathology it can be a gradual progressive loss of vision (cataract), inability to see distance (lens related myopia), difficult in seeing near (presbyopia) and difficulty in near and far (aphakia). Accommodation due to the lens is usually symmetrical in both eyes. If it is not, a local pathology should be looked for. The acuteness of the decrease in vision can give a clue to diagnosis and should be asked in every patient. Sometimes patients with mature cataract can come with a sudden loss of vision noted when he accidently closes one eye. Patients with cataract can complain of glare, photophobia and difficulty in night driving. This is due to the scatter of light by the opacities in the lens. Acute pain in the eye is the next common complaint and is related to sudden rise in intraocular pressure (IOP) due to any of the lens-induced glaucoma. A history of trauma, use of steroids, family history of early cataracts, etc. should be asked for in patients with cataract. Past uveitis as a cause of cataract may be indicated by a history of recurrent redness of the eye. History of systemic diseases like diabetes, calcium metabolic disorders, Wilson's disease, etc. should be elicited for special forms of cataract. In children besides hereditary causes maternal infections like rubella can also be a cause and should be explored.

Before cataract surgery one should also see if patient has any breathing difficulty, cardiac problems, is on anticoagulants etc. History of claustrophobia and inability to tolerate drapes during surgery should be explored.

12.3 Examination

A general examination to look for systemic conditions like Marfan's syndrome, Weil Marchesani syndrome etc. can give a clue to the cause of the lens pathology and should be part of the examination. Even prior to surgery on the lens, systemic co-morbidities need to be looked for and appropriate precautions taken. The lens is easy to examine and its examination is not complete without dilating the eye.

12.3.1 Vision

Examination of the lens begins with the vision assessment. A sincere effort to get the best corrected vision should also be made. During retinoscopy dark areas in the reflex suggest media opacity which could also be due to cataract. In children the amount of obscuration of the red reflex will give an idea of the disability caused by cataract. A more myopic central reflex compared to the rest of the lens periphery suggest an index myopia due to nuclear sclerosis. A central ring reflex suggest an anterior lenticonus. When patients have near vision problems with the dis-

tant correction in place the near vision and amplitude of accommodation should be measured in patients where this is indicated, like in patients with trauma or those who have used medications in one eye. Amplitude of accommodation should normally be the same in both eyes normally. The simplest way to examine the amplitude of accommodation of the lens is to see how close the patient can read keeping the distant correction in place. The reciprocal of the nearest distance at which the patient can read the N6 or equivalent, in meters give the amplitude of accommodation. So if the patient can read at 20 cm from the eye the amplitude of accommodation is +5.00 dioptres. RAF (royal air force) rule if available in the clinic is also a simple tool to measure the amount of accommodation. If the near vision is less than what is expected for that age and if the problem is unilateral, one should look for a local cause like trauma or instillation of medicines that affect accommodation like atropine. If both eyes are affected, one should suspect systemic toxicity like botulinum poisoning.

With distant and near vision correction in place if the near vision is affected more than distant vision then a posterior subcapsular cataract or opacification should be suspected.

12.3.2 Torchlight Examination

With the torchlight one should assess the depth of the anterior chamber. A very shallow anterior chamber (AC), or an irregular AC, may suggest a lens subluxation. Shallow chambers may be seen in angle closure where there is a relative pupillary block due to the enlarging lens. The pupil has a slight greenish grey colour normally. A whiter colour suggest lens opacity. A jet black pupil suggests aphakia or pseudophakia. Table 12.1 shows the clinical differences between the two. In black cataracts the pupillary area appears brown.

Aphakia is the absence of lens from the patella fossa of the eye. Therefore the patient can be aphakic when the human lens is in the vitreous. In pseudophakia one will see a glassy reflex from the surface of the polished intra-ocular lens

Table 12.1 Differences between aphakia and pseudophakia

Feature	Normal	Pseudophakia	Aphakia
Unaided vision	Better that 6/60	Better that 6/60	Counting fingers
Limbal scar	None	Yes	May be absent
Anterior chamber (AC)	Normal	Deep	Deep
Iridodonesis	Absent	May or may not be present	Present
Pupil colour	Greyish green	Jet black	Jet black
Purkinje 3 image	Normal	Glassy reflex	Absent
Disc size	Normal	Normal	Small (due to the absence of magnification of the lens)
Disc colour	Red	Paler than normal (due to lack of absorption of blue light by human lens)	Paler than normal

(IOL) in the pupillary area when a light is shown into the eye. This is best elicited by moving the torchlight from side to side and observing the pupillary area. When the cornea is cloudy or AC is hazy a faint glassy reflex may be the only hint of an IOL in the eye.

In the olden days when slit lamp was not readily available and cataract surgery was done only after the cataract was mature, it was important to assess with the torchlight if the patient had a mature cataract or not. The shadow of the iris on the lens was looked for in these cases. If the cataract is mature, it meant the lens is full of cataractous material and there was no gap between the lens cortex and the iris to enable a shadow formation. In immature cataract an iris shadow is seen. With today's surgical methods the mature cataracts are more difficult to do compared to immature cataract!

12.3.3 Slit Lamp Examination

Examination of the lens is best done with the slit lamp. Before dilatation one should see if the lens is covering the entire pupillary area. One should also look at the pupillary sphincter for tears suggestive of trauma. White dandruff like flakes is (Fig. 12.2) seen on the lens surface in *pseudo-exfoliation syndrome*. The pseudo-exfoliative material is arranged in a radial manner on the surface of the lens that is in contact with the iris. It is thought that the con-

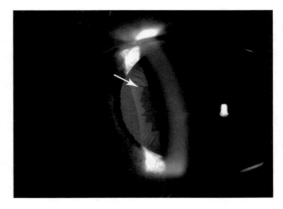

Fig. 12.2 Lens showing pseudo-exfoliative material (white flakes) arranged in a radial pattern on the lens surface (white arrow)

stant rubbing of the lens causes these deposits. Pseudo-exfoliative material can also be seen on the iris especially at the pupillary border. *Iridodonesis* is a fine tremulousness of the iris that is best seen soon after a blink or when the eye is moved from side to side. Iridodonesis suggest subluxated lens or lax zonules as seen in microspherophakia. This is also seen in aphakia. With lens subluxation the unsupported lens hit the iris due to the vitreous coming and hitting the lens. In aphakia the vitreous itself comes forward and hits the iris and causes the tremulousness.

Examination of the lens is best done after dilatation of the pupil. After noting the amount of dilatation, the surface of the lens is inspected

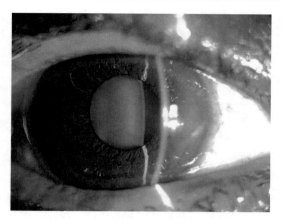

Fig. 12.3 View of cross section of a cataractous lens using the slit beam of slit lamp

with the diffuse light. Isolated brown pigments or while dandruff like material arranged in a circle in the mid pupillary may be seen on the surface of the lens in pseudo-exfoliation. White spots may be seen as sub-epithelial spots (*glaucoma fleckens*) in patients who have had angle closure attacks in the past. A thin slit beam focused on of the lens giving a cross-sectional view of the lens (Fig. 12.3) can locate the exact position of the lens opacities.

With the slit beam one should move across the pupil to see if the thickest part of the lens is in the centre of the pupil. If there is subluxation, this will shift. The edge of the lens should not be seen normally even with pupillary dilatation. If the edge is seen in a localised area, it suggest *lens subluxation*. If the edge is seen inferiorly and is associated with a notch, a *lens coloboma* should be suspected. If the margins are seen all around, then a *microspherophakia* should be suspected. Here the lens will appear more spherical than the normal biconvex lens shape. Direct and retro-illumination will reveal the zonules attached to the micro-phakia in these cases.

With the slit beam one should make an assessment of the curvature of the front and back surface of the lens. In *anterior lenticonus* there will be a sudden increase in the curvature of the central part of the lens and is suggestive of *Alport's syndrome*. On scanning the posterior curvature one may see a deficiency of the posterior capsule at the posterior pole with or without a posterior

protrusion of the lens matter. A small *posterior polar cataract* looking like stacked onion peel is seen invariably with this defect. Site of injury to the capsule may also be seen as an irregularity as you look at the curvature. In microspherophakia the lens edge will be circular. When scanning the lens with the slit beam one should not only look at the slit beam illuminated area but also the surrounding structures as the indirect illumination may also give some information.

After looking at the surface and curvature of the lens, one should look specifically at sub-epithelial areas. Multiple white large spots may be seen like an *anterior capsular cataract*. This is traditionally seen in glass blowers but may be seen in sun bathers and who use tanning machines without eye protection. When lens opacity is noted, its location, colour and morphology may give a clue to the aetiology of the cataract. Multiple blue dots (*blue dot cataract*) in the lens substance is congenital in origin. A zone of white dots may be seen just outside the nuclear area with clear lens within and without this area. This is again a *congenital zonular cataract* due to intrauterine stress and does not affect vision. The nucleus becomes brown in *nuclear cataract*. Opacities usually seen as multi-coloured spots just inside the posterior capsule is called *posterior subcapsular cataract*. These cataracts can be secondary to old uveitis or use of steroids. In Wilson's disease a *sunflower*-shaped greenish yellow cataract may be seen in the anterior capsular area. Following trauma a whitish flower-like cataract with feathery margin called *rosette cataract* is seen in the posterior subcapsular region. Assessment of the type of cataract and the stability of the lens is important in deciding on the type of cataract surgery that need to be done.

Retro-illumination (see chapter on slit lamp examination) is a useful method to examine the lens and also study the integrity of the zonules. Here the lamp housing is made coaxial with the microscope and the red reflex is looked at. Subtle lens opacities especially in the posterior subcapsular location can be seen well as blackish areas against the red glow of the retro-illumination. The intensity of the blockage of light gives us an idea of the significance of the opacity. In subtle lens subluxations the edge of the lens will be seen on retro-illumination as an arch. In small lens colobomas, depression in the equator can be seen on retro-illumination. The zonules holding the lens can be seen as fine radial lines against the red background on retro-illumination. Absence of these in certain segments will suggest break in zonules there. In coloboma of the lens the absence of zonules can be seen well as clear gap. In microspherophakia the entire lens border with long zonules can be seen.

In *pigment dispersion syndrome* one can see pigment in the zonules at the lens equator. To see this, one needs to use a gonioscope and look into the space between the iris and the lens.

In aphakia if there is no history of surgery or trauma one needs to look into the posterior segment with an indirect lens to look for a dislocated lens.

12.4 Examination of a Post-cataract Surgery Patient

As important as doing good surgery is the post-operative evaluation of a patient who has had a surgery for cataract. Post-operative evaluation is necessary irrespective of the surgery being complicated or not. Table 12.2 gives the checklist for the examination and the findings.

Table 12.2 Post-operative evaluation of cataract surgery

Examination	Normal finding	Abnormal finding	Possible causes
Vision with and without pinhole	Should be 6/12 or better with pinhole	Worse than 6/18 with pinhole	Look for fundus pathology if cornea clear
Wound	No leak	Leak	Poor wound construction, IOL haptic in wound, tight sutures, iris prolapse
Slit lamp Anterior chamber reaction	Clear, 1+ flare; rare cells,	Plasmoid aqueous, hypopyon, hyphema	Suspect infection, TASS, excessive surgical manipulation
Pupil margins	Round	Peaked	Vitreous in AC, sphincter rupture, capsular tag, lens cortex tag, iris prolapse, iris tuck, anterior synechiae
IOP	Up to 20 mm Hg	Corneal haze, epithelial oedema, IOP '25	Retained viscoelastic, missed glaucoma, Trabeculitis
A C depth	Deep	Shallow	Wound leak, Choroidal effusion Malignant glaucoma Air in PC, posterior synechiae, anterior synechiae, tilted lens
Intra-ocular lens (IOL)	Good glassy reflex, IOL centred will with no lens tilt	– Edge of IOL seen – Lens haptic seen – Tilted lens, absent IOL	– Decentred lens due to broken/bent haptic or haptic in the vitreous. IOL too small for the sulcus diameter. – Lens not inserted into the PC
Fundus examination	Good view	Hazy view	Corneal haze, Endophthalmitis, vitreous haemorrhage

KP Keratic precipitates, *TASS* toxic anterior segment syndrome, *IOP* intra-ocular pressure, *PC* posterior chamber

Clinical Evaluation of Glaucoma Patient

13

In a general ophthalmic practice majority of patients who are diagnosed as glaucoma or glaucoma suspects do not present with complaints related to glaucoma but are picked up in the clinic during their routine eye check-up or when they come for their glass prescription including presbyopic glasses. A high index of suspicion is therefore the key to pick up patients with glaucoma before they become symptomatic. In these days of 'cataract hunting' it is not uncommon for people to miss obvious glaucoma-related eye changes and seeing only a cataract. By the time the patients with primary chronic glaucoma are symptomatic reversing the symptoms is not possible at this present time. Early diagnosis and prevention of disability is therefore the key in management of glaucoma.

Three decades ago people had little doubt that glaucoma was a disease cause by raised intra-ocular pressure (IOP). Today that has changed. While reducing intraocular pressure (IOP) is still the mainstay of treatment, the definitions of glaucoma have changed. More than one-third of patients with primary open angle glaucoma have normal IOP.

13.1 Definitions

Glaucoma: Glaucoma is a chronic optic neuropathy characterised by typical disc and field changes (described later) where 'elevated' intra-ocular pressure is the primary and only modifiable risk factor. A very humbling definition, saying in effect that we do not fully understand glaucoma. Imagine if we defined Cholera as 'a disease characterised by watery stools that can result in death and eating outside is a known risk factor'!

Pre-perimetric glaucoma: This is a condition where there are glaucomatous changes in the disc with normal visual fields on standard testing. This definition implies two things. First, that field changes occur only after some amount of nerve damage. It is said that field changes occur only after 20–30% of ganglion cell loss. The second implication is the importance of clinical evaluation of the disc in the diagnosis of glaucoma/pre-perimetric glaucoma.

Angle closure disease (ACD): This is the spectrum of conditions where the iris at the angle of the eye is in contact with the trabecular meshwork, preventing drainage of aqueous through the trabecular meshwork and ciliary body. This in turn can cause rise in IOP and lead to glaucomatous changes.

Though according to definition glaucoma is associated with disc and field changes, the term glaucoma is also used when IOP is very high and field changes are yet to be demonstrated. Acute angle closure glaucoma, malignant glaucoma and other secondary glaucomas are some of the examples.

© Springer Nature Singapore Pte Ltd. 2020
T. Kuriakose, *Clinical Insights and Examination Techniques in Ophthalmology*,
https://doi.org/10.1007/978-981-15-2890-3_13

13.2   Applied Anatomy and Physiology

Being a gel- and water-filled sphere, the eye needs an intraocular pressure to keep the eyeball inflated. To exchange nutrients and keep the eyeball filled, the eye produces aqueous humour and also has a mechanism to exchange this fluid. Aqueous humour is produced by ciliary body in the posterior chamber. The production of this aqueous is by a combination of active and passive secretion and can be effected by many chemicals. The aqueous from the posterior chamber passes through the pupil and reaches the anterior chamber. The aqueous exits at the angle of the anterior chamber via two pathways (blue track in Fig. 13.1). About 80% of the aqueous gets out via the trabecular meshwork and Schlemm's canal. 20% of aqueous drains via the uveo-scleral pathway on the anterior surface of the ciliary body. From the Schlemm's canal aqueous drains into the systemic circulation via the aqueous veins on the sclera. The trabecular

meshwork lies anterior to the scleral spur to which it is attached. This meshwork has pillars of tissue covered with cells that transport the aqueous to the Schlemm's canal which lies on the outside. Blockage of space between the mesh can raise the IOP. From the Schlemm's canal the aqueous escapes via collector channels to the episcleral veins lying outside the sclera. From here it mixes with the venous blood and leaves the orbit via ciliary veins, superior ophthalmic vein to the cavernous sinus.

The iris is thinnest at the root of the iris near the ciliary body. Any build up of aqueous in the posterior chamber due to a block in the flow of aqueous through the pupil results in the peripheral iris bowing out before the pupillary iris is lifted up. This bowing out of the iris occludes the angle, cutting off both the trabecular meshwork and uveo-scleral out flow of aqueous. If the occlusion covers a significant part of the angle then there is a sudden acute rise in the IOP.

The angle structures start anteriorly at the Schwalbe's line, which is the junction between

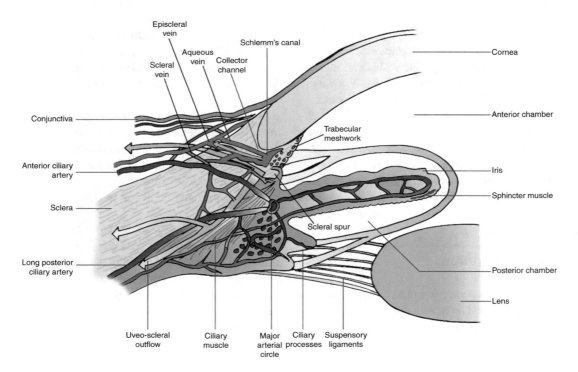

Fig. 13.1 Angle structures showing the site of aqueous production at the ciliary body and the outflow pathways

the cornea and the sclera (Fig. 13.2). The Schwalbe's line is dark in colour. Just posterior to that is the trabecular meshwork. The trabecular meshwork extends from the Schwalbe's line to the scleral spur. The anterior part of the trabecular meshwork is normally white in colour.

The middle functional part of the meshwork is more brownish and gets darker with time. The posterior part of the mesh merges with scleral spur. In conditions like pigmentary glaucoma or uveitis the entire meshwork can be coloured with the central part being the most pigmented. Posterior to the trabecular meshwork and just anterior to the ciliary body is a more whitish tissue that is the sclera spur. The trabecular meshwork inserts on the scleral spur which in turn is attached to the ciliary body. On the posterior limb of the angle is seen the ciliary body band from which arise the iris further medially. From the iris arise fine iris processes which go over the ciliary body to reach up to the scleral spur and trabecular meshwork. The angle structures thus appear as a dark, light, dark, light, dark area at the angle.

The optic nerve head receives the nerve fibres which are the non-myelinated axons arising from the ganglion cells of the retina. Since the axons from all over the retina has to pass in an orderly manner through the optic nerve head (ONH) without compromising the function of the macular region, they follow a curvilinear pattern to reach the optic disc (Fig. 13.3). The arcuate fibres from the retinal ganglion cells (RGC) which reach the superior and inferior

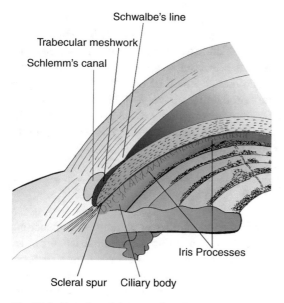

Fig. 13.2 Drawing of the normal angle structures

Fig. 13.3 Nerve fibre layer arrangement of the retina and optic disc

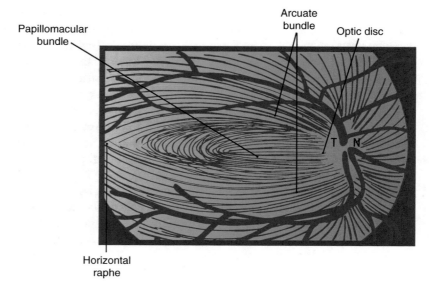

margins of the optic disc either seems to be more susceptible to glaucomatous damage or damage in them is more easily detectable by clinical methods. The vertical diameter of the average ONH or disc is about 1.5 mm. In coloured race it can be larger.

The blood supply to the optic nerve head is from the four posterior ciliary arteries arising from the ophthalmic artery before it branches. The short posterior ciliary arteries are multiple small branches of the posterior ciliary arteries given off just behind the globe. They penetrate and supply the prelaminar, laminar (part of the optic nerve at the lamina cribrosa of the sclera) and postlaminar parts of the optic nerve. Some fine branches of the central retinal artery (CRA) also supply the prelaminar branches of the ONH. The inner layers of the retina including the ganglion cell layers are supplied by the CRA.

Besides the RGC axons numbering 1–1.5 million the optic nerve has glial tissue, extracellular matrix and blood vessels. The space that is not occupied by the axons appear as a depression on the optic disc and is called the **optic cup**. The axons of the ganglion cells get out of the eye by going through a posterior sieve like defect in the sclera called lamina cribrosa. The connective tissue beams of the lamina cribrosa can be seen clinically if the cup is very deep. The scleral rim through which the nerve enters the eye is just outside the rim of the optic nerve and should not be mistaken for the optic disc rim.

13.3   Types of Glaucoma

An understanding of the types of glaucoma is necessary to understand the clinical features of the various clinical types. Though the role of IOP is not as central in glaucoma now as it used to be in the past, due to historical reasons and for treatment strategies, glaucomas are still classified using IOP and their reasons for elevation as the basis for classifications.

Traditionally glaucoma have been divided into childhood glaucoma and adult glaucoma. Adult glaucoma is further divided into primary

glaucoma and secondary glaucoma. Each of the primary and secondary glaucomas can be divided into open or closed angle glaucomas. Table 13.1 gives the classification with their characteristics.

The prevalence of glaucoma or pre-test probability of glaucoma shows racial variation. In the population over 40 years of age the prevalence among Caucasians is about 1–2%. It increases in coloured population to up to four times that value. Therefore doing, only an investigation on the population to diagnose glaucoma would make no sense. A combination of history and clinical examination should be used first to take the pre-test probability above 40% at least so that any further investigation carried out will be useful and increase the diagnostic post-test probability significantly.

13.4   History

Since a good number of patients with glaucoma go to the ophthalmologist/optometrists for other reasons, history tailored for glaucoma suspects may have to be asked after the examination has started and the doctor has found something suspicious. Family history of glaucoma should be asked routinely to patients in the eye clinic. For patients who may not be aware of the diagnostic entity, questions like anybody being blind in the family, or was told to have raised eye pressures needing eye drops every day, can give us a hint. Patients should be asked for presence of systemic diseases associated with glaucoma. Thyroid eye disease, migraine, use of systemic steroids, history of taking antihypertensive medication (causing low blood pressure at night), snoring at night and ocular trauma are all risk factors for glaucoma and patients should be quizzed about them. It will only be a relative who can tell you about the snore while sleeping! Old ocular trauma is easily forgotten and so one should ask about the games played, involvement in an accident or fist fights, etc. History of severe blood loss in an accident or during surgery may explain a field loss with no other evidence of glaucoma. History of intermittent haziness of

Table 13.1 Types of glaucoma and their characteristics

Disease type	Characteristics	Prototype disease
Primary glaucoma		
Primary open angle glaucoma (POAG)	Typical disc and field changes with no ocular or systemic causes that raised IOP. Open angles on gonioscopy	Age related POAG
Normal tension glaucoma (NTG)	Like above but with no recording of raised IOP	Age related NTG
Juvenile open angle Glaucoma (JOAG)	Like POAG in patients between 5 and 35 years of age	JOAG
Ocular hypertension (OHT)	Elevated IOP but no disc and field changes as yet	Age related OHT
Primary angle closure suspect (PACS)	Iridotrabecular contact of at least 270° on gonioscopy, normal IOP, disc and visual fields	PACS
Primary angle closure (PAC)	Iridotrabecular contact of at least 270°, with either raised IOP and/or PAS but with normal disc and visual fields	PAC
Primary angle closure glaucoma (PACG)	PAC with evidence of disc and field changes	PACG
Acute angle closure glaucoma	Acute rise in IOP to levels high enough to make the patient have headache or eye pain with congestion of the eye	Acute angle closure attack
Sub-acute angle closure glaucoma	Brief episode of raised IOP with above symptoms, narrow angles	Intermittent angle closure glaucoma
Chronic angle closure glaucoma	Elevated IOP with disc and field changes. Angle closed with areas of peripheral anterior synechiae in the angle	CACG
Secondary glaucoma		
Secondary open angle glaucoma	Angles are open with raised IOP due to outflow obstruction caused by underlying ocular or systemic causes	– Pigmentary glaucoma- pigment blocking the trab-meshwork – Angle recession glaucoma – Carotid artery fistula with raised episcleral venous pressure
Secondary angle closure glaucoma due to pupillary block	Pupillary block due to causes like posterior synechiae causes peripheral iris bowing and angle closure with raised IOP	– Seclusio pupillae due to exudates in the pupillary area – Phacomorphic glaucoma
Secondary angle closure glaucoma with no pupillary block	Angles close due to pushing of the iris by the ciliary body or pulling up of the peripheral tissue by fibrous tissue	– Post scleral buckling – Neovascular glaucoma
Plateau iris syndrome	Narrowing of the angle because iris root abnormality and not pupillary block	
Childhood glaucoma		
Primary congenital glaucoma	Dysgenesis of trabecular meshwork	Buphthalmos
Glaucoma with congenital anomalies	Raised IOP associated with ocular malformations Raised IOP associated with extra-ocular malformations	Peters anomaly Sturge-Weber syndrome
Secondary glaucoma in childhood	Raised IOP with either open or closed angle, secondary to an ocular pathology	Retinoblastoma associated raised IOP

vision with headache may be suggestive of intermittent angle closure glaucoma. History of transient ischaemic attack or cardiac problems may explain some of the field defects due to embolic phenomenon in the branches of central retinal artery. Before starting medications one should take a history of obstructive pulmonary airway disease (contradiction for use of beta blockers) and allergies to sulpha group of drugs to which carbonic anhydrase inhibitors belong.

Patients already diagnosed as glaucoma can be asked for previous reports, especially disc photographs and fields. This will give a clue to the progression of the disease. These patients should also be asked about any visual disability like bumping into things, involvement in any accidents, etc. Rarely patients seek help only when they are visually handicapped, in which case an assessment of their functional capabilities with respect to their vision should be done. Many of these patients have an associated cataract.

Patients already on medications should be asked for the list of medications they are on and how they are tolerating their drops. A direct question regarding compliance with the use of drops will seldom give a correct answer. Question about how long a bottle takes to finish, how often drops are missed or under what circumstances one may miss using a drop should be asked. A person who claims to never ever miss a drop is a suspect and is best if a relative corroborates. Side effects of the drops if any should also be enquired into.

13.5   Examination

13.5.1 General Examination

Glaucoma, especially the secondary glaucomas, may have systemic associations that can give a clue to the diagnosis. A cafe au lait spots or swellings all over the body is suggestive of phacomatosis like neurofibromatosis where patients are prone to develop raised IOP. A very tall stature compared to other family members could suggest Marfan's syndrome, the subluxated lens can cause secondary angle closure glaucoma. Obesity if present should be noted and could be a pointer to sleep apnoea. A reddish discoloration on one side of the face with or without hypertrophy is suggestive of Sturge Weber syndrome. Here the raised episcleral venous pressure causes glaucoma.

Thyroid eye disease (TED) is a predisposing factor for glaucoma. Mild lid retraction, prominent eyes and ocular discomfort can all be early indictors of TED.

The upper cheek being pulled back due to maxillary hypoplasia along with microdontia is suggestive of Axenfeld Rieger syndrome which is associated with malformation in the eye and glaucoma.

Having a recording of patient's blood pressure and pulse rate is useful if the patient has never had them checked.

13.6   Ocular Examination

Examination of all parts of the eye have relevance in the diagnosis and management of patients with glaucoma. Of these, measurement of IOP, evaluation of the angle and examination of the ONH is most important.

Vision and refraction should be done not only to get an idea of the patient's disability but also to make sure that the fields are done with the appropriate correction. For patients with very high refractive errors like in aphakia, appropriate contact lens is needed for field assessment.

Hypermetropia is associated with angle closure glaucoma and nanophthalmos. High myopia may be associated with tilted disc which may mimic fields similar to glaucoma. Index of suspicion for glaucoma should be high in a myope. Myopia only in one eye, associated with trauma, may indicate a subluxated lens.

13.6.1 Face and Ocular Adnexa

Before doing the slit lamp examination, the lids, surrounding areas and the face should be examined with a torchlight or bright sunlight. It is worth standing back and looking at the face as a whole. The patient is also asked to open the mouth to look for dentition and high arch palate. On the lids look for any red patches, hyperpigmentation or areas of bogginess giving the upper lid an S-shaped contour. Red patches suggest a haemangioma, hyperpigmentation of the lids and the sclera on one side is seen in nevus of Ota. S-shaped lid with or without nodules on the face is suggestive of neurofibromatosis. All of these conditions can raise IOP on the side of the lesion. A prominent eye or proptosis may be due to thyroid eye disease. Proptosis with redness of eye and orbital pulsation would suggest a carotid cavernous fistula. Keeping the bell of the stethoscope on the globe may give a bruit. Any scars on the face due to trauma may suggest an ocular injury that was probably ignored at the time of injury. A floppy, easily evertable lid is suggestive of floppy eyelid syndrome with possible sleep apnoea. Abnormally long lashes and sunken eyes are seen in patients who have used prostaglandin analogues over a long time.

13.6.2 Ocular Surface

A combination of slit lamp and torchlight should be used to examine the ocular surface. If the patient is not on any medications mild congestion of bulbar conjunctiva with papillary reaction of the tarsal conjunctiva suggests ocular allergy and patient should be asked about use of topical steroids. Allergy to topical medications including antiglaucoma medications also show a similar picture. Scarring of tarsal conjunctiva suggest old allergies or trachoma. Small stain positive areas on cornea can also be a sign of toxicity to topical medications.

Dilated blood vessel under the conjunctiva in one eye is suggestive of a carotid cavernous fistula or an arterio-venous malformation. A dilated subconjunctival anterior ciliary artery (sentinel vessel) could point to an underlying melanoma and associated glaucoma. A featureless limbus with hypoplastic iris is aniridia that is associated with raised IOP. The presence of a localised elevation of the conjunctiva or scarring in the upper limbus suggestive of a past filtering surgery should be looked for. The conjunctiva may be boggy and elevated in the region of a functioning filtering bleb. There may be an associated defect in the iris in the periphery suggestive of a peripheral iridectomy. If the conjunctiva over the bleb is avascular and thin, a Seidel test (see chapter on examination of cornea) is done to see if there is any bleb leak. Before trabeculectomy the conjunctiva should be

examined for limbal scars so that the surgery can be sited in an area away from the scar.

13.6.3 Cornea

Corneal size and clarity should be first looked at with the torchlight before a slit lamp examination is started. A cornea measuring more than 11 mm in the horizontal axis is not normal and glaucoma should be suspected.

Storage disorders like muco-polysaccharidosis show cloudy corneas, this and congenital hereditary endothelial dystrophy (CHED) should be ruled out before diagnosing congenital glaucoma. Storage disorder will show collection of material in the stoma of the cornea. The stroma will be thick in CHED.

Using slit lamp the corneal epithelium is examined for punctate erosions to rule out toxicity to drops. In patients with very high IOP there may be epithelial oedema that can be made out with retro-illumination or sclerotic scatter (see Chap. 6).

Examination of the endothelium will give many a clues to the cause of secondary glaucoma. A copper beaten appearance of the endothelium with pigments is seen in irido-corneal endothelial (ICE) syndrome. Keratic precipitates (KPs) seen as white or brownish white dots on the endothelial surface of the cornea is seen in Posner Schlossman syndrome and other uveitic glaucomas including viral uveitis. Pigment dusting on the endothelium vertically in the form of a cigar (**Krukenberg spindle**) is seen in pigmentary glaucoma. Stellate KPs diffusely scattered on the endothelium point to a Fuchs heterochromic iridocyclitis.

The Schwalbe's line move more centrally (**posterior embryotoxon**) in developmental glaucomas. A horizontal break of the endothelium (**Haab's striae**), best seen on retro-illumination, is seen in congenital glaucoma.

Thickness of cornea should be assessed, though it can be measured with a slit lamp, it is more accurate when measured with an optical biometer or ultrasound pachymeter. Thin corneas measure IOPs artificially low and is a risk factor for glaucoma progression.

13.6.4 Sclera

The sclera can be pigmented in Nevus of Ota. In long-standing cases of high IOP the sclera stretches and the underlying uveal tissue bulges (**staphyloma**) at the limbus or at the region where the anterior ciliary artery pierces the sclera. This should be looked for by lifting the lid.

13.6.5 Anterior Chamber

Anterior chamber (AC) should be examined first with the torchlight and then with the slit lamp. An initial assessment of the depth of the anterior chamber is made using the flash light.

In **flash light test** the light is shown from the temporal side parallel to the Iris plane. This is best done by resting the rim of a 1–2 inch diameter torch on the zygomatic bone laterally (Fig. 13.4) Light from the temporal side should fall on most of the nasal iris if the entire iris is in one plane. If however the central iris comes forward as it happens in shallow anterior chamber, the temporal half of the iris will cast shadow on the nasal iris and it will not be illuminated. Based on the assumption that the amount of iris under the shadow has a relation to the depth of the chamber it has been divided into four grades. Grade 1 is no iris shadow, grade 2 less than one-third, grade 3 is shadow covering one-third to half and grade 4 is shadow covering more than half of the nasal iris. Grade 4 shadow is a poor indicator for angle closure. Its **usefulness is in its negative predictive value**. That is, if the shadow does not cover more than half the iris, then it is unlikely that there will be an angle closure on gonioscopy.

Van Herrick method is another method of assessing the AC depth using slit lamp. Here a

thin slit is shown just inside the temporal limbus keeping the lighthouse about 5–10° from the microscope. The corneal thickness is compared to the distance from the endothelium to the iris. If the corneal thickness is equal to the AC depth, it is graded as 4, grade 3 is if the AC depth is half the thickness of the cornea. If AC depth is quarter the thickness of cornea, it was grade 2. Grade 1 was if the AC was less than quarter the corneal thickness. Here again, like flash light test, the usefulness is in the negative predictive value. That is, if the Van Herrick is grade 2 or more, the chance of angle closure is minimal.

Irregular shallowing of the AC may be suggestive of a lens subluxation, iris cyst or a ciliary body melanoma.

IOP may be raised in viral uveitis. So the AC should be looked at for cells and flare in cases the raise in OP is unilateral. Posterior synechiae causing iris bombe can be seen uveitis.

Anterior chamber should be checked to see if it is clear and there is nothing hindering the view of the iris. Hyphaema (collection of blood in the AC), hypopyon (collection of white blood cells inferiorly with a horizontal pus level), inverse hypopyon (white emulsified silicon oil seen floating near the upper limbus) with the horizontal demarcation line blow the emulsified oil can all cause raised IOP. Using slit lamp one should look for vitreous in the AC in cases of trauma and in aphakic patients. Vitreous in AC is identified by looking at the dispersed pigments or cells in the anterior chamber. If the pigments are stationary in the AC and not moving along the aqueous currents, it means they are trapped in the vitreous in the AC. In fact the pigment may show a vibratory movement along with the vitreous in which it is entangled. If the vitreous is going to the wound, then pupillary distortion caused by the pull of the vitreous will give a hint to its presence.

13.6.6 Lens

Lens abnormalities itself can be a cause of glaucoma. Careful examination will give hints as to

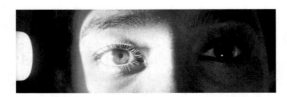

Fig. 13.4 Flash light test; the light is shown from the temporal side parallel to the eye

the aetiology of the raised pressures. This examination is best done with the slit lamp. A mature swollen lens block the pupil and causes a phacomorphic glaucoma. The AC will be uniformly shallow here. In phacolytic glaucoma the lens will be hypermature with a cloudy AC and resembles endophthalmitis; however KPs are absent. On dilating the pupil, pseudo-exfoliative material on the lens will point to a pseudo-exfoliation glaucoma (Fig. 13.5).

A small spherical lens is suggestive of microspherophakia and can cause intermittent angle closure glaucoma if the lens comes into the AC or blocks the pupil. Phacodonesis is a fine tremulousness of the lens seen when the eye makes small saccadic movement as after a blink. This is suggestive of lens subluxation and should be looked for in all shallow ACs. The subluxated lens may cause a pupillary block.

A posterior subcapsular cataract may suggest long-term use of steroids which may be the reason for the glaucoma. Sometimes localised lens opacities especially near the posterior capsule can give field defects that mimic glaucoma.

Anterior chamber intraocular lens can cause pupillary block glaucoma or UGH syndrome. Fine white plaques under the anterior capsule near the pupillary border (glaukomflecken) is suggestive of previous acute rise in IOP as seen in angle closure attacks.

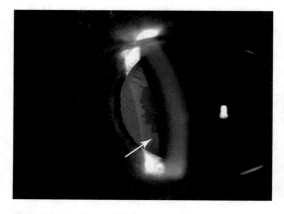

Fig. 13.5 Pseudo-exfoliation on the lens (white arrow)

13.6.7 Pupils and Iris

Relative afferent pupillary defect (see Chap. 11) should be looked for in all suspected cases of glaucoma because it is a very sensitive sign of asymmetrical optic nerve damage. Glaucomatous nerve damage is rarely symmetrical.

Pupillary sphincter rupture will be seen as small discontinuities in the pupillary margins with the torn edges going outward to the iris root. This suggests ocular trauma and may be associated with angle recession. Iridodonesis (tremulousness of iris) if present is added evidence of lens subluxation and trauma. Area of atrophy of the iris near the pupillary border and a vertically oval pupil are suggestive of past attack of angle closure glaucoma. Atrophic areas on the iris can also be suggestive of past attacks of viral uveitis which can raise IOP.

The pupillary edge of the iris should be examined for white flakes like that seen in dandruff. This suggests pseudo-exfoliation which can cause a secondary open angle glaucoma. Iris transillumination may be seen with retroillumination in pigmentary glaucoma and pseudo-exfoliation, especially in patients with light-coloured iris. In patients with heavily pigmented iris this finding is rare.

The colour of the iris in the two eyes should be noted. In nevus of Ota the iris on the affected eye will be darker. In Fuchs iridocyclitis the iris will be muddy with some loss of its features, moth-eaten appearance and lighter in colour compared to the fellow eye in pigmented iris. In light-coloured iris the affected eye may be darker. Nodules on the iris may suggest phacomatosis or uveitis, both of which can cause raised IOP.

Circular and some radial vessels may be seen at the root of the iris in 10% of lightly coloured iris. If these vessels become more prominent and more haphazard in distribution with some new vessels developing at the pupillary margin, then neovascularisation should be suspected. As neovascularisation worsens, the posterior pigmented layer of the iris migrates anteriorly and produces ectropion pupillae. The neovascularisation also causes peripheral anterior synechiae and raised IOP.

The periphery of the iris should be inspected for any laser peripheral iridotomy (PI) done in the past. Retro-illumination can help in the identification especially in pigmented eyes. In light-coloured iris, transillumination can be deceptive and one confirms the patency of PI by being able to see the ciliary body or lens capsule through the iridotomy site.

13.6.8 Gonioscopy

Assessment of the angle of the anterior chamber should be routinely done as a part of the eye examinations in most patients after the age of 40 years. Gonioscopy is one of the most difficult clinical examinations in ophthalmology; competing with indirect ophthalmoscopy for the pride of place. It is therefore all the more important that during training, gonioscopy is performed in as many normal people as possible to become good at picking out the abnormal angle. Seeing into the angle and its structures directly is difficult because the light from the angle does not come out of the eye due to the total internal reflection of the rays at the cornea air interface. The light from the angle has to travel from a denser medium to a rarer medium to be seen by us. To circumvent this a gonioscopy contact lens (gonioscope) has to be used. This contact lens made of either glass or plastic removes the cornea air interface and at the same time changes the angle of exit to allow the light rays coming from the angle to be seen.

Two broad types of gonioscope, direct and indirect, exist (Fig. 13.6). The direct gonioscope of which Koeppe lens is the prototype is a concavo-convex contact lens placed on the cornea. The anterior convexity of this lens is such that the angle of the incident light from the angle is less than the critical angle, thus allowing direct viewing. However for the direct viewing of the angle one had to view from the opposite limbus and cannot use the slit lamp for the same. This lens is used with the patient lying down and operating microscope adjusted so that one looks from the opposite side at an angle of about 80° to the cornea. This lens is useful for examination under anaesthesia and modifications of this lens like Barkan and Swan-Jacob lens can be used for surgical procedures in the angle because the image here is not inverted unlike the mirrored lenses. Fundus examination with a direct ophthalmoscope and high plus is also possible with the Koeppe lens on. To place the lens on the cornea its concave surface has to be filled with methyl cellulose or saline and quickly turned over avoiding air bubbles. The clarity of the angle is better if saline is used but it is still not as good as indirect lenses.

The indirect lenses are the more commonly used lenses in the clinic. Here the anterior surface of the lens is flatter. The diameter and the concavity of the posterior surface depends on the type of lens used. Inside the body of the lens are mirrors placed at an angle of around 62° from the line perpendicular to the iris. The mirror inside the lens redirects the reflected image to the straight ahead direction so that it can be viewed through the slit lamp microscope. Though there are many types and makes of indirect gonioscopy lenses available, only the two main prototypes of these lenses will be described here.

The Goldmann lens is a single or two mirror lens (Fig. 13.6a). The diameter of the posterior concave surface is about 12 mm with a curvature (radius of curvature 7.3 mm) steeper than the cornea. The mirrors inside (if 2, kept opposite to each other) has a tilt of about 62°. To view the angle the

Fig. 13.6 Optics of gonioscopy, (**a**) indirect and (**b**) direct gonioscopy

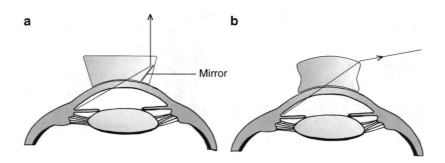

a   b

— Mirror

cup of the concave surface is filled till the brim with coupling fluid having methyl cellulose. The patient's eye is anaesthetised and chin rested on the slit lamp after explaining the procedure and patient told not to move back during the lens insertion. The patient is now asked to look down while the upper lid is held up with one hand. By looking down the patient is not intimidated by the approaching lens and the first point of contact is the sclera. With the other hand the fluid-filled gonio-lens is touched on the lower lid and quickly turned on to the ocular surface before the coupling fluid escapes. By manipulating the lens air bubbles if any that may have been trapped is allowed to escape. A block of wood or sponge may be needed to be kept under the elbow to stabilize the hand holding the lens to facilitate examination.

The angle is best examined with the room dimly lit. A slit illumination is used and the intensity is kept as minimum as possible. The height of the slit beam should be shortened so that no part enters the pupil. This is done so that light in the pupillary area does not cause a pupillary constriction and open up a normally occludable angle. The beam angle is made such that one gets a good slit view of the angle with the light extending from the endothelial side of the cornea over the angle and on to the surface of the iris. The Schwalbe's line at the junction of the cornea and sclera is made out by looking at the intersection of the lines demarcating the anterior and posterior surface of the cornea as it reaches the corneal periphery (Fig. 13.7).

Confirming this landmark is especially important in closed angles where a pigmentation on the corneal endothelium anterior to the Schwalbe's line can be mistaken for trabecular meshwork and the closed angle is missed. The corneal endothelial line and the iris line should intersect at the apex of the angle if the entire angle is being seen. If instead of an intersection one sees two separate lines it means the last roll of iris is blocking the view into the angle and one will have to look 'over the hill' to see into the angle. To do this one will have to ask the patient to look towards the viewing mirror. After confirming the position of the Schwalbe's line one will have to identify the trabecular meshwork, sclera spur, ciliary body band, peripheral iris and the iris processes.

The angle viewed through the mirror of the indirect gonioscopic lens has a left to right inversion but the antero-posterior relation is unchanged. To see parts of the angle not covered by a particular position of the mirror, the lens is rotated to bring into view the area that needs to be seen. The view of the angle is end-on. Therefore the angle estimation by looking at the angle of intersection between the corneal and iris ray is inaccurate with lot of variability. A more objective and functionally relevant way to assess the angle is to describe what part of the angle can and cannot be seen. The grading given in Table 13.2 is based on such a philosophy. Along with this one could make an effort to describe if the angle is wide open or narrow, if there is synechiae, the

Fig. 13.7 Slit illumination at the angle of a normal eye showing the meeting of anterior and posterior corneal lines at the Schwalbe's line (courtesy of Heiko Philippin, originally published www.cehjournal.org")

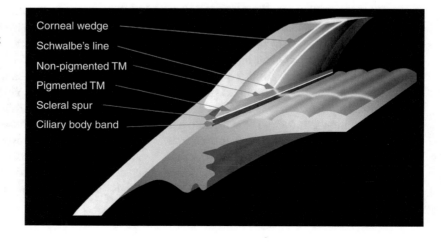

Corneal wedge

Schwalbe's line

Non-pigmented TM

Pigmented TM

Scleral spur

Ciliary body band

Table 13.2 Grading of angle (RPC grading)

RP Centre gonioscopic grading	
Grade 0	No dipping of the beam
Grade 1	Dipping of the beam
Grade 2	Schwalbe's line and ant 1/3 of trab mesh seen
Grade 3	Up to anterior 2/3 of trab mesh seen
Grade 4	Posterior 1/3 of trab mesh seen
Grade 5	Scleral spur seen
Grade 6	Ciliary body visualised

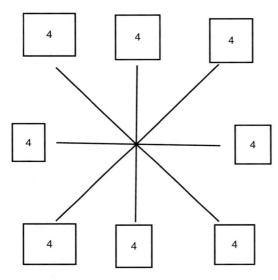

Fig. 13.8 Documentation of angle structure if the angle is open to grade 4 all around

level of insertion of the iris, the integrity of the iris process and any other abnormality seen in the angle. The extent of these findings in terms of the number of clock hours and the location can be noted as in Fig. 13.8.

With large diameter contact lens when pressure is applied to the lens it either presses over the angle and makes it appear closed or presses further into the cornea to open the angle.

The indentation gonioscope or Susman's lens was designed to circumvent some of these issues. It has four mirrors in it placed opposite to each other and at 90° to one pair (Fig. 13.9). These lenses have a posterior diameter of only 9 mm

and a radius of curvature of 8.1 mm which is flatter than the corneal curvature. Due to the flatter posterior surface and smaller diameter, there is no need for a coupling fluid and the lens can be directly placed on the anaesthetised cornea to do gonioscopy. The gonioscopy lens should only just touch the cornea. If excessive pressure is put on the lens, it will not only distort the cornea but also open up an occluded angle due to the displacement of the aqueous from the centre of the AC to the periphery as a result of the central indentation by the lens. This central indentation produced when needed is also the advantage of using the lens. If the initial inspection of the angle shows that the peripheral iris is apposed to the cornea, the next question to ask is if this is permanent due to synechiae or just an appositional closure due to forward bowing of the iris. On indenting the central cornea by applying pressure on the cornea with the lens, if iris moves away and angle opens up, it is only appositional closure. If it does not open, then one assumes it is a synechial closure. Sometimes only some areas will open up and this gives us the location of the anterior synechiae. With four mirror contact lens the lens does not have to be rotated to see all around. Shifting view from one mirror to the other would suffice. The extent of the apposition and synechiae in degrees or clock hours should be recorded.

Examination of the angles can reveal early signs of neo-vascularization of the angle. Fine vessels first appear to cross-over the sclera spur and on to the trabecular meshwork. As more new vessels develop the iris gets pulled over the trabecular meshwork to form synechiae. In contrast to this, the vessels in Fuchs heterochromic cyclitis are even finer and synechiae do not develop.

The trabecular meshwork is normally only lightly pigmented in the central part overlying the Schlemm's canal. In pigment dispersion syndrome, uveitis, trauma, following intraocular surgery, melanoma, pseudo-exfoliation syndrome etc., the trabecular meshwork can be heavily pigmented. Normally, blood will not be seen in the Schlemm's canal. Blood enters the canal if the venous pressure outside the eye is high like in

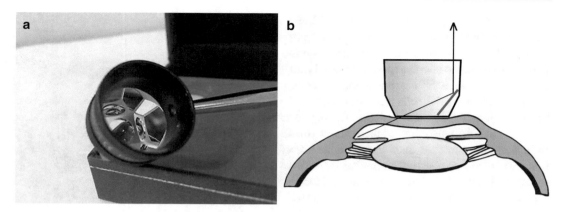

Fig. 13.9 (**a**) 4 mirror Indentation gonioscope. (**b**) Pressure on cornea opening the angles

carotid cavernous fistula or AV malformation. In hypotony when the intraocular pressure is very low, then too blood can enter the Schlemm's canal.

The thin lacy iris process should not be mistaken for peripheral anterior synechiae (PAS). The latter is more thick and broad and obscures the angle. The identification of iris process is important in making out angle recession. In **angle recession** there is disinsertion for the ciliary muscle from the scleral spur. In areas of angle recession, the iris process get disrupted and cannot be seen. On either side of the recession the iris process will be present and is a good method to identify angle recession. In addition, in a recessed angle the scleral spur will be more prominent and the ciliary body band will be wide. If in doubt the same area of the fellow eye should be compared to see the difference. In **cyclodialysis** a gap can be seen between the scleral spur and the ciliary body. The gap may be seen going inward like a cave.

Gonioscopy can also help evaluate the block excision in trabeculectomy, check for foreign body in the angle, look for micro hyphaema or hypopyon, detect early KF ring on the endothelium and pigmentation at the lens equator in pigment dispersion syndrome, etc.

To prevent transmission of infection gonioscopes should be disinfected between patients. Like applanation prisms the lens can be dipped in Daikin's solution between patients and rinsed with saline at the time of use.

13.6.9 Fundus and Optic Disc Evaluation

The techniques of fundus examination is discussed in chapter on examination of the retina. The very basis of glaucoma diagnosis is currently dependant on the clinical findings of the disc and its immediate surrounding areas. Typical field defects is the other feature to diagnose glaucoma.

In glaucoma, examination of the fundus beyond the disc helps us rule out non-glaucomatous pathology that give field defect similar to glaucoma. A branch retinal vein or artery occlusion can give rise to a glaucoma like field defect. Localised chorioretinitis patch in the arcuate area can give isolated scotomas in the Bjerrum's area of the field. A central retinal vein occlusion can be the result of raised IOP. A worsening diabetic retinopathy or laser treatment for the same can cause worsening of the field defect. Vasculitis can cause vessel occlusion and field defects. A retinoschisis or a localised retinal detachment may cause a nasal step like field defect. It is therefore obvious why examination of the entire retina is important before one comments on the field defect or its progression.

The optic disc evaluation is central to glaucoma evaluation. That glaucoma is not a single entity is clear now. It is still not clear what the primary reason for the optic nerve damage is. Is it an autoimmune disease triggered by raised IOP? Does the primary insult occur in the retinal ganglion cell, optic nerve head, postlaminar optic nerve or even in the lateral geniculate body is not clear. Loss of nerve fibre axons, ganglion cells, blood vessels and glial cells have all been noted histopathologically in these patients. The biggest problem in distinguishing glaucomatous disc from non-glaucomatous ones is the wide variation seen in normal disc of the population. Added to this are the racial variations. One should therefore be well versed with normal variations to suspect if a disc is glaucomatous even before the field defects develop. When field defect is seen, one should try and corroborate with the disc changes. It is said that 20–30% nerve is lost before field defects appear.

As has been mentioned previously the disc rim has the axons and the cup is the area devoid of axons. The disc is best evaluated with a slit lamp so that one can get a three dimensional view of the disc at high magnification. Along with the slit lamp one should use a 60 or 78 D lens to evaluate the disc. The advantage of these lenses is that the nerve fibre layer and macula can be evaluated under higher magnification. If a 90 D lens is used, the magnification of the slit lamp can be increased. When measuring the disc however, one needs to use a multiplication factor with the slit lamp measurement to get the actual measurement of the disc parameters. With a 60 D lens this is not needed. The multiplication factor depends on the lens used. With a 90 D lens if the slit lamp measurement is 1.2 mm, then that value is multiplied by 1.5 to get the actual measurement. With 78 D lens the multiplication factor is 1.1.

The disc is best evaluated after dilating the eye. To examine the right eye, the high power positive lens is held with the right hand between the thumb and index finger in front of the eye between the slit lamp and the eye (Fig. 13.10). An elbow support like with gonioscopy facilitates the examination. The patient is asked to look at the right ear of the examiner with the left eye. In case the patient is one eyed, he is asked to look straight ahead. The lens is kept parallel to the face in front of the pupil and slit lamp moved closer to the eye. As one moves in the disc will start coming into view and

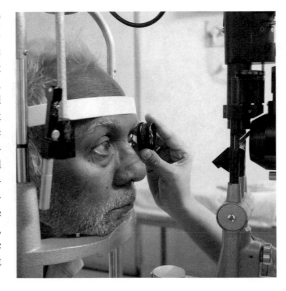

Fig. 13.10 Examination of the disc with a 78 D lens

the slit lamp is focused on the disc. The illumination should be as low as possible. The angle between the microscope and the light housing can be zero degree, 5° or greater (till binocular viewing is possible). By tilting the lens and moving the slit lamp from side to side the disc and its surrounding areas can be examined. For examination further into the periphery of the retina patient should be asked to look to the area of interest and the lens tilted a bit. To measure the disc size the slit light is made coaxial with the microscope. The slit is narrowed and shown on the disc. The height of the slit is now reduced till its edges coincide with the disc margin. The measurement on the slit lamp housing scale multiplied by the correction factor gives the size of the disc. Once the disc is seen an effort should be made to look at the disc margin, identify the scleral opening and examine the neuro-retinal rim, both the margins and the surface. The cup should be identified not only by the paler colour but also by the change in the contour of the surface that is made out on stereoscopic viewing. The dipping of the vessels on the surface of the disc at the margin of the cup will also give a clue to the edge of the cup.

Direct ophthalmoscope has many disadvantages when evaluating the disc. The high magnification restricts the amount of retina one can see at a time. The lack of stereopsis makes the evaluation of the cup unreliable. The magnification of the indirect ophthalmoscope is not high enough to see the details of the disc clearly. However indirect ophthalmoscopy is mandatory for examination of the retina up to the retinal periphery. Three mirror examination is good but the contact lens examination makes it cumbersome and view of the rest of the eye after an examination is difficult.

Normally the vertical disc diameter is about 1.5 mm. The normal cup size can be 0–0.5. The cup size is described as a proportion of the total disc diameter. The diameter of the disc is given a size of 1. A 0.5 cupping would mean 50% of the disc diameter is occupied by the cup. A cupping of more than 0.7 in either eye should raise the suspicion of a possible glaucomatous change. If an enlargement of cup over and above what is expected with age can be shown by comparing old disc photos, then one is more certain that the cupping is pathological. The area of the pallor being less than the cup area is an indication that the aetiology may be glaucomatous. One should keep in mind that larger discs will have larger cupping because there is only a fixed number of about 1.5 million axons that need to pass through the neuro-retinal rim and the rest of the space has to be made up by the cup. Measuring the disc diameter in every eye will give the examiner an idea of the relation between the disc size and cupping in their population. Between the two eyes if there is a difference of more than 0.2 in the cup size the larger cupped disc is suspect. In these cases also it is worth while measuring the diameter of the disc. If the disc size is the same and the cupping is asymmetrical, then it is more likely that there may be a pathological change. Care should be taken when evaluating a patient with tilted disc. It is easy to miss the cupping in a patient with tilted disc because the cupping is not seen 'end on'. The vertical and horizontal cup size can be different. It is usually only the longer vertical cupping that is measured.

Besides the fallacy in estimating the disc cupping in patients with tilted disc there may be artefactual field defects too in these patients.

The nerve fibre rim or the neuro-retinal rim is not uniformly thick in all around. Though not universal, in majority of the normal people, the inferior rim is the thickest, followed by superior, then nasal and the thinnest rim is temporal. This is called **ISNT rule**. In a glaucoma suspect if you find the inferior rim thinner than the nasal rim, the suspicion of a glaucomatous change should increase. More useful than the overall rim thickness is the detection of localised thinning of the neuro-retinal rim. Usually near the superior or inferior rim one may appreciate a local outward bulge of the cup in an area. This **notch** should be about 0.1 cup in size to be significant. Associated with the notch one may see a **disc margin haemorrhage** or **wedge-shaped nerve fibre layer defect** (Fig. 13.11). There could be a field defect associated with the notch. The neuro-retinal rim is normally not pale in early glaucoma. If there is pallor other causes should be thought of.

The arteriolar branches of the central retinal artery normally follows the rim of the cup on the surface of the disc. In case the cup enlarges it may lie on the bed of the cup and is called '**baring of the circumlinear vessels**'. If the cupping occurs at a level deeper to the disc surface, the vessel that is climbing to come to the surface gets pushed in and the whole arteriole on cross-section looks like a bayonet—called the **bayoneting**

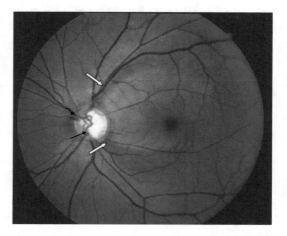

Fig. 13.11 Glaucomatous disc showing notching of the inferior cup (black arrows) along with the arcuate nerve fibre defects (white arrows) and disc margin haemorrhage (curved arrow)

sign. The number of vessel on the neuro-retinal rim is also reduced in glaucoma. Increased prominence of the lamina cribrosa was previously thought to be a pointer to glaucomatous change but does not seem to have much diagnostic value.

The presence of disc margin haemorrhage is abnormal and is thought to be a sign of glaucoma, especially the normal tension glaucoma (Fig. 13.11). Here flame-shaped haemorrhage is seen at the junction of the disc and the retina. The haemorrhage is transient and in the region of the haemorrhage one sees nerve fibre layer loss and associated field defect later. Other causes of disc margin haemorrhage like posterior vitreous detachment, diabetic retinopathy, branch vein occlusion, etc. should be ruled out.

The nerve fibre layer (NFL) of the retina is best seen with the red free light. It is seen as a white fibrillar sheen around the disc, more clearly seen near the superior and inferior pole of the disc. Wedge-shaped defects in this sheen (Fig. 13.11) starting at the disc margin is suggestive of glaucomatous nerve fibre loss. There may or may not be an associated neuro-retinal notching and a field defect corresponding to the NFL defect. The significance of the NFL defect increases if there is a corresponding visual field defect. Thin streaks of NFL defect can be normally seen in people and has no clinical significance. Sometimes with the NFL loss, before the cup enlarges fully, the glial tissue at the rim hold the vessels up. This is called the **over pass phenomenon**, i.e. the blood vessels floating over a collapsed disc below.

Peripapillary atrophy can be seen in normal people, especially the myopes. There are two morphological types seen. Alpha zone atrophy seen as an area of hypo- and hyper-pigmentation around the temporal disc (temporal crescent) is mostly in myopes and is not associated with glaucoma. Beta zone atrophy has a characteristic whitish appearance and represents the loss of choriocapillaries and retinal pigment epithelial layer in that region. This is seen more in areas where there is an associated field defect. The alpha zone lies outside the beta zone (Fig. 13.12).

With the current ease of availability of disc photography a disc photograph is the best record

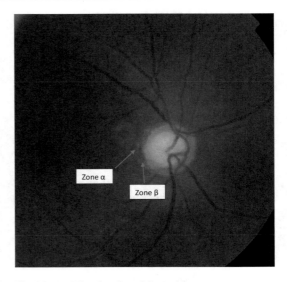

Fig. 13.12 Disc showing alpha and beta zones

for glaucoma patients. One can draw a diagram of the disc marking the cupping, notching, NFL defects, etc. on it. The size of the disc and amount of cupping should also be mentioned.

When evaluating the disc in glaucoma one isolated sign mentioned above may not have much significance. Two or more signs appearing together and matching with the rest of the finding and history should give one a better confidence in the diagnosis. One should also keep in mind other optic nerve pathologies like optic disc pit, coloboma, Drusen, myopic disc, tilted disc, etc. when evaluating a patient with suspected glaucoma.

Finally, assessing the glaucomatous disc is a pattern recognition. It is only a matter of time before artificial intelligence will classify the disc better than humans. However to pick up all other features of clinical presentation and put it together will still need doctors!

13.7　Intraocular Pressure Measurement

Measuring the IOP is central to the current management of glaucoma. However it has so many factors affecting it that the absolute number one gets when measuring IOP is not important. There is confusion as to what the normal IOP distribution pattern is. Is it Gaussian (parametric) at all? Is it skewed to the right? Is it Gaussian in some age groups? The classical teaching of the normal range of IOP being in between 10 and 21 mmHg is based on the assumption that IOP distribution in the population is Gaussian when in fact it may be skewed to the right. Due to the variability in pressures seen in patients with glaucoma, it is difficult to define normal IOP in terms of the pressure that do not cause glaucoma! Added to this is the variation of IOP with age, race, sex, the time of day it is measured, the position in which it is measured, the instrument used to measure, etc.

IOP is thought to increase with age probably due to a reduction in outflow facility. Asians and Blacks have higher IOP than Caucasians. Females after menopause are said to have higher IOPs. Diurnal variation of IOP is a story of variation in itself! Classically it is thought that most people have the highest IOP is in the morning; but peaks at midmorning, afternoon have been reported. More important than the actual peak is probably the fluctuation. A difference of more than 10 mmHg IOP during 24 h is thought to be pathological. 6 mmHg is suspect. While a 24 h measurement is ideal, practically one could take measurements in the clinic every 2 h for the whole day to get an idea. The supine position increases the IOP. The equipment used to measure the IOP also affects the reading. In spite of all this IOP is the only parameter we can control in the management of glaucoma.

13.7.1 Applanation Tonometry

The gold standard for measuring IOP is still the Goldman applanation tonometer (GAT). In all measurements of IOP the basic assumption is that the amount of deformation of the globe by whatever method is affected by the pressure in the eye. The more the IOP, more difficult the deformation will be.

In GAT the applanating cylinder/prism is touched on the cornea in such a way that a prefixed area of the cornea is flattened. The force required to applanate is dependent on the intra-

ocular pressure (Imbert-Fick principle). The applanation tonometer comes as an extra attachment to the slit lamp. Once attached, it can be moved into position before measuring the IOP. The eye is anaesthetised with proparacaine first. Then a drop of fluorescein is used to stain the tears. The applanating prism should not be used directly from Dakin solution in which it is kept to prevent transmission of infection from patient to patient. The prism is washed in sterile saline, dried and mounted on the prism holder in the applanation tonometer. It is kept in such a manner that the red mark on the prism coincides with the white mark on the holder (Fig. 13.13). The stem of the holder should be supported while inserting the prism so as to not affect the calibration. The measurement knob on the side of the tonometer is turned so that the 1 mark (not zero) on its circular scale coincides with measurement spot on the side of the applanation box. It is at the 1 reading that prism balances with the counter

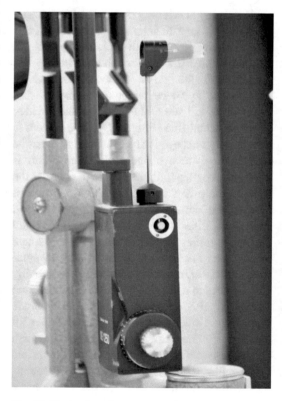

Fig. 13.13 Applanation tonometer with the prism fixed correctly

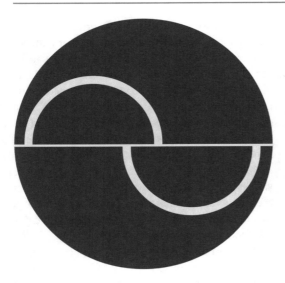

Fig. 13.14 View through the applanation prism showing the mires of the cornea

weight and is floating freely to move either side. Keeping the prism coaxial, the beam of light is made a full spot with maximum brightness. The lighthouse is kept in such a way (usually at 60° angle to the microscope) that all the light falls on the side of the prism. The cobalt blue filter is now put on and the prism viewed monocularly through the eyepiece which is aligned to the prism. One will see a blue circular disc divided by a horizontal line (Fig. 13.14). The patient is now told that his eye is anaesthetised and that he should keep the eye open while the prism is brought in contact with the cornea to measure the IOP. As the prism approaches the eye, before it touches the cornea two blue half circles will appear on either side of the central horizontal line and signifies that the prism is about to touch the cornea. These semicircles should be symmetrical. If not, make it symmetrical by moving the slight lamp up or down. Moving the slit lamp up or down after the cornea is touched can abrade the cornea. Now gently move in a bit further till the two symmetrical circles become greenish (Fig. 13.14) signifying that the prism has touched the tear film. These rings may or may not intersect with each other. Now turn the knob on the side till the two circles overlap in such a way that

the inner aspect of the two half circles just touch each other. If the circles pulsate significantly, then the circle is made to overlap in such a way that the oscillation due to the pulsation is equal on both sides of the end point. A slight pull back of the slit lamp after the measurement should disengage the prism from the cornea. If that does not happen it means the prism has been pushed in too much to take the measurement and that will underestimate the IOP. Again if the fluorescein ring is too thick due to excessive tears it will over-estimate the IOP and vice versa if it is too thin. Eye should be wiped gently or more fluorescein put to make the rings optimal. Measuring without holding the lid would be ideal. However due to reflex blinking you may need to hold the lid up. If the lid is help up by the examiner, one should ensure that the patient does not squeeze the lid and the examiner does not press on the eye as both can increase the IOP. Once the end point is reached the slit lamp is drawn back and the prism taken out after stabilising the holder with the examiners fingers. The prism is put back into the Dakin solution. Alternatively hydrogen peroxide solution can be used. The reading is measured off the circular scale. 1 corresponds to 10 mmHg and 2, 20 mmHg.

In patients with thyroid eye disease IOP is also measured in the up gaze position by asking the patient to look up; before looking up, the patient's chin is tilted down so that the cornea realigns in the straight ahead position when the patient looks up. An increase in IOP of over 6 mmHg suggests that the muscles are tight and the IOP may increase even in the sleep due to Bell's phenomenon.

If the corneal astigmatism is high, the IOP measurement in the standard horizontal position of the prism is not accurate as the mires will not be circular. To counter this one can measure the IOP with the prism line horizontal and vertical and then take an average. Alternatively there is a red line on the prism that should be aligned to the flatter axis of the cornea by using the degree mark on the prism holder.

Since the IOP measured by the applanation tonometer is affected by corneal thickness and corneal thickness by itself is a risk factor (thin corneas increase the risk of glaucoma), corneal thickness is measured using ultrasound or light pachymeters and recorded if the equipment is available. Though correction factors have been described based on the corneal thickness it is not very accurate.

13.7.2 Calibration of Tonometer

Any equipment that measures need to be calibrated regularly to ensure no additional errors due to the equipment creeps in. The applanation tonometer has a calibration rod that is fixed to a slot on the side of the applanation box to do the calibration. The manufacturer gives the instructions for calibration. Calibration should be done once a month.

In presence of corneal oedema and scars, applanation measurements are not accurate and an electronic tonometer like Tonopen is better. Since a tonopen is not available as a standard equipment in the examination cubicle it is not described here.

13.7.3 Digital Tonometry

Digital tonometry is only useful to make assessment of IOP at the extreme ends of the IOP spectrum. This is really useful only in a non-clinic situation like in a non-ophthalmology ward, emergency room or in the clinic when patient is not co-operative. Realistically only three readings are possible by this method, very low (less than 5 mmHg), very high (more than 40 mmHg) and 'in between somewhere'!

To do the digital tonometry, patients should be asked to look down (not close the eye) so that the hard tarsal plate moves down and out of the way of the upper part of the lid through which our fingers feel the globe. Now globe should be alternatively pressed with the two fingers above the tarsal plate. Essentially what one is doing here is looking at the ease of fluctuation in the globe as a surrogate for the IOP (Fig. 13.15).

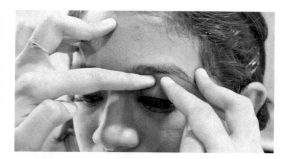

Fig. 13.15 Examination of intraocular pressure using digital tonometry

With the patient looking down the outer three fingers of both the hands is rested on the forehead to take the weight of the forearm. Now the index fingers of both the hands is kept on either side of the globe and pressed alternatively. When one finger presses the other feels the transmitted pulsation. The softer the eye greater is the movement of the globe wall. This test can really only rule out a very soft eye or a very hard eye. This is ideally useful to assess a patient in the emergency room who comes with one sided headache and vomiting to rule out angle closure glaucoma. A very soft eye in a patient after a traffic accident could suggest an occult rupture of the globe.

13.7.4 Indentation Tonometry

Indentation tonometry done using Schiotz tonometer is the other method of assessment of the IOP in the clinic without the use of expensive equipment. Schiotz tonometer has a central plunger located in the middle of a footplate of the equipment. With the footplate rested on the cornea the central plunger can move up or down. The amount of downward movement on the plunger depends on the IOP. Softer the eye the more the plunger moves in. The plunger is attached to a scale which then reads off the IOP based on a conversion table that is available with the tonometer. To get more reliable conversions, the scale readings should be within two and five divisions. To ensure this weights are added to the plunger so that any IOP measurement can be brought to this

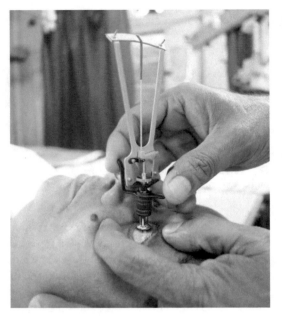

Fig. 13.16 Examination of intraocular pressure using Schiotz tonometer

reading. Since indentation is dependant on the scleral rigidity the validity of this measurement is not good.

The measurement is taken with the patient lying down (Fig. 13.16). After explaining to the patient that the tonometer will be kept on the eye to measure the IOP the eye is anaesthetised with topical proparacaine. Keeping the lid open with two fingers of one hand the tonometer is placed on the cornea using the handle of the tonometer. The reading when the footplate is fully rested on the cornea gives a value on the scale which should be then converted to the IOP reading using the conversion sheet given with the tonometer. With hand held applanation tonometer (Perkin's tonometer) and Tonopen available for patients who cannot sit at the slit lamp the use of indentation tonometer is limited to outreach work in remote areas.

In spite of all the uncertainties, because of the centrality of IOP in our management strategies it is important to measure IOP as accurately as possible. These measurements are most useful when we are measuring the IOP for the same individual with the same instrument, multiple times. It is also important to give IOP no more importance than it deserves especially considering all the variability associated with its measurements.

13.8   Field Examination

For glaucoma evaluation and management, in the present day there is no role for examining the visual fields with methods like confrontation, tangent screen, etc. Doing the same for a glaucoma patient even in exit examinations for trainees is not justified.

Investigations: Automated fields evaluation, nerve fibre layer and ganglion cell study using OCT, disc photo evaluation using artificial intelligence and electronic diurnal IOP monitors are the important investigations that will aid one in further evaluation and management of glaucoma patients. Students will need to refer to specialist books on these subject to understand the scope of these investigations better.

14.1 Introduction

In keeping with its function and importance, the retina and its support system (the choroid) are hidden far behind in a relatively dark space. Projections of lighted images are better appreciated in a dark room! In addition to the posterior segment being critical in the image processing, it is the only part in the body where we can see a part of the brain (optic nerve) directly. Direct viewing of the posterior segment is not possible and one needs special strategies for its clinical evaluation. Besides knowledge one needs to practice these clinical skills to become competent in its use.

Due to the location of the retina, examining it is more difficult and require more than a torchlight or a slit lamp. This makes the examination of the retina a little more dependant on special equipment and their use needs practice.

14.2 Applied Anatomy and Physiology

14.2.1 Vitreous

The vitreous is a transparent gel consisting of relatively small amounts of collagen fibrils, hyaluronan and 98% water. The vitreous is in the form of a gel with the water and hyaluronan interspersed between the collagen fibrils. The vitreous body is in apposition to the retina and is attached to retina around the disc, at the large blood vessels, around the macula and in a mid-peripheral ring on the posterior surface of the lens. The space inside this ring is called **Berger space**. The vitreous is also strongly attached in a non-detachable form to the vitreous base, which is an area extending from 3 mm behind the ora serrata to 2 mm in front of the ora. The Berger space is connected to the pre-macular area through a channel in the vitreous called **ciliobursal space** (Hyaloid canal/Cloquet canal). This channel may be responsible for the flow of inflammatory cytokines from the ciliary body to the macula causing macular oedema in uveitis.

14.2.2 Retina

The retina extends from the Optic disc to the **Ora Serrata** (Fig. 14.1). The retina is mainly divided into an outer **retinal pigment epithelial (RPE) layer** and an inner **neurosensory layer**. Embryologically, first the optic nerve stalk forms as a balloon, which then invaginates on itself to give an outer RPE layer and inner nervous layer. Though these layers are apposed to each other there is no tissue bridging these two layers. Thus, there is a potential space between these two layers which can be separated easily in certain retinal pathology to produce a retinal detachment. The inner neurosensory layer is transparent to let

© Springer Nature Singapore Pte Ltd. 2020
T. Kuriakose, *Clinical Insights and Examination Techniques in Ophthalmology*,
https://doi.org/10.1007/978-981-15-2890-3_14

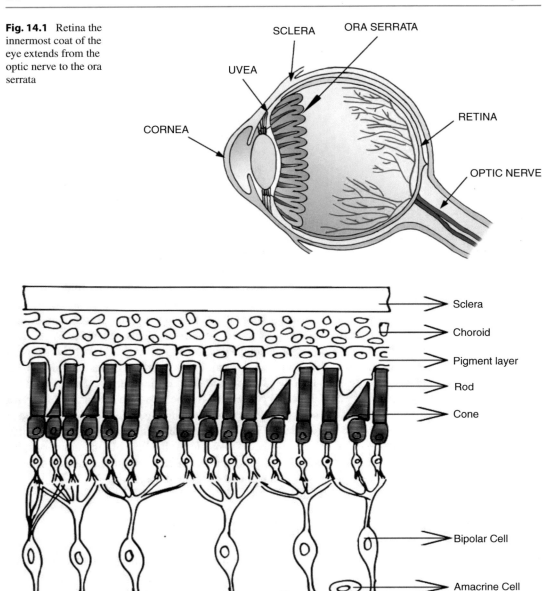

Fig. 14.1 Retina the innermost coat of the eye extends from the optic nerve to the ora serrata

Fig. 14.2 Diagrammatic cross-section of the retina and choroid

the light reach the **photoreceptor layer of rods and cones** which are the cells that first recognise light. In the macular area of the retina there is a

yellow colouration due to the xanthophyll pigments present there. The neurosensory layer is divided into nine layers (Fig. 14.2); between the

Layers   **Cells**

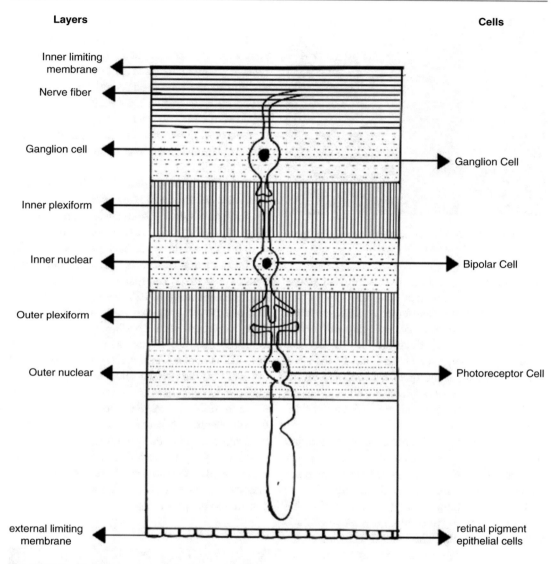

Inner limiting
membrane

Nerve fiber

Ganglion cell   Ganglion Cell

Inner plexiform

Inner nuclear   Bipolar Cell

Outer plexiform

Outer nuclear   Photoreceptor Cell

external limiting   retinal pigment
membrane   epithelial cells

Fig. 14.2 (continued)

outer nuclear layer and RPE is the external limiting membrane and the layer of rods and cones not
marked, which are essentially layers of stimulus-
processing cells sandwiched between their connecting fibres and supporting membranes. The
innermost layer is the **internal limiting membrane (ILM)**. Once the light hits the outermost
photoreceptor layer of the neurosensory retina, it
sets of a series of chemical reactions in the rods
(sensor cells that process dim light vision) and
cones (cells that process bright light vision
including colour) that eventually causes its depo-

larization and generate the first neural signals.
The glutamate released by the rod is picked up by
the bipolar cells with which they synapse.
Bipolar cells which are the first order neurons in
the visual pathway then synapse with the **ganglion cells** (second order neurons) in the inner
retina. Afferent fibres from the ganglion cells
form the **nerve fibre layer** just under the
ILM. The fibres are non-myelinated till they
become the optic nerve outside the lamina
cribrosa of the sclera (sclera outlet). The retinal
layers between the outer plexiform layer and the

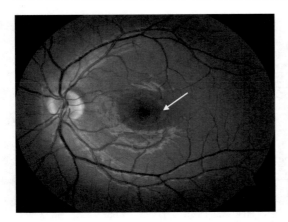

Fig. 14.3 Posterior pole of a normal retina with fovea (white arrow), centred within the macula

ganglion cell layer is like a mesh and extra-cellular blood in this area takes the shape of an ink blot. The nerve fibre layer is arranged like a fan with the nerve fibres going to the optic nerve. Blood in this layer therefore has a feathery appearance. About half of the fibres of the optic nerve decussate at the optic chiasma to join the optic tract on the opposite side and reaches the lateral geniculate ganglion from which the third order neurons arise.

The retina does not have a uniform structure over its entire surface area (Fig. 14.3). The structure and the light/image processing capability varies from the ora-serrata to the macula.

Posteriorly temporal to the optic nerve, the area surrounded by the temporal vessel arcades is called the **macula**. The central 1.5 mm of the macula has a depressed area called the **fovea** which is the area of the retina with the highest density of photoreceptors. The fovea has only cones and gives us the highest spatial visual acuity and colour vision. Besides the density of the cones, there is also a one to one connection between the cones and the bipolar cells. As one goes into the periphery, multiple photoreceptors connect to one bipolar cell. To allow unhindered passage of light the centre of the fovea has no blood vessels and is called the foveal avascular zone. Beyond the fovea, rods appear and have their greatest concentration 20° from the fovea. At the centre of the fovea is **foveola** and represents the centre of the visual field or the

zero degree. The blind spot due to **optic nerve** that lies between 15° and 20° temporal to the centre of fixation and is about 7° vertically. As clinicians it is good to learn to correlate the field position to the retinal anatomy. The **optic disc** measuring an average 1.5 mm in diameter and the retinal vein which is 125 microns diameter at the disc are used as the measuring rods of the retina. Size of retinal lesions can be described as 'so many' disc diameters.

The retina is the thinnest at the **foveola** (about 0.01 mm) where there is only a single layer of cones. Just outside the fovea the retina is the thickest at about 0.3 mm thick. As one moves away from the macula the retina becomes thinner again. At the ora serrata retina is only 0.08 mm thick. Since the retina is transparent, the colour of the fundus comes from the RPE layer and the choroid. The cherry red spot one sees in central retinal artery occlusion or in conditions like Tay Sachs disease is due to the obscuration of red reflex by the oedema or deposits in the retinal stroma around the fovea. At the foveola since there is only a single layer of cells there is not enough extracellular tissue for fluid or storage materials to collect. The foveola therefore allows the reddish hue from the RPE and choroid to be seen through as cherry red spot (Fig. 14.4). The retina at the ora is very thin, degenerated and without capillaries. At the ora serrata the retina has thin dentate processes that extend into the pars plana.

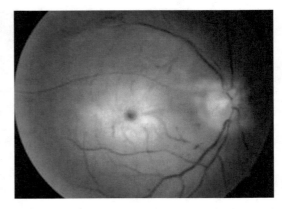

Fig. 14.4 Cherry red spot at the fovea with white oedematous macula around, in a patient with central retinal artery occlusion of the right eye

The retina has a dual blood supply. The inner neurosensory layers of the retina are supplied by the central retinal arteries via its capillaries. The outer part of the neurosensory retina including the RPE is supplied by the chorio-capillaries. Only 5% of oxygen needs are met by the central retinal artery (CRA). The CRA divides into four main braches to supply each of the quadrants. These divide and give about four layers of capillaries to supply the inner retina. These capillaries do not extend beyond the outer part of the inner nuclear layer. The retinal arteries are end arteries like the vessels of the central nervous system. Like the CNS the retinal capillaries retain a blood retina barrier with tight junctions at the endothelial cell level. In about 20% of the population there is a cilioretinal artery derived from the ciliary circulation of the choroid and supply the macular area. On angiography this artery fills earlier along with the choroidal circulation. If cilioretinal artery is present, it will be spared in cases of a CRA occlusion and central vision may be preserved. The capillaries drain into retinal veins having a similar arrangement like the artery and finally drains into the central retinal vein (Fig. 14.3).

The retinal vein is larger than the retinal artery and their ratio is 3:2. Since the retinal vein has deoxygenated blood, they look darker than the arteries. In fact what is seen as arteries and veins is the blood column within them. The AV crossing changes seen at the crossing of artery and vein is due to the blood column being hidden by the thickened vessel walls of the artery. It is for the same reason that one does not see AV crossing changes if the artery crosses under the vein. The retinal arteries are different from other arteries of other parts of the body in that they do not have the internal elastic lamina and so is not directly affected by the giant cell arteritis.

14.2.3 Choroid

The choroid is an integral part of the retina in terms of function. The retina cannot function without the choroid. Besides supplying nutrients to the outer part retina it also acts like a light, heat and waste sink of the retina. The **Bruch's membrane**, considered a part of the choroid is a five-layered structure that includes the basement membranes of the RP on the inside and the chorio-capillaries on the outside. In the centre of the membrane is an elastic layer sandwiched on either side by a collagenous layer. It is primarily a rupture of this layer that is seen in the clinical entity of blunt choroidal rupture. Outside the Bruch's membrane is the fenestrated **choriocapillary layer** that supplies nutrients to and removes waste from the outer retina. Outside the capillary layer are 'two' vascular layers with progressively larger calibre vessels called **Sattler layer** and **Haller layer**. Blood supply to the choroid is from the short posterior ciliary arteries and is a low-pressure system. The venous drainage is via the vortex veins that exit the globe behind the equator. The choroid has the highest metabolic rate and blood flow per gram of tissue anywhere in the body.

14.2.4 Normal Posterior Segment

Posterior segment starts from the back of the lens. The lens is centred in a depression on the anterior face of the vitreous called **patellar fossa** or hyaloid fossa. There is a small clear space between the lens and the anterior face of the vitreous called **Berger space**. This space is connected to the pre-macular area through a channel in the vitreous called ciliobursal space (**Cloquet canal**). Both these can be made out during the slit examination. Only part of the canal can be made out at a time. This may be the pathway for the flow of inflammatory cytokines from the ciliary body to the macula. The vitreous is transparent. Slit lamp examination will reveal a fine fibrillary structure going in the antero-posterior direction with a few isolated cells seen as glistening dots in some patients. The posterior border of the fibrillary structure in the vitreous cannot be normally made out as it is attached to the retina.

The optic disc is vertically oval and about 1.5 mm in diameter. It tends to be larger in the more pigmented race. The margin of the disc is well delineated all around. The disc has a periph-

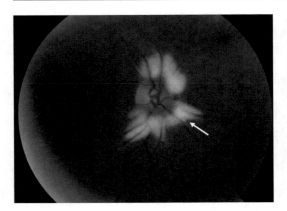

Fig. 14.5 Myelinated nerve fibres (white arrow) at the disc blurring the disc margin

eral **neuro-retinal rim (NRR)** having the nerve fibres and a central depression called the **cup** without axons. The neuro-retinal rim (NRR) is more reddish pink with mildly lighter colour temporally, compared to the central paler area. The red colour of the NRR is due to fine capillaries on the surface of the disc. The axons of the nerve fibre layer till they cross the lamina cribrosa posteriorly are not myelinated. If the nerve fibres going to the disc are myelinated, they appear as yellowish feathery patches usually at the disc margin (Fig. 14.5). This is not pathological.

In some patients the underlying choroid does not reach up to the disc margin and the sclera below will be visible as a white ring/crescent at the outer disc margin. There may be pigmentation at the border of the choroid.

The central retinal artery and vein passes through, approximately the centre of the disc. These vessels can be seen dividing into smaller vessels as they pass over the temporal and nasal half of the retina. The pulsation of the central retinal artery cannot be seen when looking at the retina because the intraocular pressure (20 mmHg) is much lower than the diastolic blood pressure (80 mmHg) and there will be a column of blood in the artery always. The tributary of the central retinal vein at the margin of the disc or the cup on the other hand shows pulsation in most people because the IOP collapses the vein when the venous pressure falls below the intraocular pressure. In people who do not

have spontaneous venous pulsations, slight pressure on the globe to increase the IOP will produce the venous pulsation. The arteries are smaller than the veins and has ratio of about 2:3. Normally the arteries cross the veins in front of them and the junction does not show any narrowing of the veins. The peripheral retina at the ora may not have any easily visible blood vessels. The large blood vessels lie just under the internal limiting membrane.

Twenty percent of the population may have an artery (cilioretinal artery) arising from the choroidal circulation that supplies the macula.

The retina is transparent, lies flat on the choroid and follows the curvature of the globe. The reddish colour of the retina is due to the reflection from the melanin and blood of the choriocapillary layer and the RPE layer itself. When the RPE and chorio-capillary is thin, like in the retinal mid-periphery the larger choroidal vessels can be seen. A flower-like pattern of large choroidal vessels can be seen just posterior to the equator of the retina and is a landmark for the equator of the globe. The central area of the flower pattern is the beginning of the vortex veins.

The macula lies temporal to the disc within the superior and inferior temporal vascular arcade. This area had got a diffuse yellowish ground glass appearance and is more obvious in the pigmented race (Fig. 14.3). In the centre of the macula, about two disc diameters from the disc lies the fovea that appears as a darker red spot with a shiny foveal reflex present in normal people. If the curvature of the fovea is disrupted due to any pathology, then the foveal reflex is absent.

14.3 History

Since the retina and choroid is a single functional unit, their clinical presentation will be similar. The retina is a transducer that converts the light energy (analogue signals) to electrical energy (digital signals). The main complaint of these patients will be some alteration in the vision. It can be reduced vision, distortion of vision, black or white areas in the field of vision or curtain coming into the field of vision, etc. The amount of decrease in vision will depend on the area of the retina involved. A 6/6 vision is only possible at the fovea. So if the fovea is normal, spatial acuity may still be normal. On the other hand, if only the foveola is affected, the vision may be 6/12 due to the light processing happening within the fovea but outside the foveola. If the fovea alone is damaged, the vision may be 6/24 to 6/60 due to the image processing possible in the macula outside the fovea. Outside the central perifoveal macula the visual potential is only about 3/60.

A history of night blindness (**nyctalopia**) and day blindness (**hemeralopia**) should be asked in patients suspected to have retinal dystrophies. This history may be taken after the initial eye examination when one is suspecting a dystrophy. Night blindness is seen in vitamin A deficiency due to nutritional or metabolic causes.

If the retina is distorted due to crumpling of the 'retinal screen' due to membranes growing over it, patients will complain of distortion of vision like 'seeing straight line appearing wavy'. If the photoreceptors are brought together due to scarring, then the same sized image will fall on larger number of photoreceptors and thus will appear larger (magnification of images). On the contrary, if the receptors are separated apart due to stretch as in central serous retinopathy (CSR), the patient will complain of minification of images.

Since the retina has no pain or touch sensation receptors, any pull or irritation of the retina will appear as flashes of light. A persisting location of this flash in a quadrant of the field that is not temporal may give a clue to the location of traction. Transient traction is mostly localised temporally by patients and may not have much localising value. If the flash of light is in the nasal half of the field, then the traction may be in the temporal retina. Pressure on the eyeball, vitreous traction, etc. will give patient a sensation of light.

Patients may complain of a curtain coming in front of the eye in retinal detachment and in cases of haemorrhage or vitreous opacities coming in the field of vision. The position of the opacity in space may give a clue to the location of the lesion. If the opacity stays in the same place when the eye is moved, then the lesion is on the retina. If the opacity moves independent of the eye movement, then it is a vitreous opacity.

Some patients may complain of missing areas in the object they are looking at (**negative scotoma**) in acute macular lesions. This can be seen in premigraine conditions and transient arterial occlusions. They can go unnoticed and can be detected on field testing. Very rarely they complain of black areas (**positive scotoma**) in their central fields.

People with unilateral retinal pathology often do not realise they have a problem till they close the good eye for some reason to find decreased vision in the affected eye.

Congenital colour vision defects are often picked late when the patient undergoes formal testing as part of a check-up or a job application. Children with hereditary problems may not complain themselves thinking that is how vision is for everybody. Colour vision defects do not need treatment and is perfectly compatible with normal life.

The acuteness of the symptoms also give a clue to the aetiology. A sudden onset of decrease vision in one eye could be a central retinal artery occlusion as opposed to a gradual loss of central vision seen in dry age related macular degeneration. Bleeding into the retina or sub-retinal space due to sub-retinal neovascularization can cause acute decrease in vision.

14.4 Examination

Vision: Best corrected vision may or may not be normal in retinal pathology. When the patient's vision is 6/9 or less, a pinhole is used to check if vision worsen it or improves it. The reduced amount of light entering the eye through the pinhole reduces the contrast. This affects the visual processing in a compromised retina and vision drops with pinhole in case of macular pathology.

Colour vision evaluation with Ishihara's chart (see Chap. 4) is a useful test especially when evaluating cases of heredomacular degeneration. Colour vision is significantly altered in cases of heredomacular degeneration. In acquired causes a 15 hue test may be more useful.

The time macula takes to recover after a bright light is shown in the eye depends on the health of the macula. Measurement of this recovery is the basis of the **Macular stress test**. This and other macular function tests are not used now by the ophthalmologist after the advent of better examination and investigation techniques. In mature cataract; pupillary reaction, RAPD, colour discrimination, appreciation of the continuity of the line with Maddox rod, etc. may give a preliminary idea of the macular function (see Chap. 4).

Since light has to reach the retina for images to be formed, all structures superficial to it, namely cornea, lens and vitreous, are transparent. This enables the examiner also to see deep into the body to visualise retina. The retina has nerves, arteries and veins that can be seen in vivo. In addition to examining the retina for eye pathology, examination of the retina gives an insight into how the body's vessels, interstitial tissues and nerves are affected in systemic diseases. With the advent of large field imaging capabilities of the retina augmented with optical coherence tomography (OCT) imaging there may be a day when one may not even have to clinically look at the retina but only see its images captured by electronic devices. Combine this with artificial intelligence (AI) learning; even the interpretation of these images may be done better by machines than humans. Until that day comes and the machines are available in every clinic one needs to know the classical methods of examining the posterior segment. A clinical examination also affords the human touch that is sometimes so important in the healing process, both physical and psychological.

14.5 Direct Ophthalmoscopy

The earliest equipment to examine the fundus was the direct ophthalmoscope. It is still a very useful tool to examine the patient by the bedside and is still widely used by general physicians as part of their physical examination. The direct ophthalmoscope is a reflecting light source kept almost in line with the examiner's line of vision. Keeping the examiner's eye close to the ophthalmoscope preferably resting scope on the upper

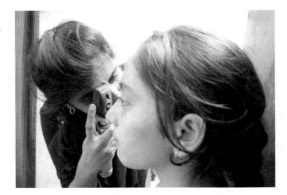

Fig. 14.6 The positioning and holding of the direct ophthalmoscope to examine the retina

medial angle of the orbit (Fig. 14.6), one can peer into the patient's eye through the pupil. The light from the scope diverges from the pupillary area to illuminate the retina. The reflected light from the retina is parallel in an emmetropic eye and gets focused back as a point on the retina of the emmetropic examiner enabling him to see the retina of the patient. Thus, to see the patient's retina one only uses the optics of the patient and the examiner. In case patient or the examiner has a refractive error, the series of lenses incorporated into the direct ophthalmoscope's wheel can be rotated into the viewing hole to compensate for the refractive error. If the patient has a refractive error of minus 3.00 dioptre (D), then the −3.00 D lens in the scope is turned into place. If the patient has a −3 D and the examiner has a −7 D refractive error, then a −10 D lens is put in place. The examiner can also wear his glasses and do ophthalmoscope. This is especially useful when the examiner has astigmatism of over 1 dioptre. The problem with using glasses is that one cannot get as close to the patient pupil as would have been possible without glasses, thereby reducing the amount of retina one can see at a time. The closer you are to a key hole (pupil), the more you can see the room (retina) you are looking into! In patients with very high refractive errors, direct ophthalmoscopy can even be done with patient's glasses on. The problem here again is that one will be further away from the key hole (pupil) and the field of view reduces further.

Since ophthalmoscopy is done uni-ocularly, depth perception is not possible. Height of lesion is estimated by the difference in the power of the lens required to focus the top and base of the lesion. Size of lesion can be estimated using the graticule provided in the scope. Good ophthalmoscopes have filters in the light path to give red free light and cobalt blue filters. A slit beam light is also provided to evaluate macular hole lesions. Red free light is used to study the nerve fibre layer and blood vessel lesions. Blood vessel lesions will look black (it has no red light to reflect) in a greenish background and so highlighted better. Nerve fibre layer defect will also be demarcated as a darkish fan-shaped area. If the patient reports a break in the slit beam projected on the fovea, a full-thickness hole should be suspected. A normal eye for all practical purposes has a dioptric power of +60 dioptres. The magnification produced thus is 60/4 or 15 times when one does direct ophthalmoscopy. The downside of the high magnification is the field of view which is only 5° (size of the disc).

With direct ophthalmoscopy one can see up to the equator with the eyes dilated. If the flash light test (see Chap. 13) does not show a very shallow anterior chamber, one can dilate the pupil of the patient with the short-acting mixture of tropicamide and phenylephrine. It takes about 30 minutes for one drop of the combination to dilate the pupil in pigmented iris. In poorly pigmented iris the dilatation is faster.

14.5.1 Performing Direct Ophthalmoscopy

The patient can be seated or lying down for the examination. The examiner rests the ophthalmoscope in the angle between the superior and medial margins of his orbit and looks through the peephole to ensure his eyes are in line with the peephole. The right eye of the examiner is used to examine the right eye of the patient and the left eye for the left. Failing this the nose will come in the way of the examination! The light of the scope is now shown into the patient's eye from about half a meter from the patient (**distant direct ophthalmoscopy**). If the media of the patient is clear, the examiner will see a bright glow in the pupillary area of the eye being examined. Media opacities will appear as dark shadows in the red glow. Dark shadows which are transient and seen only in some positions should not be mistaken for media opacities. Shadows which move with the movement of the scope belong to the cornea. Those which move in the opposite direction belong to the lens or vitreous. It has to be kept in mind that this test has a poor specificity to detect media opacities.

Once the distant direct ophthalmoscopy is done, the patient should be asked to continue to look straight ahead with both eyes open as you come closer to the eye. When examining one-eyed patients, they should be asked to imagine they are looking at a distance when the scope covers their eyes.

As one comes closer to the patient's eye, the first thing one sees should be the disc provided the patient is looking at the distance. If a vessel is seen instead of the disc, then one should trace the vessel to the side with the larger diameter to reach the disc. The size of the disc, its colour, margins and the cupping is now noted. From the disc the vessels are followed to look for the calibre of the arteries and veins (AV). AV crossings should be examined to look for AV crossing changes suggestive of atherosclerotic changes of the vessels. AV crossing assessment is done at the third crossing of the artery and vein. The area in between the vessels should also be noted for any red or yellow spots suggestive of bleeds or exudates. The focus in now shifted to the macular area to look for changes in the macular area. The foveal reflex is best examined by asking the patient to look into the light. The foveal reflex and the surrounding macula are better seen this way. The foveal reflex will be seen at the centre as a bright spot in normal patients and is due to the concave mirror effect of the fovea. If the pupil is not dilated, then pupil will constrict when patient looks at the light making examination of the macula difficult.

After examining the posterior pole the light can be swept up, down, and to the sides to examine the retinal periphery up to the equator. The patient can be asked to look up to see the upper retina better.

Except for bedside examinations an ophthalmologist seldom uses the direct ophthalmoscope in the eye clinic today. The indirect methods of examination of fundus is used in the clinic now because it offers stereoscopic view of the retina and a greater field of view. However one should keep in mind that most of the retinal lesions including retinal holes causing retinal detachments were first described using the direct ophthalmoscope!

14.6   Binocular Indirect Ophthalmoscopy

With indirect ophthalmoscopy the examiner is not looking at the retina directly but at an image of the retina in space. Lack of stereopsis, small field and inability to see up to the ora serrata were the big disadvantages of direct ophthalmoscopy. At the cost of magnification (reduced from 15 times to five times) indirect ophthalmoscopy overcame all these limitations. Seeing large areas of the retina at a time (possible with indirect ophthalmoscope) is very helpful in making a diagnosis by seeing the overall pattern of the pathology. If one were to see close up one stone alone of a wall, it will be difficult to say which building it belongs to. However, if one were to move back and see more of the building at a time, the recognition is easier. The axial magnification, i.e. the magnification in the antero-posterior direction, is highest with indirect ophthalmoscope. With the axial magnification and stereopsis, elevated lesions like central serous retinopathy is better made out with indirect ophthalmoscope.

The indirect ophthalmoscope consists of a headband with a light source and a set of lenses and prisms to bring the examiners pupils close together so that the light source and the examiner's pupil are at the entrance pupil of the patient (Fig. 14.7). The light illuminates the retina. The reflected light from the retina passes through a condensing lens of around +20 D held by the examiner in front of the eye (Fig. 14.8) and gets focussed as an **inverted image in space** between the headband and the condensing lens. It is this indirect image of the retina that is viewed by the examiner. Presbyopic examiners would therefore **need plus lens addition** to the eyepiece of the headband to facilitate viewing of this image in space that is focused around 25 cm from the examiner. Since the examiner holds the condens-

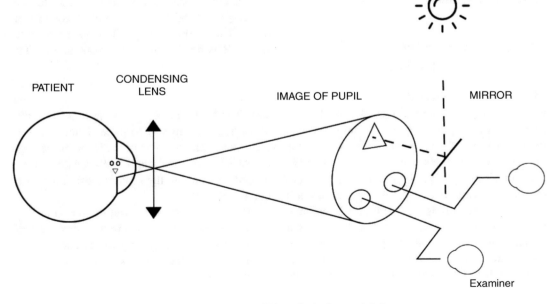

Fig. 14.7 Line diagram showing the viewing system of binocular indirect ophthalmoscopy

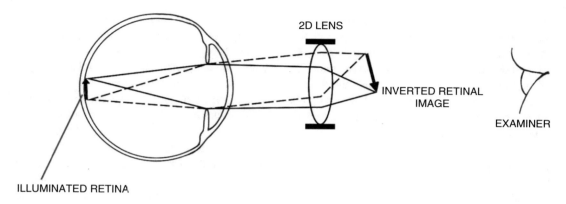

2D LENS

INVERTED RETINAL
IMAGE

EXAMINER

ILLUMINATED RETINA

Fig. 14.8 Ray diagram of the image of the retina seen by indirect ophthalmoscope

ing lens with one hand, the other hand is free to work with on the eye or draw the fundus picture as it is seen.

Indirect ophthalmoscopy is not as easy as direct ophthalmoscopy to perform. There has to be coordination between the examiners head, his hand holding the condensing lens and the patient's eye to enable view of the retinal image constantly. As one starts doing indirect ophthalmoscopy one will only get intermittent view of the retina. Initially the area of the retina seen and the amount of time you can see the retina will seem beyond the control of the examiner. The first exercise when learning to do indirect ophthalmoscopy is to learn to keep the image of the disc constantly in view. Once the disc can be constantly held in view irrespective of small movements of the patient's eye, the next exercise is to learn to follow a vessel by which it means that from the disc a vessel is followed out to the periphery. Once this head, hand, eye co-ordination is achieved and the retina can be comfortably seen up to the equator, the final step is to learn to depress the patient's peripheral sclera so that the retinal periphery up to the ora-serrata can be seen. Indirect ophthalmoscopy is the best way to clinically see the retina all the way up to the ora serrata. The idea of depressing the retinal periphery is to bring the area of retina anterior to the equator into the pupillary axis so that it can be viewed from outside. Normally the ora is facing in and posteriorly. Depression makes the retina point inward towards the pupil so that it can be seen from outside (Fig. 14.9).

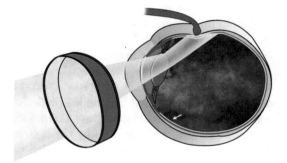

Fig. 14.9 Normally posteriorly directed peripheral retina (white arrow) points anteriorly with depression so as to facilitate viewing through the pupil

14.6.1 Performing Indirect Ophthalmoscopy

Positioning the headset of the indirect ophthalmoscope correctly facilitates the examination. The first thing to ensure when the headband is placed is to make sure one is binocular or seeing with both eyes. This is done by closing one eye and looking at an object about 30 cm in front of you. The object should be in the centre of the field or the light beam. Now close the first eye and see through the other. If the same object continues to be in the centre of the field of the fellow eye, then one is binocular. If not, the eyepiece of the indirect is moved till the object is in the centre.

The next step is to ensure that the light is falling on the upper part of the field of view. For this hold up the closed fist with thumb pointing up in front of the eye. The position of the light is adjusted so that it falls on the upper part of the thumb while the whole fist is in the field of view. At the beginning of the examination the intensity of the light should be kept the lowest possible to reduce the patient discomfort. As the patient's photoreceptors get bleached, the light intensity could be increased if needed.

Indirect ophthalmoscopy is best done with the patient lying down supine. One cannot see the ora serrata all around if the patient is not lying down. To do the actual ophthalmoscopy the indirect lens is held with the thumb and the index finger, preferably in the non-dominant hand. The lens is placed a finger length in front of the eye and the light from the headband shown through the lens into the eye (Fig. 14.10). The dominant hand can help with the retraction of the lids of the eye being examined if needed. It can also be used to depress the eye, hold the cryo probe during surgery and to do retinal drawings. If holding the lens with the non-dominant hand is difficult, one can start with the dominant hand and then switch. The light is first shown to the mid-periphery of the retina so that the patient gets used to the bright light. Then the posterior pole can be looked at. To examine the inferior retinal periphery, the patient should be asked to look inferiorly and anterior globe depressed with a cotton bud or metal depressor through the lower lid. Patient should be warned about the discomfort due to the depression. To

depress the medial and lateral part of the globe one may have to anaesthetise the conjunctival sac with proparacaine and the depression is done gently over the conjunctiva in the medial and temporal periphery because the lid cover in this area is not possible. Moving the depressed area during the examination highlights the relationship of the lesion to the rest of the retina and the vitreous. The area of the depressed retina will look white compared to the rest of the retina and this change helps to study the retinal relationships better. In retinal detachment, with depression, the white colour change of the retina does not occur, but in retinoschisis white with pressure/depression occurs. Depression can also help localise the position of the retinal lesions with respect to sclera. If the retinal lesion is on the mound raised by the scleral depression, it means the lesion overlies the clock hour of the sclera depressed.

The image seen with indirect ophthalmoscope is inverted both horizontally and vertically. This can confuse the examiner initially. The spatial inversion makes the orientation of lesions difficult to comprehend. To circumvent this problem, while drawing the retinal diagram (recording the findings) the drawing sheet/paper is kept on the patient's chest, so that the examiner is looking at the sheet the right way when the examiner is standing at the head end and looking towards the feet of the patient. In other words, when looking from the foot end the chart will be vertically and horizontally inverted. In this position of the drawing chart, one can draw as one sees it and there is no need to mentally reverse the positions.

Recording the finding: Charts with pre-drawn circles depicting the area of the equator, ora serrata and the anterior border of pars plana are available (Fig. 14.11). The chart also has radial lines that depicts the clock hours of the fundus. The radial lines stop outside the arcade and do not reach the centre. The equator is identified by the vortex veins. The centre of the circle depicts the fovea. The disc is drawn as a small circle on the right side of the fovea for the right eye and on the left side of the fovea for the left eye. In the right eye the disc is drawn at the centre point of the space between the lines from the one and five clock hour points. The retinal features seen is

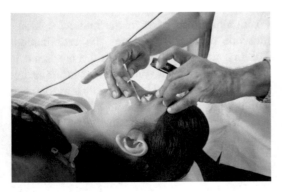

Fig. 14.10 Examining a patient with indirect ophthalmoscope, two fingers hold the lens, one finger retracts the lid and the last two fingers steady the hand by resting it on the forehead, the fellow hand can be used to depress the sclera

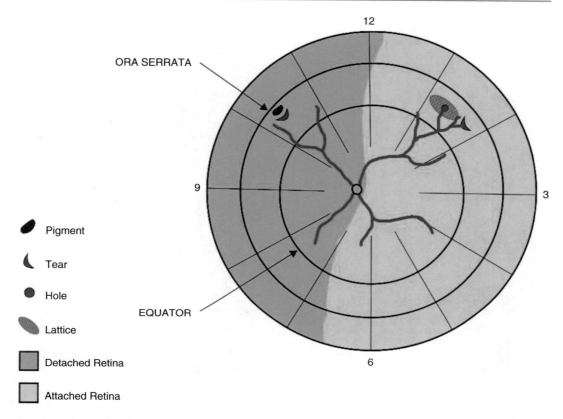

12

ORA SERRATA

9

3

Pigment

Tear

Hole

EQUATOR

Lattice

Detached Retina

6

Attached Retina

Fig. 14.11   Retinal drawing sheet with depiction of a partial retinal detachment drawn

drawn on this sheet. Figure 14.12 gives the colour coding for the various lesions commonly encountered in the fundus.

Accurate retinal drawing is most useful for patients with retinal detachment. It helps not only in the diagnosis and documentation but also in planning of surgery. When drawing the retina the first thing to see is the extant of the detachment and mark it. Next the veins are drawn with its branching. The veins should be marked as seen till it reaches the peripheral holes so that it can be used to track all the holes during surgery. Arteries need not be drawn. Though it has been suggested that each dentate process at the ora serrata be seen and marked, this is not something that is practical to do. Only the dentate processes associated with a peripheral hole or tag need to be marked. While training seeing all the dentate process may be a good exercise to gain mastery over the examination technique.

14.7   Bio Microscopic Examination of the Posterior Segment

Examination of the fundus with slit lamp (biomicroscopic examination) is now the default method to examine the posterior segment. Examination of the fundus with the Hruby lens that comes attached with the Haag Streit slit lamp did not become popular due to the poor quality of images and the difficulty in its use. With the advent of the high power plus lenses, examination of the fundus with the slit lamp became popular.

The two most popular non-contact lenses to examine the fundus are the +78 dioptre (D) and +90 D lenses. The pupils have to be dilated to get a good view of the retina. The 78 D lens has a larger magnification and is more useful to see the details. The +90 D, on the other hand, gives a larger field of view at the cost of magnification

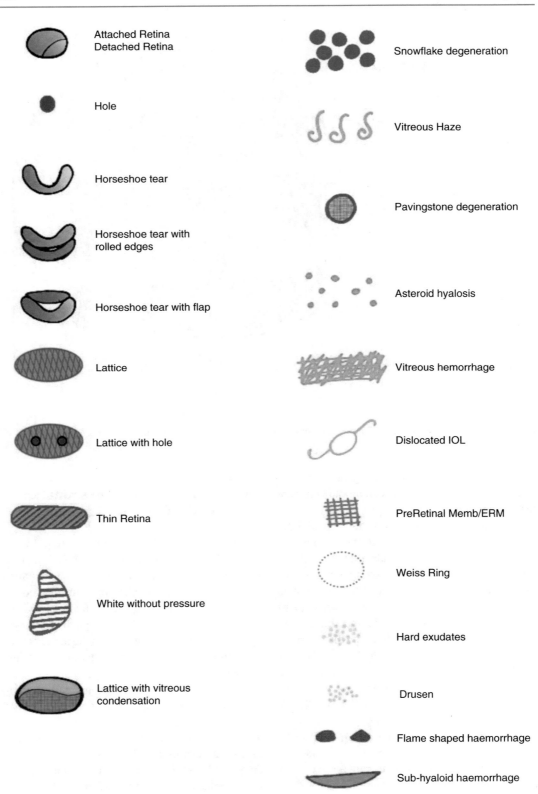

Fig. 14.12 Depiction of pathology seen for retinal drawing

and one can see beyond the equator almost up to the vitreous base in most cases. To see vitreous base, ora serrata and pars plana, one needs to depress the periphery and use the indirect ophthalmoscope. Like indirect ophthalmoscopy the retinal image seen with +78 dioptre and + 90 D lens is also inverted. Magnification of the slit lamp can be used with +90 D lens if more magnification is required.

To view the fundus, the patient's chin is kept on the chinrest like in anterior segment examination. If the right eye is being examined, patient is asked to look at the examiner's right ear with the patients left eye. The light source is either kept coaxial or at 5° to the microscope and moved as far back from the patient as possible. Now the lens is held with the examiners left hand between the thumb and index finger in front of the eye. The slit lamp is now moved in till the disc can be seen clearly. The disc margins, the neuroretinal rim, the cupping, vessels on the disc, etc. are examined. Tilting the lens to the sides, up and down enables one to see a bit more into the periphery. To enable one to see more into the periphery the patient has to look in the direction the fundus need to be seen. To study the inferior retina the patient should be asked to look down. To see the macula well the patient needs to look at the light, but this produces glare. For better viewing of the macula, the light housing is tilted to a slant and the light beam is made horizontal. This reduces the glare and one can appreciate subtle details in the macula. To keep the hand steady and to reduce strain, a block of wood or foam can be kept below the elbow of the arm holding the lens. Examiner's left hand is used to examine patient's right eye.

Red free light of the slit lamp can be used to study the nerve fibre layer of the retina. The retinal nerve fibre layer is seen as a brightly reflecting layer with a radiating pattern from the disc. Loss of nerve fibre will appear as dark gaps in this layer. Red free light will show microaneurysms as black dots against the green background. Though theoretically it may appear to be a better modality to look for micro-aneurysms, it does not make much difference clinically.

14.8   3 Mirror Examination

3 mirror contact lens examination is a direct ophthalmoscopy using the slit lamp. The 3 mirror lens is plano concave (Fig. 14.13) and has an anterior flat surface and a posterior curved surface that stays over the cornea and the limbus with the help of a coupling fluid. Inside the lens, located around the central clear area are three mirrors angled at about 73, 67 and 59°. The central part of the lens is used to examine the posterior pole, about 30° of the fundus. From 30° to the equator the 73° mirror is used. Beyond equator the 67° lens is used. The 59° lens is used to look at the angle of the anterior chamber. The image of the central 30° is **not** inverted and can be seen directly. The steadying of the globe with the contact lens and the coupling fluid enables us

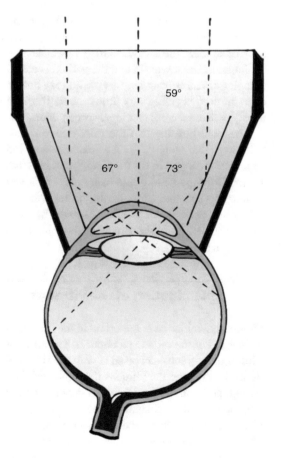

Fig. 14.13 Cross-section of the three mirror lens showing the mirror angulation and the area of the eye seen through the lens

to see the details of the retina more clearly than the 78 D lens and is useful for picking up subtle macular oedema and epiretinal membranes. Even fine new vessels or intra-retinal microvascular anomalies (IRMA) are better made out with the posterior part of the lens. The mirrors are used to see the more peripheral areas of the retina. It gives a horizontally inverted image of the opposite side retina and only small areas of the retina are seen at a time. This makes orientation and interpretation difficult. To see up to the ora is difficult even with the peripheral mirrors. If one can see the vitreous base and ora serrata easily, a choroidal detachment should be suspected.

To examine the fundus, before placing the chin on the slit lamp, the ocular surface has to be anaesthetised first. The concave surface of the contact lens is now filled with a viscous fluid like artificial tears. The patient is asked to keep the chin on the slit lamp rest after explaining to the patient the procedure, instructing him not to move back or squeeze the eyelids hard. The lens is now held against the lower lid and the patient is asked to look up. The contact lens is now quickly turned on to the cornea giving very little time for the fluid to escape from the contact lens, cornea interface.

The light housing and the microscope is initially kept like with +90 D lens examination and then can be moved in till the fundus can be seen. The microscope and light housing can be moved around to see other parts of the retina and this movement needs some practice. To see the mid-periphery all around the lens with the mirror has to be rotated.

14.9   Examination of the Vitreous

Vitreous examination is important in the diagnosis of diseases of the retina and choroid. The anterior third of the vitreous can be seen with the slit lamp alone. To examine the vitreous the angle between the lighthouse and the microscope depends on the amount of pupillary dilatation. The default angle is 5° and one gets a click when the lighthouse is at a 5° angle with the microscope in the Haag Streit slit lamp. With larger pupils the angle between the two can be above 5° and is limited by the position where the light entering the pupil is cut off by the

iris as one looks into the pupillary region with the microscope. The vitreous is examined in a dark room with the slit illumination set at the brightest. Normally, the fibrillar structure of the vitreous is seen and is devoid of cells. A few isolated cells can be normal. Unless one looks for cells it is easy to miss them. To see the deeper parts of the vitreous, the central part of the 3 mirror gives the best clarity. However a +90 D lens can also be used. To see the posterior vitreous the angulation is kept at 5° in the horizontal direction. To improve the view of the posterior vitreous the light housing is tilted forward so that the light appears as coming from below. Opacities like cells in the posterior vitreous and the posterior border of a detached vitreous (seen as a wavy line) can be made out. To the see the posterior vitreous face better one can ask the patient to move the eye up and down. The detached vitreous face seen as a bright white line can be seen to have an undulating movement. This is seen more easily in the upper part of the posterior vitreous. If the vitreous detachment is complete, this line may be seen even without the aid of the convex lens as the posterior edge of vitreous comes anteriorly in the superior part.

The indirect ophthalmoscope is a good instrument to make out larger vitreous opacities in the periphery and centre including the detached ring like fibrous condensation at the disc called **Weiss ring**. Some vitreo-retinal relationships at the retinal periphery is better made out with indirect ophthalmoscope and depression. As one observes the retina over the depressed area the vitreo-retinal relationship can be studied.

Besides cells and vitreous condensations the vitreous may have blood in it that can come from the normal or new vessels on the retina. Dense vitreous haemorrhage precludes the view of the fundus but the red blood cells can be seen in the vitreous behind the lens with the slit lamp alone. When haemorrhage is limited, one can actually see red clots in the vitreous. Over time the blood is dehaemoglobinized and appear as yellowish white clumps described as **chicken fat** appearance.

Vitreous exudates due to endophthalmitis (infection in the eye) or severe uveitis can also cause opacification of the vitreous. Here however there will be a history of surgery or trauma and the eye will be red. Slit lamp examination will show a lot of cells in the vitreous and even the anterior chamber.

A benign commonly seen pathology in the vitreous is **asteroid hyalosis**. Here the vitreous has entangled in its fibrils calcific small yellow white particles. These particles float along with the fibrils and do not settle down. Unless the deposition is very dense it does not affect vision. Though there is an association with diabetes and hypertension it has no diagnostic value.

As opposed to asteroid hyalosis, one might rarely see glistening yellowish cholesterol particles in a condition called **synchysis scintillans** or cholesterolosis. These particles settle down to the bottom and get churned up with the eye movements. This is attributed to old traumatic vitreous haemorrhage. Opacities may be seen in the vitreous in lymphoma (due to lymphoma cell infiltration) and amyloidosis (due to amyloid deposition).

Vitreous pigments can be seen in retinitis pigmentosa, old uveitis and in patients with rhegmatogenous retinal detachment.

In some hereditary vitreo-retinal degenerations like Wagner and sticklers syndrome, the vitreous cavity will be optically empty like after a vitrectomy or there will be very few fibrils seen.

Green markings on the fundus drawing depict vitreous opacities. Though drawings on oil paper pinned to the front on the retinal drawings have been suggested to record vitreous finding, it is difficult and serves little use. Often vitreous findings are recorded as texts like PVD (posterior vitreous detachment) present.

14.10   Interpreting Retinal Lesions

When a lesion is seen on posterior segment examination, first try to describe the lesion in one's mind. Then an effort is made to locate the position of the lesion both with respect to the depth of the lesion (vitreous, retinal, sub-retinal, choroidal) and location on the retina (posterior pole, equatorial, retinal periphery, pars plana). These two features along with history, will give an idea of the type of lesion one is dealing with.

Small red pinhead like dots in the retina can either be a **dot-shaped haemorrhage or a microaneurysm**. The former is a fine haemorrhage in the deeper layers of the neurosensory retina while the latter are out pouchings in the retinal capillaries. A **blot-shaped haemorrhage** is a larger haemorrhage and looks like an ink blot in the retina. These findings are seen in many retinopathies and is a very non-specific sign. Trying to remember the clinical findings of each disease condition of the retina without understanding the underlying pathology is not only difficult but also confusing. If one can figure out the type of lesion seen and understands its pathology, by putting together all the types of lesion seen, one is in a better position to postulate the possible aetiology. Table 14.1 lists the signs and the characteristics of lesions seen on the retina and its significance. Figure 14.14 shows a composite picture of some of the commoner lesions seen in the retina with their usual locations.

Unlike the anterior segment, it is not easy to make out the level of the lesion in the retina.

Table 14.1 Lesions seen in the retina and its associated significance

Clinical finding	Layer involved	Pathology	Significance	Examples of clinical conditions
Dot haemorrhage	INL, OPL	Small blood collection in the deeper neurosensory retina	Unstable capillaries	Diabetic retinopathy, vein occlusions, leukaemia
Blot haemorrhage	INL, OPL	Small blood collection in the deeper neurosensory retina	Unstable stable capillaries and venules with high vessel pressure	Diabetic retinopathy, vein occlusions, leukaemia
Flame-shaped haemorrhage	RNFL	Bleeding into the nerve fibre layer of the retina	Unstable vessels with high vessel pressure	Diabetic retinopathy, vein occlusions
Micro-aneurysm	INL	Outpouching of the capillary wall	Ischaemia	Diabetic retinopathy
Macro-aneurysm	Inner retinal layers	Localised dilation of arteriole	Atherosclerosis with hypertension	Hypertensive retinopathy

(continued)

Table 14.1   (continued)

Clinical finding	Layer involved	Pathology	Significance	Examples of clinical conditions
Hard exudate	OPL	Collection of lipids and protein in the deeper neurosensory retina	Compromised blood retinal barrier	Diabetic retinopathy, vein occlusions
Soft exudate	RNFL	Oedema of the nerve fibre layer	Ischaemia	Diabetic retinopathy, vein occlusions
Pre-macular bleed	Sub ILM	Blood between the ILM/ posterior hyaloid and RNFL	New vessels, bleeding disorder	Diabetic retinopathy, leukaemia
IRMA	INL- RNFL without ILM breach	New vessels or dilated capillaries	Retinal ischaemia	Diabetic retinopathy, Vasculitis
New vessels	INL- RNFL with ILM breach	New vessels breaching the ILM and coming into the vitreous cavity	Sever ischaemia, likely to bleed and cause retinal traction	Diabetic retinopathy, vein occlusions
Drusen	Sub RPE	Collection of lipofuscin material	Degenerative change	Age related macular degeneration

INL inner nuclear layer, *OPL* outer plexiform layer, *RNFL* retinal nerve fibre layer, *ILM* internal limiting membrane, *RPE* retinal pigment layer, *IRMA* intra-retinal microvascular abnormalities

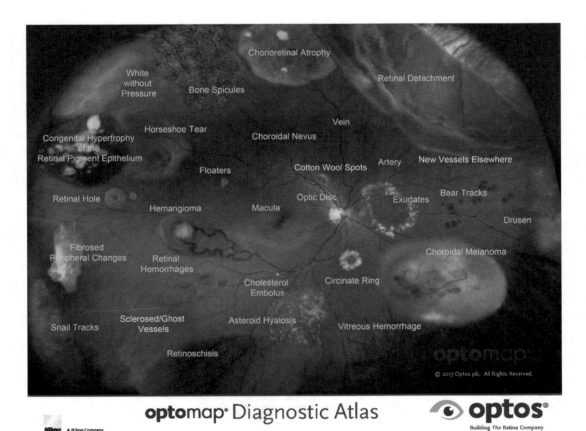

Fig. 14.14   A collage of the retinal lesions seen on fundus examination (courtesy Optos inc)

The slit illumination (lighthouse) and the microscope cannot have an angulation above 15° when examining the retina. The thin retina (1/5th thickness of the cornea) precludes a good optical cross-sectional view. However the retinal blood vessels and the RPE layer act as reference points based on which an assessment of the depth of the retinal/choroidal lesion can be made. It is here that the optical coherence tomography (OCT) scores over clinical examination of the retina.

A pre-retinal lesion will cover/hide the retinal blood vessels. A classic example of this is the pre-retinal **sub-hyaloid bleed** between the ILM and nerve fibre layer. Sometimes gross oedema of the retinal nerve fibre layer (RNFL) can hide the blood vessels, as seen in papilloedema. Lesions that are crossed over by the retinal blood vessels can be intra-retinal of sub-retinal. The architecture of the tissue around the lesion shapes the lesion and gives a hint to its location. Haemorrhages of the retina at the nerve fibre layer have a triangular feathery pattern (**flame-shaped haemorrhage**). Oedema of the retinal nerve fibres is described as **soft exudates** and can be transient. Deeper haemorrhages have an ink blot-like pattern (**blot haemorrhage**). White centred blot haemorrhage (Roth spots) in not specific for bacterial endocarditis. In fact it is seen in any condition that causes large, relatively superficial blot haemorrhages, like leukaemia, central retinal vein occlusion, severe anaemia etc. Hard exudates are collections of proteins and lipids in the deeper layers of the neurosensory retina and do not disappear easily.

Oedema or deposits (seen in storage disorders) in the retina makes it loose its transparency and the underlying RPE/choroid layer will not be seen clearly. At the fovea, since there is no other tissue other than the photoreceptors for the oedema to collect it remains transparent and the RPE layer is seen through as 'cherry red spot'. As the retinal oedema clears the underlying choroid can be made out. If the oedema is localised like seen in diabetic macular oedema localised swelling with greying of the retina can be made out. In acute retinal detachment, in addition to retinal oedema, the retina is thrown into folds due to the smaller retinal surface area needed. This gives the retina the cloudy wrinkled appearance in fresh retinal detachments. Sub-retinal blood will occupy much larger areas compared to blot haemorrhages and will obscure the RPE layer. The white discolouration seen in the area of the bleed as time passes is due to the dehaemoglobinization of the blood and the consecutive fibrosis as seen is wet age related macular degeneration. Lesions at the RPE layer causes a decrease in the reddish reflex and pigmentary hypertrophy (seen as black spots) as seen in retinitis pigmentosa or dry macular degeneration. **Drusen** is a yellowish pinhead like lesion seen at the level of the RPE due to deposition of lipofuscin material in the Bruch's membrane. If large areas of RPE is atrophic, the underlying large choroidal vessels will be seen clearly. In conditions where the RPE and the chorio-capillaries get atrophic large choroidal vessels and the sclera will be seen through, e.g. myopic macular degeneration with posterior staphyloma. In sub-RPE lesions RPE layer will look intact but pushed forward like in pigment epithelial detachment. In cases of choroiditis the inflammation may cause large deep yellowish discolouration in the choroid. Some choroidal lesions can cause secondary changes leading to RPE atrophy and pigment hypertrophy and should be kept in mind when assessing these lesions.

While in the early stages of choroiditis the RPE is still visible, in retinitis the yellow exudates and oedema mask the RPE and the finer retinal vessels. In the later stages even the larger vessels can be covered. As opposed to the smaller sized exudates seen in diabetic retinopathies inflammatory exudates are large and the vitreous will have inflammatory cells.

A wrinkling of the retinal surface as evidences by increased tortuosity of retinal surface capillaries and radial lines at the macula, suggest presence of early epi-retinal membranes. As the membrane matures and becomes thicker, it will cover the surface blood vessels. A bright sheen on the retinal surface seen more clearly with the red free light may also suggest the presence of an early epi-retinal membrane.

Full-thickness neuro-retinal holes will look red against the surrounding paler retina. The red colour is due to the RPE being seen through the retinal defect. In the very lightly pigmented Caucasian race retinal holes especially in the retinal periphery may be difficult to make out due to the lack of pigmentation in the RPE layer. Macular hole (retinal hole seen at the fovea) seen at the posterior pole is easily seen even in the Caucasian race because of increased pigmentation of the RPE in this region. Since the posterior pole is more easily amenable to biomicroscopic examination, slit lamp examination will show an actual depression in slit over this area. This type of depression in the slit can also be seen if there is an epiretinal membrane around the fovea (**pseudo hole**). To distinguish a pseudo-hole from a true hole, a slit beam can be shown vertically over the fovea and patient asked if there is a break in the beam of light (**Fischer's test**). If patient sees a break in the beam, it is a true macular hole.

Examination of the peripheral retina can show degenerative lesions restricted to the periphery. The commonest and potentially troublesome degeneration seen in up to 10% of the population is the **lattice degeneration** and appears like a thin piece of lace cloth kept circumferentially on the retinal periphery. For those who may have seen the path of a snail, this degeneration has also been described to have snail track appearance. Retinal pigmentation can be associated with this degeneration. Vitreous condensation can be made out at the border of the lattice degeneration when the lesion is depressed. There may be atrophic holes (defects in the neuro-retina) within the degenerative area or tears (breaks in the neuro-retina due to pull of vitreous) of the retina at the border of the degeneration. If lattice degeneration occurs radially, they are posteriorly located and more pigmented.

Small round atrophic areas of the retina with large choroidal vessels and sclera seen at the base of the lesion is a harmless degeneration called **cobble stone degeneration**.

In the pars plana region one may see pinhead sized cystic changes which are again harmless. Sometimes extending from the ora in line with the dentate process are ridges (**retinal tuft**) that come into the peripheral retina. At the end of these retinal tufts may be seen cystic areas that can be associated with tears and retinal detachment.

At the posterior border of the vitreous base one may have small elevations of the retina called **retinal tags** that tear if there is a vitreous detachment. This can cause retinal detachment.

As mentioned earlier the retinal vessel wall cannot be normally seen. However with vasculitis, the blood vessel walls appear yellow due to exudates that may cover the blood column. The vasculitis patches can be segmental. Later on in the disease process pigment hypertrophy may be seen around it.

Vasculitis and other vasculopathies like diabetic retinopathy, vein occlusions, etc. can cause retinal ischaemia that triggers compensatory mechanisms that need to be looked for.

In central vein occlusions, to bypass the block, veins at the disc margin called **optico-ciliary shunts** may be seen to dip into the choroid by the side of the disc. These vessels should not be mistaken for new vessels on the disc. In branch vein occlusions shunt vessels may be seen crossing the horizontal raphae to anastomose with the venous system of the functioning side. These vessels should not be mistaken for intra-retinal microvascular anomaly (IRMA) which are abnormal vessels within the retina that form in response to ischaemia. IRMA vessels are more localised and branching compared to the long, larger calibre shunt vessels. The IRMAs should also be distinguished from new vessels which are tufts of fine vessels that grow out of the retina into the vitreous. New vessels are seen at the disc or on the retina elsewhere. Detailed stereoscopic examination with three mirror will help distinguish the two, failing which, a fluorescein angiogram will show leakage with the new vessels.

When retinal detachment (RD) is suspected, one needs to first ensure that the retina is actually elevated and it is not the white colour of the retina one is mistaking for a detachment. With stereoscopic vision of indirect ophthalmoscope one can actually appreciate the elevation. Once the retinal surface is seen elevated, the question to ask is, is it a RD or retinoschisis? If it is a RD what type of RD is it? Is there an associated choroidal detachment?

Retinoschisis is a split in the inner layers of the neuro-retina and the whole neuro-retina does not get detached from RPE. In retinoschisis the inner retinal layer is very transparent. The schisis is usually located in the inferotemporal part of the fundus. The schisis margins are more circular and meets the ora in an acute angle compared to the obtuse angle of RD. A field test with the fingers may reveal an absolute scotoma if the schisis comes posterior enough. When peripheral retina is depressed, white discolouration with pressure is seen as with normal retina. This white with pressure is absent with RD. Rarely retinal tears can be seen in the outer or inner layers of the retinal schisis. If both layers have a hole, then an associated retinal detachment may be present.

If RD is confirmed, then one needs to distinguish between a rhegmatogenous (due to retinal hole) RD, tractional RD and exudative RD. In rhegmatogenous RD a retinal hole as described above will be seen. In non operated primary rhegmatogenous RD. The location of the hole can be found out more easily using the Lincoff's rules shown in Table 14.2. One should also be aware that there may be more than one hole and the detachment caused by the primary hole may open up new holes. Every effort should be made to find and localise all the retinal holes. In acute RD the retina is cloudy white with surface wrinkling of the retina seen. In long-standing retinal detachments the retina may be transparent due to atrophy and may have retinal cysts. If the RD is not total, then the margins of a long-standing detachment will have a pigmented border (body trying to wall of the detachment) called **demarcation line**. The RD may extend beyond the demarcation line in which case it may be seen under the newly detached retina. When examining a rhegmatogenous RD one should also look for con-

traction of the retina due to **proliferative vitreo-retinopathy (PVR)** that is essentially a reparative/scarring process of the retina. Signs of PVR changes include star folds on the retina, surface membranes making the retina stiff and immobile, yellowish white band on or under the retina and mid-peripheral retina coming towards centre and closing like an umbrella over the disc. If signs of PVR are present, it should be recorded in the diagram. The vitreous examination is a must in the evaluation of RD. With rhegma it will show brownish pigments (tobacco dusting) in the vitreous that are the RPE cells which have migrated into the vitreous through the retinal hole (**Shafer sign**).

If the fundus cannot be seen clearly, a low intraocular pressure (IOP) compared to the fellow eye suggest a rhegmatogenous RD. The explanation for the low IOP is supposed to be the flow of aqueous out the eye via the rhegma and the underlying mild uveitis that may be present.

In tractional retinal detachment, classically seen in proliferative diabetic retinopathy, one should be able to see fibrous bands pulling up the retina. The tip of the pulled up retina is pointed and the rest of the elevated retina has a concave surface unlike the convex surface of a rhegmatogenous detachment. Tractional RD is localised and do not reach the ora. If tractional RD is associated with rhegmatogenous RD, then the surface will be convex in areas, with surface wrinkling. The RD may reach the ora serrata.

Exudative RD is the most difficult to distinguish from rhegmatogenous RD if a cause for the exudation cannot be found. A repeated examination of the retina should be done to rule out a hole in the retina before labelling it an exudative detachment. Renal failure, melanomas or secondaries in the choroid, pan uveitis, thick sclera

Table 14.2 Lincoff and Gieser rules to locate the primary hole in primary rhegmatogenous retinal detachment (RRD)

Rule 1: In superior, temporal or nasal detachments: The primary break is within 1.5 clock hours of the highest border of RRD (in 98% of cases)

Rule 2: In total detachments or superior detachments that cross the 12 o' clock meridian (vertically above the disc): The primary break is at 12 o' clock position or within a triangular area whose apex is at ora serrata at 12 o' clock meridian and base intersects the equator at 11 o' clock and 1 o' clock position (in 93% of cases)

Rule 3: In inferior detachments: The side with higher level of fluid will have the break (in 98% of cases). If both sides are of equal height then the break is likely to be at 6 o' clock position (vertically below the disc)

Rule 4: In bullous inferior RRD the primary break should be looked for above the horizontal meridian

are some of the commoner causes of exudative RD. History therefore is very useful. One may have to go back to the history after the examination to rule out an underlying cause. Exudative detachments behave like rhegmatogenous detachments. Since the sub-retinal fluid is less viscous with exudative detachment, they have been described to shift easily. This is neither easy to make out nor very specific. Like rhegmatogenous RD these also reach the ora serrata. One should examine the vitreous carefully for cells and look beyond the retina to the choroid to see if there is any choroidal mass causing the exudation.

Rarely the retinal elevation is so very shallow that it is difficult to make out an elevation. In such cases one will have to use ultrasound or OCT depending on the indication to make out the elevation.

Rhegmatogenous detachments can be associated with choroidal detachments and can affect the prognosis of the patient. It should therefore be a practice to ask yourself if there is a choroidal detachment or not. Besides the fundus examination there are other findings that will hint at the presence of a choroidal detachment. The intraocular pressures can be very low or unrecordable. The anterior chamber can be shallow due to the rotation of the ciliary body anteriorly as a result of the choroidal detachment. On fundus examination if the ora serrata is seen easily one should suspect a choroidal detachment. With a little experience one will be able to appreciate that the RPE layer has come forward closer to the detached retina in early stages of the choroidal detachment. In large choroidal detachments the retina may seem attached to the choroid and the choroid will appear like four to five mounds in the periphery. The depressions in the choroid is due to fibrous strands attaching the choroid to the sclera and also allowing vessels to pass out of the eye.

Chalk white colour seen below the level of the retina is usually the sclera. The sclera is seen when the overlying RPE and choroid is atrophic or absent. The choroid can be absent in any area extending from the inferior pole of the disc to the periphery of the retina due to a developmental anomaly called **coloboma**. This occurs due to the improper closure of the optic cup. Where the closure is deficient the choroid and RPE is absent and the sclera will be seen clearly through the retina. If these patients develop detachments and the hole is in the retina over the colobomatous area, it is very difficult to make out the retinal hole against the white background. A careful three mirror examination is required to find the hole.

14.11   Optic Disc

Optic disc examination is more fully discussed in the Chaps. 13 and 15. The optic disc is normally flat with a central depression. Sometimes the remnants of the primary vitreous will persist in the centre of the disc as a fibrous tuft of tissue called **Bergmeister's papillae** and should not be mistaken for a neovascular front. Neovascularisation will appear as fine blood vessels at the margin of the disc early in the course of the disease. Later fibrous tissue grows in and spread along the vessel arcades to cause tractional detachment.

Black pigmented, round lesion abutting the disc and the retina known as melanocytoma is a benign lesion and should not be mistaken as a melanoma.

The paler central or paracentral depression on the disc is invariably the cupping of the disc. However in larger abnormal looking disc with a large cup one should suspect a **disc coloboma**. At times a depression may look grey with inability to see the floor of the depression. Here one should think of an **optic disc pit**. These pits are usually situated at the temporal part of the disc and causes localised recurrent macular RD that can be mistaken for a CSR.

Neuro-Ophthalmology Examination

15

15.1 Introduction

Many neurological diseases affecting the eye have their origins in the central nervous system (CNS). The ocular symptoms more often than not is secondary to a diffuse neurological problem like a demyelinating disease or a localised lesion in the brain or meninges. A neurologist or a neurosurgeon will also be needed to co-manage the cases seen in the clinic. The ophthalmologist role is primarily to understand and interpret the ophthalmic symptoms and signs we see. The first thing an ophthalmologist needs to do is to rule out an ophthalmic cause for the symptoms and signs before the neurologist can intervene. Referring an uncorrected hypermetrope with headache to a neurologist would be a big disservice to the patient. Ophthalmologists have to make sure the patient does not have an ocular condition like amblyopia before referring him to the neurologist for evaluating the visual symptoms. The neurologist relies on an ophthalmologist to monitor the patients while on treatment. The ophthalmologists are in the unique position to see the nerves and vessels of the CNS in vivo (the optic nerve is an extension of the brain and the central retinal artery has all the characteristics of CNS vessels including having a blood brain barrier).

Sometimes a clinical sign can be due to multiple reasons. Lesions in multiple areas may give a similar clinical sign, e.g. a field defect. The exact localization will then depend on looking for the function of the nearby structures that may be affected. An ophthalmologist should therefore be able to do a general neurology examination to localise the lesion.

One could question the role of a time-consuming examination in this age of imaging. There are three reasons for spending the time doing the examination. First, to order a sensible imaging request one should have an idea of the possible lesion and its location. Second, examination would reveal patient's other difficulties which they may not be aware of or mention, thereby enabling us to give advice to cope with them. Finally, as mentioned in the beginning of this book, who would want to give up a chance to be a Sherlock Holmes and pass the opportunity to do real-life detective work of localisation and diagnosis of the pathology!

Neuroanatomy and physiology is not something that an ophthalmologist revises daily. Even if one were to read up after the last neuro-ophthalmology case seen in the clinic, the subsequent case invariably comes soon after you have forgotten what was read for the previous case! Unfortunately there is no escape from understanding the relevant anatomy and physiology to make a diagnosis and monitor progress. One should not only be aware of all the nerves and centres controlling the visual system but also know about its support systems like the blood supply, coverings, etc.

© Springer Nature Singapore Pte Ltd. 2020
T. Kuriakose, *Clinical Insights and Examination Techniques in Ophthalmology*,
https://doi.org/10.1007/978-981-15-2890-3_15

It is clear from the embryological development of the brain and eye that the eye is an extension of the brain and is the only place in the body were the central nervous system can be seen in vivo.

15.2   Applied Anatomy and Physiology

In processing vision the analogue image of objects in the real world fall on the photoreceptors (first order neurons). Stimulation of the photosensitive chemicals/pigments in the rods and cones sets of a series of chemical reactions which eventually convert the light signals into digital/electrical signals. These signals are partly processed in the retina by bipolar cells (second order neurons), amacrine cells and horizontal cells to be eventually transmitted to the ganglion cells of the retina. The third order neurons (part of the central nervous system) via its axon transmit signals to the cells in the lateral geniculate body (LGB) of the thalamus via the optic nerve, chiasm and the optic tracts. Part of the fibres from the optic tract reach the pre-tectal nucleus without synapsing in the LGB. A part of these nerve fibres are thought to be from a set of light-sensitive ganglion cells (coniocellular) in the retina. The clinically relevant arrangement of fibres in the visual pathway is given in Table 15.1.

The axons in the optic nerve comes from the eye on the same side. The optic nerve reaches the chiasma where the medial fibres representing the temporal field of vision crossover to reach the optic tract posteriorly (Fig. 15.1). During the crossing a small knuckle of fibres from the supero-nasal part of the optic nerve is thought to reach the junction of the opposite optic nerve through the chiasma. This is supposed to be the explanation for defects in the opposite eye in lesions at the junction of the optic nerve and chiasm. The uncrossed and the crossed fibres from the opposite side then travel posteriorly via the optic tract to reach the LGB. In the lateral geniculate body the fibres representing the similar areas of the field from both eyes come together and synapse with the neurons in the LGB in a layered

Table 15.1   Nerve fibre arrangement of visual pathway

1. Macular fibres is temporally located at the optic nerve (ON) head
2. Macular fibres become central on reaching the chiasm
3. Nasal half of the fibres cross at the macula
4. A small knuckle of the upper nasal fibres go to the junction of the ON and chiasm before crossing
5. Upper fibres (lower field) rotate to lie medially in the posterior part of optic tract
6. Lower fibres lie laterally in the LGB
7. Fibres from same region of the field in both eyes come to lie close together at the LGB. The fibres representing the left half of the field from both eyes reach the right LGB
8. After synapsing in the LGB fibres representing lower retina (upper field) travel via temporal lobe to reach the lower half of the calcarine cortex (V1)
9. After synapsing in the LGB fibres representing upper retina (lower field) travel via parietal lobe to reach the upper half of the calcarine cortex (V1)
10. Fibres representing the central field (macula) end in the posterior tip of the occipital cortex
11. Fibres representing peripheral retina end progressively more anteriorly
12. Upper part of the calcarine fissure get fibres representing the upper retina or lower fields and vice versa for the fibres representing upper fields

fashion (Fig. 15.1). The fibres representing both eyes are still not as close to each other in the LGB as compared to the cortex. So much so lesions here do not give as much a congruous field defect like cortical lesions. Some fibres from the optic tract bypass the LGB and synapse in pre-tectal nucleus. These fibres from the light-sensitive ganglion cells sub-serve the pupillary reaction. Some of these fibres get projected to the hypothalamus to help in the circadian rhythm of the body.

Axons from the LGB neurons travel backwards as the optic radiation to reach the primary visual cortex (striate cortex). The optic radiation travel via the temporal (Meyer loop) and parietal lobes to reach the visual cortex. Therefore lesions in these lobes can affect the visual field. The fibres sub-serving the upper part of the field go via the temporal lobe and those sub-serving the lower part of the field go via the parietal lobe. All the fibres from the LGB synapse in the V1 area (postero-medial part of occipital cortex). In the V1 area the macular fibres reach its most poste-

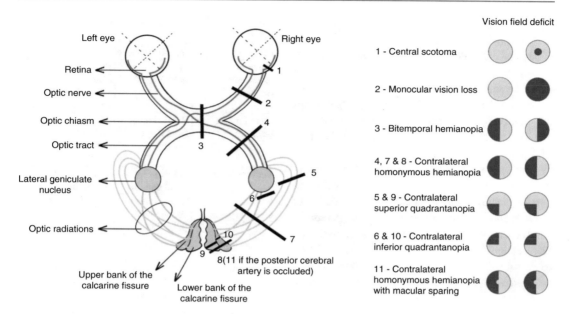

Fig. 15.1 The visual pathway with locations of potential pathology and the field defects they create

rior part. The peripheral fibres are represented more anteriorly in the calcarine fissure. From the V1 fibres project to the V2, V3 and other association areas of V4 and V5 of the parieto-occipital cortex. V2 and V3 areas are visual integration areas and respond to 3D images. V4 area is concerned with colour vision. V5 area deals with movement and direction. This area may be responsible for pursuit movements of the eye. V5 also receives direct input from the LGB.

Visual processing is not fully understood. After the initial processing by the V1 to V5 areas, there are associative areas in the temporal and parietal lobes which does more processing that helps us interpret what we are seeing and where in relation to space we are. The former is subserved by the so-called ventral pathway and the latter by the dorsal pathway.

The fibres representing the corresponding areas in the field of both eyes gradually come closer together as they travel to the visual cortex and is closest at the occipital cortex. Thus, the more congruous (similar) the field defect of both, the more likely the lesion is closer to the occipital cortex. Both eyes send information to either half of the visual cortex. However, the most peripheral temporal fields of each eye is only repre-

sented in the anterior most part of the visual cortex on the contralateral side.

The primary visual cortex is supplied by the distal branch of the posterior cerebral artery (PCA). The posterior most part of V1 area is also supplied by the middle cerebral artery. Thus, the tip of the occipital cortex has a dual blood supply and this is given as the reason for macular sparing that is sometimes seen in PCA blocks. The posterior circulation also supplies most of the centres that control the eye movements. Only the optic nerve and the blood supply to the anterior part of the lll, lV and Vl nerve are supplied by the branches of the internal carotid artery.

Like the visual pathway, the understanding of the intricacies of eye movement control is also far from complete. The control of eye movements can start and be controlled from multiple centres in the brain. For the perfect functioning of a vehicle, besides the start system, we need accelerators, breaks, steering, gears and feedback systems to make midway corrections. It is beyond the scope of this book to describe in any detail the pathways that is currently thought to be involved in all these. Only the pathways that may have relevance in deciphering the clinical findings will be mentioned here. The clinician should be aware that multiple pathways are involved in eye movements and when they are abnormal it may not always be possible to explain the exact abnormality one sees. Recording the abnormality is the first step and one should not be put off if the finding cannot be explained. Since multiple pathways are involved, evaluation of the eye movements can give an insight into pathology in many areas of the brain.

The two main reasons to control eye movements are a) to fix on the object of regard when needed and b) to maintain fixation irrespective of the movement of the object or the self (person).

To fix on the object of regard, first there should be a recognition of the object to fix and a volition to fix on the object. The volition to move the eye (**saccades**) does not always have to be based on an object to be fixed. The person can move the eye up, down or to the sides by one's own will or follow a command.

Once the object is fixed the eye should be able to follow the object if it moves. This is called the pursuit movement and is a **conjugate** movement. Fixation should also be maintained as the object moves close to us or away from us. This is achieved by convergence or inhibition of the same.

If the object does not move but our body moves, then the eye should still be able to continue to fixate on the object irrespective of the position of our body. To achieve this, feedback on the position of the head is given by our vestibular system which is then connected to the eye control systems.

From the previous description it is obvious that the afferent input for initiation of eye movements can be multiple. Table 15.2 gives a bird's eye view of the various eye movements function, the probable centres and pathways involved.

The supranuclear input for saccades come from the parietal lobe (visual reflex) or the frontal lobe (volitional). Afferent from here reach the superior colliculus and basal ganglion. It was originally thought that saccades and pursuit movements had distinct origins. Now it seems there is significant overlap. From the supranuclear centres impulses reach the superior colliculus (SC). From SC messages are relayed in the

Table 15.2 Types of eye movement and its control centres

Function	Initiation centre	Pathways involved
Voluntary lateral gaze (saccade)	Frontal eye field (area 8)	SC, BG, thalamus, brain stem network, PPRF, MLF
Visual reflex (saccade)	Parietal lobe, frontal eye fields	SC, BG, thalamus, brain stem network, PPRF, MLF
Vertical gaze	?Midbrain, basal ganglia	riMLDm, midbrain centres
Following objects (pursuit)	Visual cortex and area 19 (V3, V5)	SC, BG, Pontine nuclei. Cerebellum, vestibular nuclei, sup colliculus
Convergence	?Centre, nasal retinal disparity the trigger	Occipital cortex, LGB, midbrain
Maintaining eye position on moving head	Vestibular nucleus	Vestibular nucleus, MLF, cerebellum

SC superior colliculus, *BG* basal ganglia, *PPRF* parapontine reticular formation, *MLF* medial longitudinal fibres, *LGB* lateral geniculate body

centres in the brainstem and pons to initiate the movement. Message from here go to the cranial nerve nucleus of the third and sixth cranial nerves to initiate the lateral movement. Communication between 3rd CN and 6th CN in the pons occur via the medial longitudinal fasciculus.

The smooth pursuit movement originates in the V5 area of the parietal lobe where it receives input from the primary visual cortex and vestibular cortex. Information from here reach the pontine nuclei, SC and basal ganglia (BG). From the pons projections reach the cerebellum and vestibular nuclei. Smooth pursuit system is a double decussating system and is finally ipsilaterally represented. Impulse generators from the pons and brainstem finally send impulse to the nuclei of the cranial nerves controlling the extraocular muscles.

It is believed that the brainstem controls the vertical eye movements and pons control the lateral movements. Rostral interstitial nucleus of the medial longitudinal fasciculus in the midbrain generate the impulses for vertical eye movement. Midbrain damage can be associated with vertical gaze problems, light near dissociation, skew deviations and convergence retraction nystagmus. The pontine paramedian reticular formation in the pons is thought to generate the impulses for the lateral movement of the eye.

Medial longitudinal fasciculus (MLF) are two bundles of nerves that run from red nucleus in the midbrain to the spinal cord. This is the main internuclear connector channel in the brain stem. Majority of the input into this comes from the vestibular nucleus and shows the importance of this input in the functioning of the other systems. The MLF decussates in the pons. This enables the sixth nerve on one side to work in partnership with the third nerve on the contralateral side to move the eye in unison. If there is a MLF lesion one gets an inter-nuclear ophthalmoplegia. In a right-sided MLF lesion, on attempting to look to the left there is an adduction deficit in the right eye and the abducting left eye has a nystagmus (the lateral movement is initiated in the sixth nerve nucleus and from there message goes to third nerve).

Neural integrators in the brainstem ensures the additional neural input for sustained lateral gaze. The integrators are affected in metabolic conditions like alcohol consumption, anticonvulsant therapy, etc. and is the reason for the inability to sustain lateral gaze and gaze evoked nystagmus. When the gaze cannot be sustained, the eye drifts to the rest position and the patient has to make a refixation movement to compensate.

The ocular motor system takes input from the vestibular system to adjust eye position according to one's position in space. Likewise, inputs from the cerebellum is necessary to make adjustments so that the output matches the input.

The cranial nerves (CN) important for the ophthalmologist are optic nerve (ll), oculomotor nerve (III), trochlear nerve (IV), trigeminal nerve (V), abducens nerve (VI), facial nerve (Vll), and the vestibular nerve (VIII). The optic nerve has been dealt with as part of the visual pathway. The ophthalmologist should have broad overview of the rest of the neuroanatomy too and will not be dealt with here.

The third nerve nucleus is a set of subnucleus situated in the midbrain. All the nuclei except those supplying the superior rectus have ipsilateral innervations. The fibres from nucleus of the superior rectus crossover in the midbrain and join the third CN going out on the contralateral side. So a lesion in the nucleus affects the crossover fibres from the other side too to cause bilateral superior rectus palsy. The third nerve goes through or near the red nucleus to come out ventrally between the cerebral peduncles in the midbrain (Fig. 15.2). It then passes between the posterior cerebral artery and superior cerebellar artery, traverses the subarachnoid space with the posterior communicating artery to reach the petrous bone. The fibres in the third nerve are topographically arranged, the pupillary fibres are located superficially in the dorsomedial part and can be affected easily by compression. It is for this reason that pupillary dilatation is one of the earliest sign of uncal herniation in raised intracranial tension (ICT).

The third nerve at the apex of the petrous bone pierces the dura. It goes along the roof of the cavernous sinus and exits anteriorly passing through the superior orbital fissure and enters the orbit through the annulus of Zinn. Before entering into the orbit it divides into the superior and inferior branches. Superior branch supplies the superior rectus and LPS. All other supply is by the inferior branches. The inferior branch gives off the parasympathetic fibres which synapse in the ciliary ganglion. The fibres to ciliary body is 10 times more than those supplying the pupil and may be the reason for the light near dissociation seen in Adie's pupil.

The fourth CN (trochlear nerve) starts from the trochlear nucleus in the dorsal midbrain just caudal to the third nerve nucleus. Its fibres then crossover in the medullary velum to exit dorsally on the brain stem. It is the only cranial nerve to exit out on the dorsal part of the brain stem. After exiting its fibres sweep around the brain stem to come anteriorly. In the subarachnoid space it travels under the tentorium to reach the insertion of the tentorium. Here it pierces the dura and travels along the lateral wall of the cavernous sinus inferior to the third nerve to exit out of the superior orbital fissure. It enters the orbit above the annulus of Zinn to supply the trochlear mus-

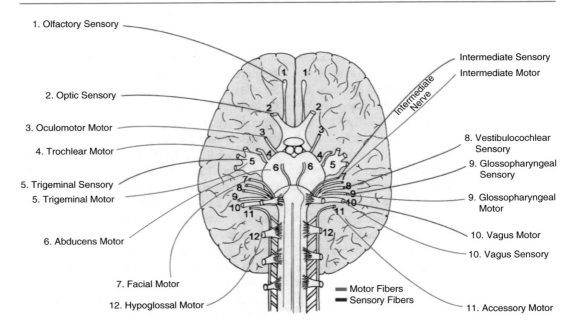

Fig. 15.2 Cranial nerves and it relation at the base of the brain

cle. Trochlear nerve has the longest intracranial course of all cranial nerves and thought to be one of the reasons for damage in head injury.

The sixth nerve (abducens nerve) nucleus lies under the floor of the fourth ventricle in the pons. Fibres from here contains both motor neurons and interneurons (connecting to third CN). Due to this, lesions of the sixth nerve nucleus can also cause gaze palsies. Motor neurons exit ventrally through the caudal pons to enter the subarachnoid space. It traverses this space to reach the clinoid ligament near the petrous tip and pierces the dura here. It enters inside the cavernous sinus (the only CN to do so) and travels forward within it to exit at the superior orbital fissure. Cavernous sinus infection therefore affects this nerve before the other nerves are affected. The nerve finally enters the orbit through the annulus of Zinn.

The fifth nerve (trigeminal nerve) has a sensory and motor component unlike the above three. The nuclear complex of the fifth CN starts in the midbrain and extends up to the cervical spinal cord. The main sensory nucleus (receives touch information) and the motor nucleus (supplies muscles of mastication and other muscles) lie in the pons. The spinal nucleus extends up to the cervical vertebrae 4 level and receives pain

and temperature sensation. Sensory nucleus via the thalamus send messages to the sensory cortex. Likewise, motor nucleus receives inputs form the motor cortex. The fifth CN pass ventrally via the pons and traverses the subarachnoid space to reach the petrous pyramid. There it penetrates the dura to lie on the floor of the middle cranial fossa. The trigeminal ganglion is located here and receive sensation from the V_1, V_2 and V_3 braches of the trigeminal nerve. These branches synapse in this ganglion before sensory inputs are sent to the brain.

V_1 branch runs on the lateral wall of the cavernous sinus and exits in the superior ophthalmic fissure. Before exiting it divides into the frontal, nasociliary and lacrimal branches. The frontal and lacrimal branches enter the orbit superior to the annulus of Zinn. These branches receive sensation from the upper lid and the area of the face above the lateral canthus. The nasociliary nerve enters via the annulus of Zinn and traverses through the ciliary ganglion to receive sensation from the eye through the short and long posterior ciliary nerves. The nasociliary nerve also receives sensation from the nasal mucosa, tip of the nose and ethmoid sinus via the anterior and posterior ethmoidal nerves. This is thought to be the reason for (**Hutchinson sign**) blisters seen on the tip of the nose also in herpes zoster eye disease. V_1 also receives sensation from the meninges of the anterior cranial fossa and part of middle cranial fossa and may be the reason for the pain around the eye in migraine. Complete anaesthesia of the cornea affect the corneal epithelial integrity due to the absence of neurotrophic factors released by the fifth CN.

The V_2 branch exits through the foramen rotundum in the middle cranial fossa. After giving of branches to the various areas in the sinus and mouth, the terminal branch goes through the infra-orbital canal in the floor of the orbit to exit in the infraorbital foramen as the nerve of the same name. This nerve gets sensation from the lower lid and the skin over the cheek. Fracture of the floor of orbit causes injury to the nerve and loss of sensation to the cheek area.

V_3 branch also contains the motor branches and exits through foramen ovale to innervate the muscles of mastication. It also receives sensation from the jaw blow the angle of the mouth. Besides causing loss of sensation on the same side the jaw deviates to the same side in case of fifth CN motor paralysis because the action of the lateral pterygoid which keeps the jaw straight is not there.

Facial nerve (seventh CN) is the last cranial nerve which is closely connected to the eye. This too has a motor and sensory component, but unlike fifth CN it has got a bigger motor component and a small sensory component. The motor nerves arise from the facial nucleus located ventral to the sixth nerve nucleus in the caudal pons. The facial nucleus receives input from the motor cortex. The dorsal part of the nucleus receives input from both the right and left motor cortex while the lateral subnucleus representing the lower half of the face receives input only from the contralateral precentral (motor) cortex. Upper motor lesions therefore affect only the lower half of the face. The facial nucleus receives additional input from the basal ganglion and is responsible for the spontaneous blink rate. Disorders of the basal ganglia like Parkinson disease reduces spontaneous blinks.

From the facial nucleus fascicles go dorsally, winds round the sixth CN nucleus and come back ventrally to exit on the ventral side of the brain stem. The nerve exits on the ventro-lateral side of the pons along with the nervus intermedius which contains the sensory fibres to the anterior third of the tongue. The nerve pass forwards and enter the internal auditory meatus along with the eighth CN. In the petrous bone it gives of the nerve to the stapedius muscle, the sensory nerve to the anterior third of the tongue and the parasympathetic fibres to the submaxillary gland. The motor fibres finally exit through the stylomastoid foramen behind the ears to reach the parotid gland. Sandwiched between the parotid gland it gives of the five branches to supply the muscles of the face.

15.2.1 Autonomic Nerve Supply

Besides the sensory and motor supply, the body also has the autonomic nerve supply. The sympathetic activity originates in the hypothalamus. The sympathetic fibres to the eye and orbit travels down the anteromedial column in the brain stem and the intermediolateral column in the spinal cord to synapse in the cilio-spinal centre of Budge. Postsynaptic second order nerves leave the spinal cord through the ventral rami of C8, T1 and T2 to form the para-vertebral sympathetic plexus. The plexus loops around the innominate artery of the right and subclavian artery on the left near the apex of the lung to reach the superior cervical ganglion near the bifurcation of the common carotids in their respective sides. From the superior cervical ganglion third order neurons go with the internal carotid to the cavernous sinuses. Just before entering the cavernous sinus the branches to the lacrimal gland leaves to form the vidian nerve. The branches to the pupil join the nasociliary nerve in the cavernous sinus and go through the ciliary ganglion without synapses to supply the dilator pupillae which lie in the iris periphery. The fibres supplying the Muller muscle reach there via the frontal and lacrimal branches. These branches also supply the skin around the eye. Anhidrosis and ptosis are clinical features of sympathetic dysfunction (Horner's syndrome) caused due to the disruption of the sympathetic supply.

The parasympathetic supply starts from the brain stem. The fibres that supply the pupillary fibres start from the Edinger Westphal (EW) nucleus which is part of the third CN nuclear complex. Input to this nucleus is from the pretectal nucleus on both sides (the reason for simultaneous pupillary reaction in both eyes). EW nucleus receives input from pupillary fibres in the optic tract which bypasses the LGB to reach there. EW nucleus receives inhibitory and other input from areas of the brain like the hypothalamus, reticular activating system, etc. It is this that causes pupillary constriction during sleep and change in pupillary size with emotions. The parasympathetic fibres travel in the third nerve (lying on its surface) to reach the orbital apex where it enters the orbit in the nasociliary nerve. The parasympathetic nerves goes via the inferior branch of the nasociliary nerve and leaves it to reach the ciliary ganglion where it synapses with the neurons in the ganglion. Postsynaptic fibres leave via the branch supplying the inferior oblique to reach posterior ciliary nerves. It pierces the sclera and reaches the ciliary body to supply the ciliary muscles for accommodation and the sphincter pupillae muscle for pupil constriction.

Para sympathetic fibres to the lacrimal gland originates in the superior salivatory nucleus. It receives input from the fifth CN and hypothalamus. Fibres from here run with the nervus intermedius to join the seventh CN and runs with it into the petrous bone. In the petrous bone these fibres go via the greater superficial petrosal nerve, vidian nerve and come out via the foramen rotundum to enter the pterygo-maxillary space. Here fibres synapse in the sphenopalatine ganglion. Postganglionic fibres reach the lacrimal gland via the inferior orbital fissure.

15.3   History Taking

There are special points in history taking one needs to keep in mind when dealing with a patient with neurological symptoms. Some time spent talking about general stuff like weather, politics, etc. will give a clue to the thinking process of the patient. One should reconfirm the history from a relative as memory, consciousness, etc. may be affected in these patients. This reconfirmation may have to be done without the presence of the patient at times. History of alcohol dependence, sex with multiple partners (to rule out sexually transmitted disease), etc. will need tact to elicit the true story. A useful rule when taking history is to take seriously the more bizarre and unusual symptoms patients describe. There will be a temptation to ascribe it to functional or imaginary causes! Patients may not volunteer symptoms like hallucination or such bizarre symptoms and may need directed questioning. When patient complains of decreased vision, the onset and character should be explored. When there is a history of diplopia one should ask if the diplopia is present even if one eye is closed (monocular diplopia). The position of the two images and the gaze in which diplopia is maximum gives us clues as to the muscles/nerves involved. As mentioned before the ultimate aim of history is to make a provisional diagnosis or a set of differential diagnosis. A directed examination based on one's clinical suspicion will make the life of a clinician and patient much easier.

15.4   Examination of the Optic Nerve and Fundus

Examination of the vision, colour vision and fields is integral to examination of the optic nerve and is discussed in the chapter on vision examination (see Chap. 4). Looking for a relative afferent pupillary defect can sometimes be the only sign of optic nerve disease and suggest early asymmetrical function of the nerves in the two eyes. Examination of the disc is the next important thing in assessing the optic nerve and technique is described under the section on fundus examination and glaucoma (see Chaps. 13 and 14). As ophthalmologist, in the clinic the disc is usually examined binocularly with the slit lamp. This and the indirect ophthalmoscope examination offers a larger field of vision and stereopsis unlike the direct ophthalmoscope. The stereopsis enables us to actually see the elevation and the oedema rather than the just the blurring of the disc margins seen with the direct ophthalmoscope. Blurring and elevation of disc margin is best seen in the upper and lower poles of the disc. Since the nerve fibres are already crowded in the upper and lower margins of the disc, any oedema there causes significant elevation of the margin and also blurring. The down side however is that in normal people this crowding makes the margin less clear compared to the nasal and temporal margins. Clinicians have therefore suggested that blurring of the nasal margin of the disc is a better indicator for papilloedema (disc oedema due to raised intracranial pressure). While there are no studies comparing these two positions, it is likely that the blurring of the superior and inferior margins is a more sensitive test and the nasal margin blurring is a more specific test for the diagnosis of papilloedema.

Other findings suggestive of early papilloedema is a cup that becomes smaller and the neuro-retinal rim pinker than normal. The veins on the disc also appears more dilated and tortuous in papilloedema.

When the disc oedema gets worse, all margins gets more blurred and elevated. With direct ophthalmoscope it becomes difficult to even locate the disc. The retinal vessels tend to come from within the oedematous tissue and there will be splinter haemorrhages on the disc margin. Due to the disc swelling, the surrounding tissues are thrown into folds running parallel to the disc and is called *Patten lines*.

As the papilloedema resolves, the disc may become pale if the oedema was chronic. The disc gets a muddy colour and appears to have some fibrous tissue on the surface. Disc oedema can be due to inflammatory causes like optic neuritis or neuroretinitis. Therefore examining the vitreous for cells especially in front of the disc becomes important. Looking for retinal vasculitis should also be part of this examination. Retinal vacuities appears like sheathing of the vessels. Colour of the neuro-retinal rim is another feature that needs to be evaluated. Normally the central cup and the temporal rim looks paler than the rest of the neuro-retinal rim (Fig. 15.3a). If the rim also becomes pale, one should suspect pathology. The region of the pallor should be noted as it gives an idea of the aetiology. For example, a pallor in the form of a bow tie affecting the temporal and nasal part of the optic nerve is suggestive of a chiasmal compression as seen in pituitary tumour. It is important to know that the disc looks pale in patients who are aphakic or pseudophakic because the normal blue filter of the natural lens is absent. The additional blue colour in aphakia gives a more whitish colour to the disc. If the disc is pale, it is suggestive of optic atrophy. In pri-

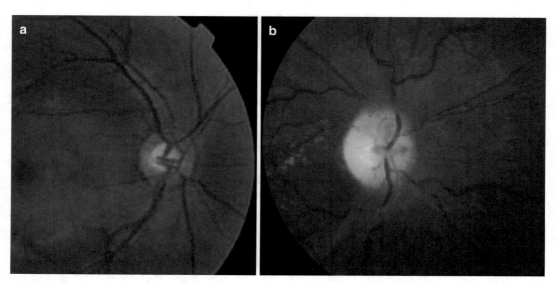

Fig. 15.3 Normal optic nerve head (disc) (**a**) and pale disc (**b**) secondary to papilledema

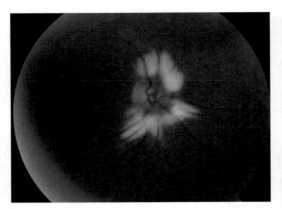

Fig. 15.4 Myelinated nerve fibres on the disc

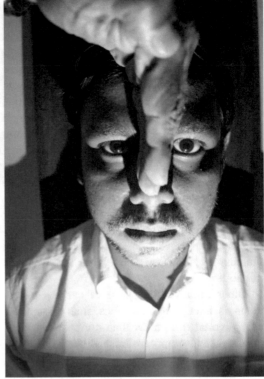

Fig. 15.5 Illuminating from below at the level of the chest to make pupil more visible in pigmented eye

mary optic atrophy (due to a primary optic nerve disease) the disc margins are sharp and the disc is pale. In consecutive optic atrophy (secondary to papilloedema) the disc is more greyer, with the surface of the disc appearing dirty due to the resolved oedema and gliosis (Fig. 15.3b).

Ruling out disc oedema can be difficult. If there is venous pulsation of the central retinal vein in a patient with suspected disc oedema, one can rule out disc oedema.

High hypermetropia with small crowded disc and patients with myelinated nerve fibres can mimic papilloedema. The latter is easy to make out because the myelinated fibres look very yellow and is usually localised (Fig. 15.4). Appearance of the disc can be subjective. When in doubt it is best to do a FA to rule out disc oedema. Leaking and staining of the disc is suggestive of disc oedema.

15.5 Pupil Examination

Chapter 11 also deals with the examination of the iris and pupil (the space formed by the surrounding iris). The long and complex pathway of the nerve fibres sub-serving pupillary reaction both within and outside skull make it amenable to be affected by multiple neurological problems. Pupil reaction is an objective test of visual function without the need for patient cooperation. It is these characteristics that make the examination

of the pupil in neurology useful. One has to keep in mind that ocular causes can also cause pupillary abnormalities. Due to the importance of pupil examination, it is worth repeating some salient features of its examination in neurology patients.

In coloured patients it is difficult to make out the pupillary margins due to lack of contrast between the black pupil and brown iris. To see the pupil well it may be useful to ask the patient or clinical assistant to shine a torch from below the nose so that scattered light illuminates the iris without inducing a pupillary reaction (Fig. 15.5). The patient should be asked to look at the distance when the pupils are inspected. Difference in the size of the pupil between the eyes (anisocoria) if any should be the first thing noted. Difference of up to 1 mm may be physiological. If significantly different, the next thing is to figure out which is the abnormal pupil. For this the pupils should be re-examined in bright light and very dim light. If the anisocoria increases in bright light, then the larger pupil is the pathological. If anisocoria is more in dim light, then the smaller pupil is the pathological one. Presence of ptosis should be looked for in anisocoria. If there is associated ptosis, then that is the affected eye (ptosis with constriction of pupil is Horner's syndrome and ptosis with dilated pupil is third nerve paresis). If anisocoria does not change with illumination, then a local cause should be suspected (drug induced, trauma, Holmes-Adie pupil, physiological, etc.).

In the extremes of age (infancy and old age) the pupils are very small and examination of pupillary reaction can be difficult. This should not be mistaken for any pathological conditions.

Once the size of the pupil is assessed one should look at the pupillary reaction. Pupils react to light and also to near viewing as part of the accommodative reflex. Examination of the pupillary reaction is best done in a very dimly lit or dark room with the patient looking at a distant target of a dimly lit red light. This relaxes the accommodation and causes maximal pupillary dilatation. Once the pupil is fully dilated, a focused torchlight is shown into each eye one after the other to see if the pupil constricts to light shown directly into the eye. This is the direct pupillary reaction. Along with contraction the speed of contraction should also be noted; a brisk contraction of the iris with the pupil reaching to about 3 mm or less in diameter suggests a normal pupillary reaction. If the light of the torch being shown is scattered, one should place the palm of the hand between the nose to prevent light reaching the opposite eye (Fig. 15.6). If direct reaction is absent in an eye, there are two possibilities. Either the afferent pathway (retina, optic nerve, chiasma, optic tracts, etc.) has a pathology or the efferent pathway (third CN, Iris tissue) has an issue.

Rarely, lesions affecting the tectum of the midbrain can compress the pupillary reflex fibres crossing the periaqueductal area and abolishes the light reaction in both eyes. This is associated with preserved vision and loss of upward gaze (Parinaud syndrome).

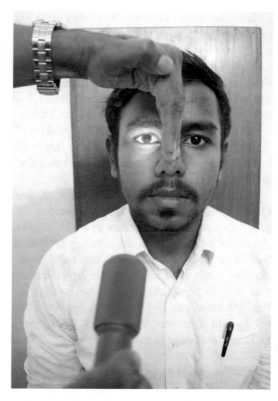

Fig. 15.6 Isolating the light from falling in the fellow eye during pupillary examination

When the retina or optic nerve is significantly damaged, the direct pupillary reaction if present will be very sluggish and incomplete. Sometimes there is an initial sluggish contraction followed by dilatation (escape phenomenon). This is due to the fact that the weak signals are made even weaker by sustained light which bleaches the retinal pigments.

In lesions of the optic tract it has been suggested that focussed light shown from the unaffected half of the field gives a better pupillary reaction (Wernicke pupil) compared to the opposite field. This test is more theoretical and is not really worth doing because it is very difficult to elicit this sign due to light scattering within the eye. There is no point trying to elicit it after the field test shows a homonymous hemianopia and imagining a Wernicke's pupil because there is no virtue in eliciting a sign which has no role in changing your post-test probability.

It is also useful to remember at this stage that pupillary reaction is also sub-served by light-sensitive ganglion cells that directly go to the Edinger Westphal nucleus to sub-serve pupillary reaction. Patients with intact ganglion cells and no vision (due to photoreceptor destruction) at all may still show a weak pupillary reaction. Patients with cortical blindness will have a normal pupillary reaction as the fibres subserving the pupillary reaction only goes up to the LGB and does not go to the cortex.

If direct reaction is present in both eyes, then checking for consensual reflex (checking for pupillary reaction in the fellow eye when light is shown in one eye) does not give any additional information. If, however, one eye pupil is not reacting, then while shining the light into the non-reacting pupil the fellow eye can be observed for consensual reaction. If present, then the efferent system is at fault in the non-reacting pupil and not the afferent system. On the other hand, if consensual is also absent, then the afferent pathway including the optic nerve and the retina could be at fault. This can be confirmed if there is a consensual reaction in the said eye when light is thrown into the other eye. It is not a must to do consensual reaction after the direct reaction because the information got from consensual pupillary examination can be deduced by checking for a relative afferent pupillary defect (RAPD). In pigmented eyes the lack of contrast makes checking consensual reaction with an additional torch a laborious task.

Relative afferent pupillary reaction (RAPD) can sometimes be the only sign of optic nerve pathology. To check for RAPD patient should be looking at the distance in a dim room. The walls of the ever shrinking consultation room often hinders distance viewing. A better instruction would be to ask the patient to look at the ceiling. This will give a more consistent distance viewing. Focussed light is now shown into one eye from below the pupillary border and patient's pupillary reaction and size is noted. After the pupil has stabilised (takes 2–3 s) the light is quickly swung to the fellow eye by passing the torch below the nose to the opposite side and light shown from below. Besides the ease of doing the test an additional advantage of shining

the light from below is that the same part of the retina (upper retina) is illuminated in both eyes. By asking the patient to look up the examiner standing in front of the patient will not hinder the patients view. One needs to shine the light in the first eye for 2–3 seconds till the pupil stabilises because in normal patients as soon as the light fall into one eye both pupils constrict. Immediately after the constriction there is a mild dilation of the pupil and then a smaller constriction before it stabilises. This stabilization after the initial constriction and dilatation takes 2–3 sec. If one moved the torch to the fellow eye too quickly we will catch the fellow eye dilating as part of the initial pupillary constriction and mistake it as an afferent pupillary defect. In normal people as soon as the torch is moved quickly to the fellow eye there may be a small additional constriction of the pupil or it remains the same. If on the other hand there is any dilatation it indicates there is an afferent pupillary defect in the eye that had the light directed on it. This means that the afferent pathway of the eye which is dilating when light is shown in it is affected compared to the fellow eye. This also means if both eyes are equally affected by the disease there will be **no RAPD**.

15.5.1 Examination of Pupil in Special Neurological Conditions

Light near dissociation: To check light near dissociation, classically once pupillary light reaction is checked, the patient is asked to look at the distance for the pupil to relax. Then patient is asked to look quickly at the pencil/pen kept in front of the eye near the nose. In normal patients one can see the pupil constrict in both eyes along with the convergence of the eye. There are neurological conditions where the light reaction is absent/markedly decreased in both eyes but the convergence (accommodative) pupillary reaction is present. **Argyll-Robertson** pupil is the classical prototype of this defect. However this is not specific and a similar picture is seen in diabetes, encephalitis, pinealomas, etc. The pupil here however is not so constricted as seen in the classical neuro-syphilis where Argyll-Robertson pupil was first described. Though it was initially postulated to be due to specific destruction of light reaction pathway it does not explain the pupillary constriction seen. Another explanation is that the accommodative pupillary fibres are more in number and stronger. When a lesion affects both, all the light reaction fibres get affected while some of the accommodative pupillary reaction fibres still remain. It is for this reason there is **no clinical condition where the convergence reaction is absent and light reaction is present**. So if light reaction is present there is no need to check pupillary reaction for near. In the distant past reverse Argyll-Robertson pupil has been described. Here the associated convergence of the eye is absent and sign is due to pre-tectal lesions.

15.5.2 Use of Pharmacological Agents to Localise Lesions

To distinguish third nerve lesions due to denervation at or distal to ciliary ganglion in conditions like Holmes-Adie pupil from more proximal lesions, one can use 2% methacholine drops. Due to denervation hypersensitivity, patients with lesions in the ciliary ganglion will show pupillary constriction. Patients with third CN lesions will not show any constriction because the acetylcholine esterase will hydrolyse the methacholine.

In sympathetic lesions affecting the pupil (Horner's syndrome) localising the site of lesion can be done with pharmacological agents. It is easier however to see the associated symptoms these patient have to localise the lesion. For example, patients with lesions distal to the superior cervical ganglion will not have anhidrosis because the fibres to the vessels of the face leave before that. Central lesions will affect the sweating of the entire side of the body. Cranial and sensory nerves involved may indicate the site of lesion.

Lesions distal to the superior cervical ganglion cause post-denervation hypersensitivity. Dilute adrenaline (1:1000) drops will cause a significant dilatation in these patients. In patients with more central lesions dilute solution will

have no effect because the amine oxidase present in the nerve endings of these patients break down the adrenaline.

Cocaine drops, on the other hand, blocks the action of amine-oxidase in patients with more proximal lesions. The adrenaline present along with amine-oxidase then causes the pupil to dilate.

Since chemical tests are difficult to organise and there are better imaging methods to localise and characterise lesions, these tests are more of historic interest than of any clinical value now.

15.5.3 Examination of Pupils in an Unconscious Patient

Examination of the pupil in unconscious patients is also done with a torch like in other patients. It can give a clue to the aetiology. Since the eye of the unconscious patient is closed if needed the help of an assistant can be sort to keep the lids open while examining the pupil. Alternatively the examiner can use his thumb and middle finger of one hand to pry both eyes open and shine the light using the fellow hand.

Majority of patients with no history of trauma and having a symmetrically reacting pupil have a metabolic cause for the coma.

Pupillary size, symmetry and reactions should be noted. Opiate overdose causes a constricted pupil but so does pontine haemorrhage. Presence of other CN palsy should also help in the diagnosis. Relatives should be asked about the use of any topical drops in the eye that may affect pupillary size or reaction, e.g. pilocarpine (pupil constriction) and atropine (pupil dilatation).

Since pupil size is an important parameter to monitor an unconscious patient, use of dilating drops to examine the fundus should be avoided if possible.

15.6   Visual Field Examination

This has been described more fully in the section on visual function examination (see Chap. 4). With the advent of automated perimetry, the role of the classical examination of the field (confrontation method) or one of its variants is restricted to people who cannot do an automated field test or need an assessment of the field by the bedside or facilities are not available. While the specificity of confrontation test (provided the patient is not a malingering) is high, its sensitivity is far from desirable. In other words, it is easy to miss a field defect when it is present if one did only a confrontation field test. To make it more sensitive using a red 2 mm ball mounted on a thin needle/pin as a target helps. Since confrontation field testing is crude test, trying to compare the field of the patient with that of the examiner does not give too much clinically useful information both for diagnostic and for follow-up purposes. When using red-topped pins, the red colour appearing drained out (lighter) in one half of the field compared to the other indicates optic pathway pathology.

Non-organic field defect like in hysteria or malingering is best made out using different targets in an automated perimeter. The fields remain the same irrespective of the size of the target in normal people. In malingering the field will keep on getting constricted with each test. If one has access to tangent screen one can demonstrate that in malingering the size of the field remains constant irrespective of the distance of the patient from the chart. Normally the size of the field on the tangent screen gets smaller as one comes closer to the chart.

15.7 Examination of the Cranial Nerves (CN)

An ophthalmologist is an operating physician and should be able to do a neurological examination that will help him make sense of the ophthalmic manifestation of the neurological condition. Besides CN examination one should be able to do an examination of the motor, sensory and cerebellar systems.

15.7.1 Olfactory Nerve (CN 1)

Meningiomas in the anterior cranial fossa can compress the optic nerve in addition to affecting the olfactory nerves. Trauma and orbital lesions may also affect the olfactory nerves.

To examine the olfactory nerve on one side, the patient is asked to close his eyes and then the nostril on the opposite side is closed by pressing the alae of the nose against the septum with a finger. A familiar odour like coffee powder, lime, etc. is presented near the nose but not close enough that the patient feels something is being kept near the nose by way of touch, air movement, noise, etc. The patient is asked to respond if he can smell anything at all. Care should be taken not to use chemicals like spirit, ether, etc. which can irritate the mucosa and thus the fifth nerve, which again will make the patient respond. Identification of the odour is not a must as that is a higher function related to memory, familiarity with the substance presented, etc. If the substance can be identified, it is an added information.

Watering from only one nose especially after trauma is suggestive of a cerebrospinal fluid (CSF) rhinorrhoea.

15.7.2 3rd (Oculomotor), 4th (Trochlear) and 6th (Abducent) Cranial Nerves

The third, fourth and sixth cranial nerves (CN) supplies the muscles that move the eye. The eye movements are controlled with the help of the higher centres to aid our visual needs. To examine the cranial nerves we use uni-ocular eye movements called ductions. When performing ductions, if one is not comparing the eye movement with the fellow eye, closing the fellow eye will help elicit the full range of eye movement in the eye of interest. Besides ductions one should check for binocular eye movements of versions (both eye moving together in the same direction) and vergence (both eye moving in the opposite directions). These movements are controlled from centres in the brain stem and above and need to be tested.

Diplopia is a common complaint in patients with muscle nerve palsies. Provided the affected eye is not the fixing eye, the outer of the two images seen by the patient belongs to the paretic eye. The image separation becomes more in the direction of the action of the muscle. This can therefore be a surrogate method to find out paretic muscle.

The third nerve in addition to supplying the extra ocular muscles also supplies the constrictor pupillae muscles which contracts the pupils. Due to the drooping of the eyelid in third CN lesions diplopia may be absent. The extent of the normal eye movement is described in the chapter on ocular motility (Chap. 8). When examining the ocular motility it is good to ask the patient to report diplopia when they notice it. Often the perception of diplopia is more sensitive in revealing a faulty eye movement.

The third CN supplies all the extraocular muscles except the lateral rectus and the superior oblique. When examining the third nerve if the pupil is covered by the lid, then the lid is raised to examine the ocular movements. The position of

the eye is noted first. An eye with third nerve palsy is deviated out (exotropic) and down. The patient is then asked to look at a target like the tip of a pencil and asked to follow it. To be sure all positions of gaze is being checked it is best to start moving the target from the centre to the six cardinal positions of gaze, the up and down movement and note the extent of movement (Fig. 15.7). In the cardinal positions of gaze the action of muscles can be isolated and examined independently without the influence of other extra ocular muscles. Limitations of eye movement is noted. In third nerve palsy there may be varying amounts of limitations of eye movement in all directions except the lateral gaze. In the lateral gaze patient may even report the disappearance of diplopia if the sixth CN is normal. The amount of ptosis and the action of the levator palpebral superioris (LPS) is also noted. The ptosis is assessed by looking at the difference between the height of the palpebral fissure in the two eyes.

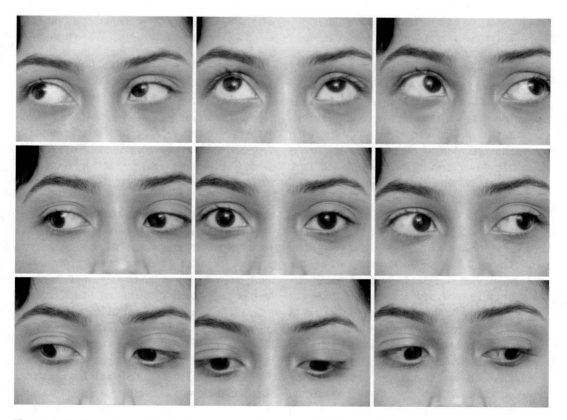

Fig. 15.7 Positions of gaze to test for eye movements in neuro-ophthalmology disorders

In isolated third nerve palsy the difference in the inter-palpebral fissure (IPF) height is enough to assess LPS function. This could be measured with a transparent millimetre scale for objectivity and followed up (see Chap. 7). Since the cornea will not be central in both eyes, the region of the largest fissure height can be measured. From the anatomy it should be clear that at the nuclear level the supply of the LPS comes from a central nucleus. So in nuclear lesions, all the extraocular muscles supplied by the third CN on the same side are affected and so is the LPS muscle on the contralateral side.

The limitation of the eye movement can be quantified by the prism cover test described in the chapter on ocular motility. Hess chart (beyond the scope of this book) is another equipment that can be used both for diagnosis and quantification of the palsy and is based on the perception of diplopia by the patient. This gives a more objective assessment.

Examination of the eye and lid movement should be followed by examination of the pupil. The direct pupillary reaction will be absent due to the efferent pathway pathology. Both direct and consensual pupillary reaction will be absent on the side of the third CN palsy. If the pupillary reaction is intact in the presence of extraocular muscle palsy, then the cause of the palsy is probably due to a medical cause, e.g. diabetes mellitus. The pupillary fibres running more superficially is spared by the vascular aetiology in these cases. When there is a complete third CN nerve involvement the aetiology is more likely to be a surgical cause like a tumour, trauma, etc.

A **fourth CN palsy** could be isolated or be seen in association with a third nerve palsy. The fourth CN or Trochlear nerve supplies only the superior oblique muscle. In isolated fourth CN palsy the patient will have a head tilt to the opposite side along with the depression of the chin to compensate for its muscle action namely intorsion and depression. On examination of the eye position, the affected eye will be deviated up. This deviation is exaggerated (confirmed by prism cover test) when the patient looks to the side opposite to the eye with the palsy and when the head is tilted to the same side. There will also

be a limitation of eye movement in the down gaze when the eye is adducted.

In the presence of third CN palsy the downward movement of the eye in adduction cannot be tested. The patient is therefore asked to look down with the eye in the abducted position (the position of the eye when sixth CN is intact); while doing so, the examiner looks at the radial vessels at the medial limbus to see if the eye is intorting which is the action of the superior oblique muscle in this position. Absence of intorsion suggests that the fourth nerve is also affected along with the third nerve.

The **sixth CN** (supplying the lateral rectus muscle) **palsy** is clinically suspected when both eyes are open and the patient is turning the face to one side (the side of the palsied nerve) to compensate for the lack of movement of the lateral rectus on that side. Sometimes the patient may close one eye (usually the eye with palsy) to keep the head straight. The head is turned or the eye is closed to avoid diplopia. In abducens nerve (sixth CN) palsy the affected eye will be esotropic (provided it is not the fixating eye). When examining the ocular movement one finds that abduction towards the side of the palsy is limited due to the paralysis of the lateral rectus.

After examining the three cranial nerves supplying the eye, in patients where it is indicated the vergence and versions should be tested. The vergence tested is convergence were the patient is asked to look at a pencil kept about 75 cm from the nose and brought slowly to the tip of the nose.

Versions are of two types. Saccadic movement and pursuit eye movements.

Saccadic movement helps us fix at a point we want to see and facilitates shifts of gaze from one point to the other. To check saccadic eye movement index fingers of the two hands of the examiner is kept about 75 cm apart (see Chap. 8). Patient is now asked to look at the left and right fingers alternatively while the examiner notes the ability to shift the gaze, the speed at which it can be done and the ability to maintain the fixation. The frontal eye fields of the frontal lobe mediates the saccadic eye movement to the opposite side, lesion on the right side prevents saccadic movement to the left. Fibres from the frontal eye fields

Fig. 15.8 Frontal eye fields along with the pathways controlling saccadic eye movements

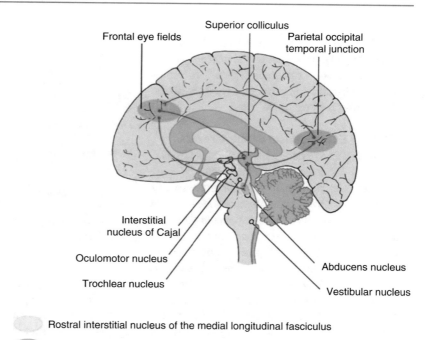

Frontal eye fields

Superior colliculus

Parietal occipital temporal junction

Interstitial nucleus of Cajal

Oculomotor nucleus

Trochlear nucleus

Abducens nucleus

Vestibular nucleus

Rostral interstitial nucleus of the medial longitudinal fasciculus

Paramedian pontine reticular formation

project to the pons along with the cortico-bulbar fibres to control the lateral gaze (Fig. 15.8). Projections also go the parietal lobe which can override the action of the frontal eye fields. The vertical saccade seems to be controlled by pathways via the basal ganglion and areas near the superior colliculus. Defects in the horizontal saccades can be picked up only in the acute phase of the disease as compensatory mechanisms kick in within a couple of hours. Some patients with diffuse frontal lobe disease will not be able to look voluntarily to any side and may have to move the head instead of shifting the gaze. Diffuse disease is also complicated by dementia. Some patients will not be able to hold the gaze and will have nystagmoid movements. Saccades can also be tested in the vertical direction by the examiner holding one hand up and the other down. The patient is then asked to alternatively move fixation from one hand to the other.

Pursuit eye movements are tested by asking the patient to look at a target like the tip of a pen kept about 40 cm from the nose. Once fixation is locked on to the target the patient is asked to follow the target as it is moved keeping the head fixed. The examiner may need to hold the head so that only the eye moves. The target is moved from the centre of the patient to one side first and then the other. The same is then done for the up and down position. The speed of movement, inability to move to any particular side, abnormal movements and a lag in the movements are all noted. The efferent pathway of the pursuit movement starts in the visual cortex and then relayed to the parieto-occipital cortex from where there are projection to the midbrain and pons. The parietal cortex of the left side moves the eye to the right side. Some projections also go to the frontal eye fields. Due to the involvement of parietal cortex there is usually a hemi-field defect too. Care should therefore be taken to move the target for pursuit slowly within the seeing half of the field so that it does not go out of view. This examination is also a good time to look for inter-nuclear ophthalmoplegia (abduction of the eye on the side of lesion present but limited abduction of the fellow eye). Optokinetic nystagmus (see Chap. 16) can also be used to check for parietal lobe function. Here a cloth or drum with 2 cm broad vertical stripes drawn 3 cm apart is moved slowly horizontally across the field of vision. Normally a person will follow a strip till it moves out of sight and then refixes on the next strip causing an optokinetic nystagmus (OKN). In lesions affecting, parietal lobe, cerebellum and vestibular pathway this OKN can be affected.

15.7.2.1 Examination of Nystagmus

Examination of a patient with nystagmus (spontaneous rhythmic eyeball movement) can be quite confusing. The movement is sometimes so fast that it is difficult to decipher the components of the movement. Sometimes the components that took time to decipher in the first place seem to change character with change in position of the eye! Added to this is the poor localising value of this sign since multiple aetiologies including drug intake can give nystagmus. All this however does not absolve the clinician of examining the patient and recording the findings. Nystagmus of recent onset may be accompanied by the patient complaining of objects in front of the eye shaking (**oscillopsia**). This also causes a decrease in vision.

To examine, the patient is asked to look straight ahead and the eye is observed in the resting position. Spontaneous movements should be observed. If spontaneous movements are observed, one should note if the movement is in the horizontal direction, vertical direction or the eye is oscillating in the antero-posterior axis (torsion). Torsional nystagmus can be easily missed with the naked eye and one may need to observe the radial vessels near the corneal limbus with a slit lamp to visualize the eye intorting and extorting alternatively. Fundus examination may also reveal fine intorsion movement as evidenced by the movement of the retinal vessels. The following points should be noted when examining a patient with horizontal nystagmus. Is the nystagmus pendular (oscillating slowly with equal speed to both sides), jerky (has a fast phase in one direction and a slow phase in the other) or rapid in both directions (saccadic oscillation)? In jerk nystagmus, by convention, the nystagmus is said to be in the direction of the fast phase (corrective eye movement). The pathology however causes the slow movement. The other points to be noted are the variation of nystagmus with eye position

Table 15.3 Types of nystagmus and probable localising potential

Type of eye movement	Possible pathology
Unilateral pendular eye movement (Heimann-Bielschowsky phenomenon	Blind eye from child hood
See-saw nystagmus	Parasellar lesions
Downbeat nystagmus	Cervicomedullary junction
Upbeat nystagmus	Posterior fossa, medullary region lesions
Convergence retraction nystagmus	Pretectal region
Periodic alternating nystagmus	Cerebellar nodules

(congenital nystagmus does not change character even in up or down gaze), positions in which the nystagmus is absent (**null point**), change in nystagmus or induction of nystagmus on occluding one eye (**latent nystagmus**), does both eyes move together (**conjugate**) or separately (**disjugate**), monocular or binocular and finally change in the beating pattern of the nystagmus over time (**periodic alternating nystagmus, intermittent nystagmus**). Some types of nystagmus are associated with head nodding (**Spasmus Nutans**) and should be looked for. When looking for change in nystagmus with eye position, the gaze should not be taken to the extreme as that in itself can produce **gaze evoked nystagmus**. Gaze evoked nystagmus in otherwise normal patients do not have any significance unless it is asymmetrical.

When confronted with a vertical nystagmus one should look to see if it is a downbeating or upbeating nystagmus and if there is a see-saw pattern. Patterns of nystagmus that may have some localising/diagnostic value (sensitivity/specificity about 50%!) is given in Table 15.3. It is this poor localising value of nystagmus that prevents clinicians from trying to observe this clinical sign in any great detail.

Nystagmus should not be confused with **nystagmoid movement** one sees in extremes of gaze. In extremes of gaze the gaze cannot be held long especially in older people and the starts to slip towards midline. Soon there is a corrective movement to put back the eye in the extreme gaze position giving rise to a nystagmus like movement. This is normal and has no clinical significance.

15.7.3 Trigeminal Nerve Examination

The fifth CN or trigeminal nerve has both a sensory component and a motor component. Besides helping in localising the lesion, the sensory supply to the ocular surface is important for the health of the cornea and ocular surface. Neurotrophic factors mediated by the sensory nerves from the fifth CN are important in maintaining the integrity of the corneal epithelium. The facial sensation is checked in the three areas supplied by the three main sensory braches of the Trigeminal nerve (ocular, maxillary and mandibular). To examine the sensation, patient is touched with a wisp of cotton on the hand and made to understand what it feels like to be touched with it. Then he is instructed to count each time he is touched with the cotton wisp. The patient is then asked to close his eyes and count each time he feels the cotton touching his face. The area above the eyebrow, chin and anterior mandible area is touched one after the other on both halves of the face and patient asked to count. If the patient responds to all the touches correctly, he should be asked if there is a difference in the touch sensation between the two halves. Examining the corneal sensation again with a thin wisp of cotton (made by twirling the cotton between the thumb and index finger) is useful to assess the effect on the cornea and also to make the test more sensitive. In the past with the intention of avoiding the transmission of herpetic infection from one eye to the other it was suggested different ends of cotton tip be used. With the current understanding of herpetic keratitis this is not needed. If the right cornea is to be tested, patient is asked to look up and to the left and the cotton tip is brought from the temporal half so that patient is not intimidated by the approaching cotton tip. The response to the corneal touch is the blink reflex mediated by the seventh CN. If the seventh CN is also affected on the same side, the blink reflex (a bilateral reflex) on the contralateral side is looked for.

The motor part of the fifth CN is tested by asking the patient to open his mouth. In case of palsy the jaw moves to the contralateral side due to the underaction of the muscle that would have kept the jaw straight when the mouth is open. Feeling for the tightening of the masseter muscle when clenching the teeth is another method to assess the motor function of the fifth CN.

15.7.4 Facial Nerve Examination (Seventh CN)

The seventh CN supplies the muscles of facial expression and lid closure. It also has a sensory component that mediates taste from the anterior half of the tongue. The upper part of the face is supplied by both the cortical hemispheres. So supranuclear lesions of the seventh CN will affect only the lower half of the face. To examine the seventh CN, observe the blink of the patient as you are talking to the patient. On inspection, the wrinkles on the forehead will be less on the side of the palsy, the palpebral fissure will be wider and the blink will not be effective on the side of the facial nerve palsy. The angle of the mouth will be deviated away from the side of the lesion along with the drooping of the angle of the mouth on the affected side. Ask the patient to close the lids tightly. In complete lower motor neuron palsy, the eye on the affected side will not close. If the eye can be closed, try to pry open the lids on both sides. If there is a palsy, the eye will open easily on the affected side. To examine the lower half of the face the patient is asked to close his mouth and blow. The cheek should balloon out equally on both sides without escape of air. One could also gently tap on the cheek to see if the air can be held in and not allowed to escape. If the muscles are weak air may escape when the weaker side is tapped. If only the lower half of the face is affected, then the lesion is an upper motor lesion (UML). Getting the patient to smile naturally is the best way to elicit the deviation of the angle of the mouth in a UML lesion. Checking the taste sensation on the anterior half of the tongue is difficult in the eye clinic and does not really add any value for the ophthalmologist in the examination of the facial nerve.

15.7.5 Examination of the Audio-Vestibular Nerve (Eighth CN)

The eighth CN has an auditory (hearing) and vestibular (balance) component. The clinical testing is usually done for the auditory component and is enough for the ophthalmologist. The simplest way to assess hearing is to rub the thumb and index finger at the external auditory meatus (external ear) of each ear separately and ask patient if he can hear it. If he can, then the same auditory stimulus is presented in both ears simultaneously using both the hands. If there is a difference in perception, it should be noted. If one has access to a tuning fork, then a vibrating tuning fork of 512 frequency is kept at the centre of the forehead. If the patient can hear the vibration on both sides equally, then one waits for the sensation to cease. When the patient cannot hear the sound of the tuning fork on the forehead, it is kept in front of both the ears one after the other and the patient should be able to hear it. If on placing it on the forehead the patient says he can hear it only on one side, then the auditory nerve on the opposite side the affected. Moving the tuning fork to the ear is to make out if there is hearing impairment due to a conduction defect (external and middle ear pathology) and is not really concerned with the ophthalmologist.

15.7.6 Examination of the Ninth and Tenth Cranial Nerve

The last four cranial nerves rarely concerns the ophthalmologist. In some rare cases, lesions affecting the orbit and the sinuses may also affect these nerves as they traverse the base of skull.

The ninth CN (glossopharyngeal) and tenth CN (vagus) can be examined together. The patient is asked to open the mouth and say 'Ah' if the upper palate does not move on one side

and the uvula is deviated to the opposite side, then the vagus CN which supplies the muscles of deglutination on that side is paralysed. With the mouth open touch the posterior pharynx on either side of the midline one after the other with a cotton bud, a resultant gag reflex on either side suggests that the ninth CN which mediates the sensation from that side is intact. Due to the discomfort of this test, it is not commonly performed.

15.7.7 Examination of the Accessory Nerve (11th CN)

To examine the 11th CN the patient is asked to turn the head to one side against the resistance offered by the examiners hand to the cheek. The force exerted on the examiners fingers should be equal on both sides in normal patients. Weakness of movement to any one side suggests a palsy of the opposite side 11th CN which supplies the sternocleidomastoid muscle. In patients where the neck cannot be turned, the patient can be asked to shrug the shoulders against resistance offered simultaneously by the examiner. Weakness on one side suggest palsy on that side.

15.7.8 Examination of the Hypoglossal Nerve (12th CN)

To examine the 12th CN that supplies the muscles of the tongue, one asks the patient to protrude the tongue. One should look for wasting of the tongue, fasciculation and deviation. If the tongue deviates to one side, the nerve on that side is affected.

15.8 Motor, Sensory and Other Examination of the Body

Complete examination of the motor and sensory system of the rest of the body is not indicated as far as an ophthalmologists is concerned. A quick comparison of the motor function on both halves of the body will be useful. The patient is asked to grip each of the hands of the examiner with his hands and squeeze tightly. The difference in the grip strength should be noted. It has to be kept in mind that the grip of the left hand may be weaker in a right-handed person. A marked difference in the grip strength suggests motor weakness.

Eliciting the knee jerk reflex is easy and can be done in the office. The test is useful in conditions like Holme-Aide pupil were there may be an isolated absence of the knee reflex. The patient is asked to sit on a chair and keep one leg over the other so that the feet is off the ground. The clothing over the knee need not be exposed if the contour of the leg can be made out. The knee cap can be palpated over the clothing and the patellar tendon can be identified just below the lower border. Strike a knee hammer over the tendon and look for the reflex forward thrust of the lower leg. Both legs are tested this way. For a quicker comparison of the two knees one can get the patient to rest both the thighs of the patient on the examiner forearm so that the thigh can be lifted to get the feet above the ground. Needless to say, this technique will not be possible in heavy patients! If the patient is lying down, with the knee flexed and some support under the knee, the knee jerk can be elicited.

Testing skin sensation can be done like was described in fifth CN testing. The sensation that is useful to test for the ophthalmologist is the **posterior column sensation**. Many neuro-ophthalmology conditions have an associated

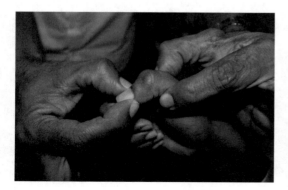

Fig. 15.9 Holding the joint of the patient when examining for joint sensation

posterior column pathology and will need it to be ruled out. In conditions like Vit B deficiency, Neuro-syphilis, Friedreich's ataxia, demyelinating disease, etc., the joint position sense carried by the posterior column is affected. The joint sensation is tested by asking the patient to close his eyes so that there is no visual clue to the joint position. The thumb joint of the feet and hand is usually tested. Thumb and index finger of one hand of the examiner should steady the proximal part of the inter-phalangeal joint (Fig. 15.9). The distal phalanx is then moved up or down and patient asked to tell the position of the distal phalanx. The phalanx should be held on the sides and not on the flexar or dorsal aspect as the pressure of the movement may give a clue.

Proprioception (Joint sensation), vestibular function and visual sensation are the three senses required for one to stand upright. At least two of three functions should be present to prevent one from falling.

The **Romberg's test** uses this requirement to diagnose posterior column dysfunctions. This is a test that is easy to do in the clinic by the ophthalmologist.

The first step of this test is to ask the patient to stand with both the feet together and observe. He should be able to stand without taking a step for at least 30 s. If that is possible, then the next step is to ask the patient keep both his eyes closed for another 30 s at least. If he sways and starts to fall within 30 s, the test is positive. With eye closed if posterior column is also not functional, then the vestibular mechanism alone is not enough to keep the balance and the patient will fall. Care must be taken to have your hands around the patient to prevent him from falling.

Cerebellar function: Patients with cerebellar dysfunction will not pass the first part of the Romberg test. To test cerebellar function a finger to nose test may be the easiest for the ophthalmologist to do. Here the examiner asks the patient to touch his own nose with the index finger and then reach out and touch the examiners finger kept within the patients arm length. This should be done by both hands of the patient. Normal people should have a smooth movement from their nose to the examiner's fingertip. If the finger of the patients sways trying to make corrective movements and finger goes past the target point (pass pointing), then the cerebellum on the side the hand was not steady is diseased.

Muscle tone: Signs of extra-pyramidal symptoms seen in conditions like Parkinson's disease may give clinician the clue to an underlying cause of dry eye. In advanced cases the walk of the patient, pill rolling tremors of the hand and poor smile will give the diagnoses. Examination of the tone of the muscles will show rigidity in patients with Parkinson's and can be elicited by a complex movement of the patients forearm. The examiner holds one hand of the patient in his own hand like one gives a shake hand. The other hand of the examiner grasps the patient's forearm at the elbow. After asking the patient to let the upper limb loose in a continuous movement now adduct and abduct the upper arm (using the hand on the elbow) and at the same time extend and flex the elbow and pronate and supinate the forearm using the other hands of the examiner. Normal patients will not show any stiffness in the movement. The examiner should learn to do this manoeuvre on colleagues before trying it on patients to get a reliable result. The movement of all three joints simultaneously in the test will prevent the patient trying to be helpful and move the joints for the examiner.

15.9 Examination of the Unconscious Patient

Since no psychophysical test is possible in an unconscious person, the first thing in the eye examination is to gently pry the eye open with the index and thumb of one hand look for the integrity of the globe especially in patients with trauma. One should also look for sub-conjunctival haemorrhage and its extent if present. Next look at the position of the eye to see if it is deviated to any side. In acute cortical damage the eyes look towards the side of the lesion because the intact side move the eye to the contralateral side. In brain stem lesion the eye looks away from the side of the lesion. **This deviation is only seen in the acute phase as compensatory mechanisms kick in later.** Slow rowing eye movements may be seen in some comatosed patients and is indicative of intact brainstem ocular motor pathways. Lesions of the pons may show a sudden downward movement of the eye with slow return to the midline (ocular bobbing).

The pupillary reaction checks the pupillary reflex pathway which bypasses the cortex. If the pupil is reacting well, then the path from the eye to the optic tract to the Edinger Westphal nucleus, to the pretectal nucleus and back into the third nerve is intact. An RAPD should be checked if the pupil is not very miosed. In patients whose pupil is miosed this may be difficult to do. The fundus examination of these patients should be done without dilating because pupillary reaction is one of the monitors for brain stem function. A direct ophthalmoscope should be used to assess the posterior pole to look for disc oedema and haemorrhages. If there is no contraindication to dilate the eye, then an indirect ophthalmoscopy is a better method to evaluate the fundus. Eye movement can only be examined by taking advantage of the vestibular pathway which control the eye movement. If cervical injury is not the cause for the loss of consciousness, then a dolls eye manoeuvre is done to elicit eye movement. Here both eyes are pried open and the patients head is moved quickly to the right and then left; the eye will continue to be in the straight head position due to the compensatory mechanisms of the vestibular system if intact. If the eye moves with the head, then either the nerves controlling the eye movements (efferent pathway) or the vestibular system (afferent) is at fault. In case of cervical trauma, if there is no bleeding in the ear, then one can irrigate cold or warm water into the external ear and look for eye movements. The convention currents produced by the cold or warmth in the semicircular canals is the afferent input for the compensatory eye movement. These tests are rarely done and may in fact be of little values now with the current advances in imaging of the brainstem area.

15.10 Examination of Neurology/Neurosurgeon Referred Case

The neurosurgeon often needs only a formal assessment and documentation of the vision including fields. When operating in and around areas along the visual pathway from optic nerve to the posterior cortex, they need a documentation of the fields and this should be done using an automated field analyser. Sometimes a visual evoked potential testing may also be in order. In patients with proptosis the neurosurgeon may want a functional assessment of the extraocular muscles along with the fields and vision.

The neurologist will need much more detailed assessment from the ophthalmologist. An idea of the thinking of the neurologist will help the ophthalmologist tailor his examination better and give sensible report.

In a patient with headache even if the symptoms are very suggestive of a migraine, underlying trigger factors like an uncorrected refractive error or a latent hypermetropia should be ruled out. The ocular motility should be done and muscle balance checked to make sure that a muscle imbalance or convergence weakness is not the cause of the headache.

In patient with suspected papilloedema confirmation of the diagnosis if needed with fluorescein angiogram should be done. Ophthalmologist may also need to follow up the papilloedema in patients with chronic diseases like benign intracranial hypertension (BIH). In patients with suspected optic neuritis, diseases like arteritic and non-arteritic anterior ischaemic optic neuritis may have to be ruled out. Evidence of retinal vasculitis (suggestive of systemic vasculitis including syphilis), vitreous cells, pan uveitis, etc. may have to be ruled out is cases that may warrant it. Sometimes vitreous cells are present only in front of the optic nerve and one should look for this with a 3 mirror or 60 D lens. Since the optic nerve and retina is an extension of the brain, there are many neurological diseases with manifestations in the eye. Often ophthalmologists help is sought to look for the ocular manifestations of the underlying disease. The phakomatosis group of disorders may have the same hamartomas on the retina or iris. Retinal pigmentation is associated with diseases like myotonic dystrophy, chronic progressive external ophthalmoplegia (CPEO), Friedreich's ataxia, etc. Cataracts may be associated with myotonic dystrophy, Wilson's disease, etc. CPEO and myotonic dystrophy are associated with ptosis. A Kayser Fleischer (KF) ring may have to be ruled out in a patient with extrapyramidal symptoms.

A complete examination of the eye is required to give a good feed back to the neuroscience colleagues who manage the parts of the nervous system the ophthalmologist do not!

One does not have to be a neuroophthalmologist to do a good ocular examination described here to support the neurosciences colleagues.

16.1 Introduction

Swetha Sara Philip and Thomas Kuriakose

Examination of a child, especially the very young, is many a young ophthalmologist's nightmare. It is a daunting task; as examining a child is not only dealing with the child but also with the parents/primary caregiver (the word parent will be used to denote both for all future references). For a child, a doctor (including an innocent ophthalmologist) is synonymous to a 'white-coat vampire', hurting and drawing blood. It may take a few visits to the hospital, especially for very young children, before they become cooperative, provided their visits each time has been pleasant. It is the experience the child has during such a hospital visit that makes a difference to the outcome of the clinical assessment. A fruitful consultation would help cut short the number of repeated hospital visits for the child and the parent. An ophthalmologist must remember that in today's world most parents are working and so cannot afford to miss work frequently for hospital appointments.

The general ambience, a waiting area that is well lit with brightly coloured wall, cartoon characters painted on the wall, lots of toys, colouring material, cartoon movies showtime, friendly receptionist and a short waiting period can enhance the 'window of opportunity'. A hungry or sleepy or sick child or a lifeless waiting room and a boring doctor will not yield a useful consultation.

A friendly examination room (Fig. 16.1) should have in addition to routine ophthalmic equipment such as the slit lamp and ophthalmoscopes; toys, audio-visual units, *rewards* (candies/stickers) to give and some free space to move around—to pick and prod. It is also a good idea for the ophthalmologist to have few colourful occluders, some loose prisms, age appropriate visual acuity charts such as the Cardiff visual acuity cards or Lea paddles or Kay pictures in his/her armamentarium. Presence of too many people in the consulting room could be

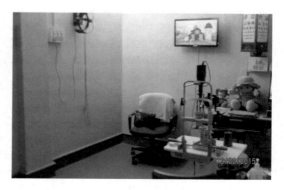

Fig. 16.1 The examination room looking like a child's play room

© Springer Nature Singapore Pte Ltd. 2020
T. Kuriakose, *Clinical Insights and Examination Techniques in Ophthalmology*,
https://doi.org/10.1007/978-981-15-2890-3_16

overwhelming and that may need to be addressed. The ophthalmologist must be an entertainer and at the same time be a confidante. He must always have new tricks up his sleeve to keep the attention of the child going and at the same time be a friend in whom a teenage patient would confide without being judged.

One has to keep in mind that unlike in adult patients, here it is the parents who are more worried than the patient (child). Does my child see? How much does he see? Why is my child's eye watering? Why are his eyes red? Why is he always complaining of headache? Why does he bump into things? The list goes on. The clinician has to adopt an empathetic approach to answer the volley of questions shot at him by the anxious parent.

16.2 Ice-Breaking Session

The last person a child wants to see is a doctor. Pretending to be primarily interacting with the parent may put the child at ease as he enters the room. Touching the child such as stabilising the head and lifting the upper eyelid for retinoscopy and fundus examination should be done at the last stages of examination and all assessments that can be done without touch should be completed before. The offer of a reward like a chocolate/sticker to the younger children, once the family is settled, may aid the process of 'breaking the ice'. As you (clinician) interacts with the parents, you may get a feel of the personality of the child. Efforts must be made for the young patient to feel like the STAR of the day especially if they are the types who enjoy that attention. Greeting them as they walk into the room and then engaging with them in some sort of general conversation like 'how are you today?' or 'what did you have for your breakfast' or 'what's your best friend name' or 'what's the favourite cartoon character' or 'which class/school are you studying in', etc. is worth the time. In a preverbal child or infant, a smile on the clinician's face or a play with a toy could be a useful exercise. Allowing a child to be comfortably seated on his parents lap or sitting away

from the clinician will aid in a satisfactory assessment. Without making it obvious, the assessment of the child begins the moment he walks into the examination room. The attitude, the ill-fitting spectacles, the facial expression, the gait... all have a story to tell. It is the keen observation of the clinician along with history taking that will unveil the story. **As the child is being entertained in a conversation or is playing with the toys, it is a must for the clinician to observe the child** for any additional clue he may get to aid in the diagnosis like watery eyes with matted lashes, ptosis (does the ptosis improve when the child is yawning or feeding on a bottle suggesting Marcus-jaw winking phenomenon), proptosis (does the proptosis increase with the child sneezing or bending to pick up a toy), facial expressions (like squeezing the eyes to see something at a distance or holding the target close to face), strabismus, nystagmus (wobbly eyes), etc.

16.3 History Taking

Breaking the ice should imperceptibly fuse with history taking. For a successful examination, history taking as a **diagnostic tool** for children assumes even more importance because the primary carer usually the mother may have noticed signs like intermittent squint that may not be obvious in the clinic. If the child is verbal and cognitively sound, it is important to explain to the parents and the patient (child) that first the history will be elicited from the patient (child) and then from the parent. The child can be asked more direct questions like 'what brought you/your family here today?' or 'what do you think is wrong with your eyes?' It is important to request the parents to hold back their input/prompting at this stage and inform them that they will be given an opportunity after the child has been spoken to. Once the child has answered all the questions posed to him by you, it is nice to inform the child that you are now shifting the question session to the parents. The parent now can be encouraged to corroborate the child's history and to get more information if any. This information from parent augments the clinical examination of the child, especially in an uncooperative child. Unlike in the adults, the history taking in children, especially in preverbal and preschool children, is challenging and needs lot of patience and skill to unearth the 'hidden diagnosis'. The history taking in children is akin to an FIR (first information report) of the parent. In olden days it is used be the mother who was the best historian. But in this day and age, with changing roles in the family, history should be ascertained from the primary caregiver. The history given by them may be coloured by their personal prejudices and those of the community around them. Making sense out of a third party history can be challenging. In older children, while it is tempting to believe the primary caregiver's history in its entirety, it is pertinent to go back to the child again and question the history or observe the reaction on the child's face. Important information like being bullied about wearing spectacles or complaining of poor vision to get spectacles to look 'intelligent' or actual story of how the injury occurred is made known when the ophthalmologist is the child's confidante. To this end it may be worthwhile talking to the child and parent separately.

In children in whom objective examination of vision may be difficult to elicit such as children with profound visual impairment, developmental/intellectual delay or cerebral palsy, the parent should be enquired about the child's visual capability, such as can the child see things on the floor, do they bump into things, does a dimly lit room immobilize the child, etc. Family history is an essential part of history taking, as many ophthalmology conditions such as retinitis pigmentosa and retinoblastoma have a genetic basis.

In some situations, like in children with special needs, it may be a good idea to review certain documents like neuroimaging before the child comes into the examining room, as some parents get upset seeing the amount of brain damage on the radiology scans. If the child has been referred for an ophthalmology check, it is important to understand what the referral is for before the child walks into the examination room.

16.4 Clinical Examination

Based on the information from history and cues from observation, the clinician should now move on to carry out the specific clinical examination. It may be useful at this point to look at old photographs of the child when relevant. **Remember, shorter the examination time, better will the cooperation from the child. A re-examination after reviewing the photos may not be a luxury especially in a child**. Once a thorough examination is done, it is worthwhile to review previous photo again to get an idea as to how the condition has changed over time especially in a child with ptosis or squint.

16.4.1 General Examination

A general assessment is more important in a child to make the relevant ocular diagnosis. As mentioned before this also should start with the child's entry into the room. Facial dysmorphia, facial asymmetry and the shape of the head including its circumference can give a clue to the diagnosis. A microcephaly may be the cause of the decreased visual function. A craniostenosis face will explain the proptosis. Hair colour and protruding chest wall seen in homocystinuria will give a clue to the cause of dislocation of the lens. An extra toe on the leg may suggest an underlying retinitis pigmentosa. These clues to the overall systemic condition of the child can have a bearing on the ophthalmic diagnosis.

Assessment of General Behaviour: Is the child hyperactive, easily distracted, inattentive, very talkative, nervous, uncomfortable in a crowded consultation room or has a speech/communication problem?

Body language: Is there a compensatory body/head movement to overcome an impaired visual function? An abnormal head position may be a sign of hidden squint or nystagmus. Abnormal ocular movement or head thrust or head nodding may be suggestive of conditions like ocular motor apraxia or spasmus nutans. Is he in pain or any kind of discomfort?

Assessment of visual behaviour: Some children may respond better if the room lights are dimmed suggesting cone dystrophy/profound visual impairment. A child may appear blind but can still easily navigate, is this malingering or is there a higher visual dysfunction? Photophobia may be due to allergy or corneal pathology or does it warrant investigation; a question the clinician needs to ask himself.

16.4.2   Vision Assessment

Trying to make an assessment of the vision in a child is not easy. This being a psychophysical test, the cooperation of the child is important. Capturing the auditory attention of the child, if required, by quietly whistling or making animal sounds or playing a nursery rhyme on the phone would increase the cooperation of the child.

The problem with assessing a young child's visual acuity compared to that of an adult is the fact that it is more subjective depending on the level of cooperation of the child. Even the acuity cards that have been validated in scientific literature give only a subjective assessment. Unlike in the adults, it may not always be reproducible even in the same sitting. Child responding to the clinician's facial expression or reaching out for toy/stationery on the table or reacting to the light from a torch gives a rough idea of the visual potential. This could be further fine-tuned by assessing the visual acuity using age-specific visual acuity cards or strategies with one governing principle that *initial assessment* especially in infants, preverbal and developmentally challenged children should be *binocular*. This not only keeps the child comfortable during examination but also provides information on the functional vision of the individual.

Uni-ocular testing is done as the next step, if possible, starting with the eye thought to have the better vision. The examiner can use his thumb or occluders to check for uni-ocular vision and employ a hide-and-seek type of game like 'peek-a-boo' or 'being a pirate' to assess the vision. If the palm of the examiner or parent is used as an occluder, care should be taken that gaps between fingers should not act as pinholes for the child to see through. Resenting occlusion of one eye or a difference in the speed or surety with which the child reaches for an object when one eye is occluded can help to rule in or rule out poor vision. Some children may be cooperative enough or may want to use their own palm to occlude one eye, which can be allowed provided it is ensured that only the palm and not the fingers is used. The clinician must be alert about the fact that children can easily fool the examiner by peeking or memorising the vision chart.

Sometimes occlusion of one eye can produce nystagmus or worsen one if already present. This nystagmus can decrease the visual acuity. In such situations it is better to use high plus lenses as occluders, so that there will be still some cues from the peripheral field that will dampen the nystagmus and help with visual acuity testing.

Visual acuity assessment involves three types of visual acuity:

- Detection acuity: to judge the presence or absence of the target.
- Resolution acuity: the spatial details contained within the target have been fully resolved, e.g. Lea grating paddle, Cardiff visual acuity cards.
- Recognition acuity: Identification of the target, e.g. Kay pictures, Lea symbols, Snellen's visual acuity chart.

According to the age of the patient, the objective of visual assessment and the facilities available, the clinician has to choose the tests most suited in the clinic for the examination of the day. A general clinic may not be as equipped as a specialised paediatric clinic. So the clinician has to choose from the tests listed below, which will yield the best visual assessment. It is also important to remember that on follow-up, same test/tests are used to assess improvement or worsening. In preverbal children more than the exact quantification it is sometimes more important to get an idea of the presence or absence of visual defects, squint, etc. If the child has a refractive correction in place, then vision should be tested with it in the first instance.

16.4.3   Vision Testing in Children Without Any Developmental Delay

16.4.3.1   3–6 Months of Age

The following sequence of testing is followed or modified depending on the clinic situation.

- *Fix and follow*: Here the target (a toy or the examiner's face) is brought in front of the child who is on the parent's lap. Keeping the child's head steady by the parent, the target is moved in the horizontal and vertical plane. Look for the child's ability to fix and follow the target. This also gives a gross idea of any abnormal ocular motility and any areas of inattention.
- *Bruckner's test*: This screening test is done using direct ophthalmoscope held at a distance of 50 cm and 3 m from the patient. It is a quick way to assess visually significant media opacities, large refractive errors or abnormal ocular alignment based on the brightness of the light reflex (light reflected from the retina hitting the examiner) in the child's pupillary area. It must be done in a semi-dark room before pupils are dilated. The child is comfortably seated on the parents lap. The examiner views through the peephole of the ophthalmoscope and throws light into both eyes simultaneously. The child is encouraged to look into the light. The red reflex from the child's eye is studied. In normal children, the red reflex from both eyes will be equal and bright. Brighter reflex is seen in deviated eye or in eyes with higher refractive error. In deviated eyes (squint), more light is reflected off the non-macular retina because the RPE pigmentation is less compared to the macula. With the refractive errors the emerging light gets focussed (in myopia) or appear to get focussed (in hypermetropia) and so, appears brighter. If there is media opacity the reflex will appear dimmer as the opacity cuts off the reflected light. The Bruckner's test has been reported to have a sensitivity of 91% and specificity of 72% in picking up significant refractive errors. In addition, this testing acts as prelude to the testing conditions that is to come and also gives clue to the examiner, the level of cooperation of the child and how to proceed with the remaining examination.
- *16 prism dioptre test*: Amblyopia (lazy eye) is one of the commonest causes of visual impairment in children. In infants and young children the routine visual acuity tests to detect amblyopia may not be easy to administer. Using prisms is a fast clinical procedure with minimal equipment to check for monocular steady fixation. The assumption is that when a child with amblyopia is given a choice, he fixes on the target with the sound eye. Conversely, a child without amblyopia will fix with both eyes. The test is performed under binocular condition with a prism (10, 12 or 16 prism dioptre) introduced base down, in front of one eye while the child is encouraged to look at a target held at 25–33 cm (16-prism dioptre prism is ideal to observe refixation movement). This induces vertical movement of a good eye due to the shift of the image upwards forcing the fellow eye also to move upwards to look at the image. If there is amblyopia and no re-fixation, no refixation movement is observed. This prism occlusion is repeated in the other eye. This test can be used in older preverbal children suspected to have amblyopia.

16.4.3.2   In children 6 months to 3 years of age

General principle used in this age group is of preferential looking. Here two targets are simultaneously presented, one with patterned target and another blank target with equal luminance. The child will preferentially look towards the pattern target. The targets could be cards or paddles.

- **Lea grating paddles**: *Principle is resolution acuity.* This test is user friendly. The paddles have alternate black-and-white high contrast gratings of different width, ranging from 0.25 cycles per degree to 8 cycles per degree, tested at 57 cm. The test begins with the examiner seated at 57 cm. In one hand is a blank paddle and other hand the grating paddle (Fig. 16.2). Both the paddles are moved and the response of the child must be noted as evidenced by an eye

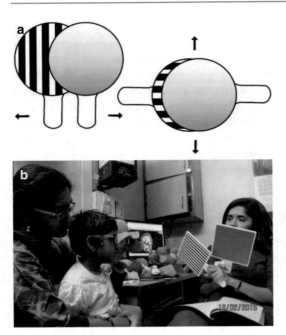

Fig. 16.2 Movement of Lea paddles (**a**) and a child being examined with Lea paddles (**b**)

or head movement. If there is no response, the distance between the examiner and the patient must be reduced. It should be done holding the paddles both in the horizontal and vertical plane. It is important that the clinician moves both the paddles out, equally and at the same time so that difference in attention is only due to the pattern and not due to a difference in the movement of the paddle. The smallest grating the child responds to give an estimate of the visual acuity of the child. It gives the examiner cues of any gaze preference, any quadrants/hemifield of neglect or visual field defect or inattention. It also helps to give ideas to the parents regarding the target size (in terms of width and contrast) that will be of visual benefit to children who are differently abled and to formulate strategies for visual stimulation accordingly.

- **Cardiff visual acuity cards**: *Principle: resolution acuity (vanishing optotypes)*. This test is very easy to administer and is a useful test in preverbal, verbal and older children with developmental delay. The test consists of single and simple recognisable pictures (fish, car, train, boat, house and duck). The target

Fig. 16.3 Cardiff card to check vision

picture is outlined as a white band bordered by black bands (Fig. 16.3). The width of each black band is half the width of the white band. All pictures are on a neutral grey background. If the target lies beyond the subject's resolution limit, it merges with the background and simply becomes invisible. The testing is done at 1 m. The pictures are located either on the top, bottom, right or left side of the card. Either the child's eye movement or verbalising or pointing towards the picture records the response. Although it is a resolution acuity testing, it also helps with detection (preverbal and children with developmental delay) and recognition acuity (verbal children). The flaw with this kind of testing is that it overestimates visual acuity in amblyopes and the low contrast between the picture and the background makes this test redundant in children with severe neurological brain damage.

16.4.3.3   In children 3 years to 5 years of age

Who are usually verbal and exposed to kindergarten training:

- **Kay pictures**: *Principle: recognition acuity.* The Kay pictures have eight familiar pictures (duck, apple, boot, apple, cup, truck, house, fish and clock) that the child can name or match. It is a high contrast visual acuity card using logarithmic progression of acuity levels. The pictures have a stroke width equivalent to Snellen's letters. It comes as crowded and uncrowded charts, which is useful to detect problems with crowding especially in children with amblyopia. It has a bit of learning curve especially for children who have yet not started kindergarten to first recognise the pictures and then match. They get easily distracted and lose interest. Another flaw in this test is that it is developed in the west and so some of these pictures are not very familiar to children in the other countries. Hence it is better to familiarise the child with the template of the pictures available and ask them to name the pictures, some say 'round' for 'clock' or 'coffee' for 'cup'. This should be accepted, provided the same terms are used throughout the examination. This test is done at 3 m and Snellen's equivalent of visual acuity can be derived from it.

16.4.3.4   In children > 5 years of age

who are now into full-time school:

- **Snellen's visual acuity chart**: *Principle: recognition visual acuity.* It is a high contrast black-and-white chart with letters or numbers. It consists of 11 lines with black and bold letters or numbers. Each letter subtends an angle of 5 min of an arc and each letter part subtends an angle of 1 min of an arc at the fovea. There are many flaws in the construction of this visual acuity chart yet is the most popular visual acuity testing chart among the medical practitioners (see Chap. 4).

16.4.4   Vision Checking for Children with Developmental Delay

In children with developmental delay a combination of tests needs to be done to assess the visual potential of the child. More than the age of the child, the visual acuity tests are based on the mental status of the child.

In infants and neonates in whom vision is a concern and there is no response to light or any toy/face, it is important to get some idea of vision and the following test could be useful.

- **Optokinetic nystagmus (OKN)**: OKN is a bilateral, reflex nystagmus that has a slow phase (pursuit) and correcting quick phase (saccade). Classically this nystagmus occurs in response to movement of the visual environment as it occurs when one is travelling in a train and looking at the passing objects. The eye follows one object for some time and then refixates on a new object in front. For testing in older children, adults with brain lesions and malingers an OKN strip consisting of alternating white and black stripes (size of which is dictated by the potential vision of the patient) on a long ribbon of cloth is used. With the head held steady, the strip is slowed moved from right to left or vice versa and the eye movement noted. Normally in patients with good vision and normal OKN reflex pathway, the slow phase will be towards the movement of the strip and the fast phase in the opposite direction. While OKN depends on directional neural mechanism, the OKN in newborn is strongly believed to be of a subcortical mechanism and is asymmetric to begin with. At 2–3 months of age, the infant views monocularly, OKN is driven by motion in the temporal-to-nasal direction. As the neonate grows, binocularity develops and OKN becomes more symmetrical resulting in the development of nasal-to-temporal OKN. This is an input of the descending pathway from cortical binocular neurons. In children less than 1 year of age and also children with neurological insults, moving the strip may not give any definite results. In such children, a way to elicit OKN is done by holding the child vertically with the head

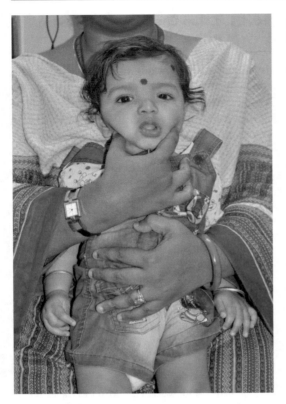

Fig. 16.4 Holding the child to elicit nystagmus. Assistant has to turn quickly with the child before the assessment

supported (Fig. 16.4) and moving the child quickly to right or left side. Normally, the eyes deviate in the direction of rotation first and then jerk back under the influence of vestibular reflex causing a nystagmus and this nystagmus is dampened in 2 s due to the fixation reflex of the child. If the vision is very poor, this dampening does not occur and the nystagmus continues for a longer time. Thus, the ophthalmologist gets the information that in spite of cortical brain damage and the child though appears blind, has some visual potential that needs to be stimulated. Spinning the child to the right and left one must look for symmetry of ocular movements.

In children who can be propped up and show some response to torchlight, Lea grating paddles would give an idea about the size of the strips child responds to. Cardiff cards or Kay pictures should be used to get a better idea of the visual acuity, the effect of crowding and contrast on vision. These

pieces of information are important for formulating visual stimulation strategies for these children.

- **'Mirror test':** *Principle: resolution acuity.* This test is simple and useful in children <9 months old and was found to have some correlation with visual acuity cards. In children, unsettled for an examination, the mirror can be turned into a fun game like 'peek-a-boo' or 'touch the person in the mirror' giving the examiner an idea of child's visual potential. It is also found to be useful in children up to the age of 3 years, with moderate developmental delay and reasonable head control, when the clinician feels that Lea and Cardiff test are not uncovering the vision potential the child possibly has. It is a good way to show parents of such children, the distance till which the child can maintain his visual attention and suggest rehabilitation strategies accordingly. The infant is held close to a wall-mounted mirror and look for the response the child gives on seeing his own reflection. The child is then slowly moved away from the mirror till fixation/interest is lost as evidenced by turning the head or eyes away from the mirror.

Evaluation of accommodation—dynamic retinoscopy: In conditions like cerebral palsy, where children have accommodation deficit, evaluation of accommodation is necessary for the management. This test helps to assess the child's ability to accommodate. It requires only a few seconds of the child's attention looking at a target suddenly brought into the visual field. Besides looking at the pupillary reaction, the examiner uses a streak retinoscope and assesses the change in retinoscopic reflex as the child shifts gaze from a distant object to the toy that is suddenly brought front of the eye. When the target is brought into the child's field of view at near, the examiner notes the constriction of the pupil and change in the retinoscopic reflex becoming more myopic.

16.4.5 Ocular motility examination

Ocular motility assessment in children is similar to that of the adults and is also discussed in the chapter on ocular motility (see Chap. 8). The important points to explore in history are birth history, family history and previous use of spectacles or patching therapy. Before motility examination one should look for facial asymmetry and abnormal head posture. If abnormal head posture is present, tests for binocular vision should be done before straightening the head.

Motility examination has to be done without the correcting spectacles (glasses) in place as the spectacle frame may obstruct visualising of the target when moved peripherally, thus falsely labelling 'restricted ocular motility'. To stabilize the head, the parent may gently place their hand over the head or hold the chin. **It is important to use a target in the form of a toy and not torchlight. It is said 'one toy one look' as the child loses interest quickly. It is therefore important to have many toys at ones disposal to keep the child focussed.** In preverbal, preschool and developmentally delayed children only VERSIONS may be possible.

Ocular motility has to be documented, including overactions and underactions. Figure 16.5 shows a described method to record deviation. While the recording strategy looks detailed and good on paper, the question one has to ask is— Does such detailed divisions change the diagnosis or management? Is it possible to make such divisions in a child whose co-operation may be difficult? How good is the inter- and intra-observer agreement of such a system of recording? Only a study looking at the questions can answer these. These questions should be asked of all recording systems clinicians come across. Clinicians should put in practice what suits him. A system given in the chapter on ocular motility can also be used.

Stereopsis: Stereopsis is about appreciating depth and 3D images. The standard tests used to assess stereopsis are:

- Titmus fly test
- Lang test
- Frisby test

Fig. 16.5 Method of recording eye movement (duction). Here the right eye is the fixing eye following the movement of the object in front of the patient. The right eyes movement is being tested. (**a**) Medial and lateral movement; (**b**, **c**) supero-nasal and infero-nasal movement

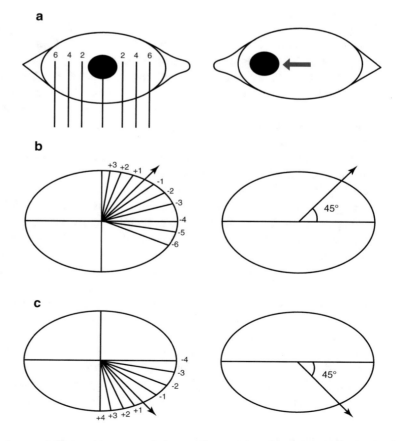

It is important that any adopted compensatory head position should **not** be corrected before checking for stereopsis as the new head position may dissociate the binocularity. Young children (usually <6 years of age) are not able to perform any of these tests well. A lack of understanding of the test or immature stereoscopic vision could be the reasons. Results of these tests depends on the level education, social upbringing, etc. Binocular single vision can be present due to peripheral fusion (due to corresponding retinal points in the periphery) and good central vision or stereopsis need not be present. Even a person with amblyopia with strong monocular peripheral cues will have some grades of stereopsis. The test retest reliability of these assessments has also been in doubt. A more useful test in children would be the 16-prism base out test to look for refixation movement. It provides a gross idea whether stereopsis is present or absent. When the child is looking at a toy, place a 16 D prism base out in front of the right eye. The eye moves to the left and so does the left eye (obeying the Hering's law). The left eye then makes a re-fixation movement to the right. When prism is removed, the eyes move to the right.

Tests like Worth 4 dot test is more applicable to children >10 years as they may be able to appreciate the number and colour of lights (details and flaws discussed Chapter 8).

16.4.5.1   Squint Assessment

When a child is brought to the clinic with complaints of squint, the first question the doctor needs to ask himself is, 'is this a true squint or pseudosquint'. Look at the facial contour, eyelid crease, epicanthal fold and nasal bridge. Before keeping the prisms in front of the child's eye, pull up the nasal bridge to iron out epicanthal fold. One should also look at the position of the corneal reflex (Hirschberg's test). As mentioned earlier, Bruckner's test is also useful. If squint is absent, then ask the parents why they felt so, how often in a day do they appreciate the squint and if it is present even when the child is well and active or more so when the child is sick/sleepy/tired. When in doubt one should also look at old photographs. Carefully look at these photos, even a small angulation of the camera can give a false impression of squint. If squint is present then one will have to proceed with measurement of squint. Place the prisms in front of the child's eyes and same trick of distracting using auditory stimulation or videos or toys have to be used. Krimsky test as described in Chapter 8 should be done in very young children whose attention span is very short or in children with uni-ocular poor fixation. In children who are uncooperative, a combination of Hirschberg's and Krimsky's test would give a rough idea of the angle of squint. Children in whom angle of squint could not be measured in the first visit will require repeated visits. Refractive error should be ruled out as the cause for squint. Cycloplegic refraction should be done in children especially if they have esotropia. A squint examination is never complete without a dilated fundus examination to rule out any retinal cause for squint. If there is a refractive error, it needs to be corrected and the squint has to be reassessed with the refractive correction in place especially before planning a surgical intervention.

16.4.6   Torchlight and External Examination

16.4.6.1   Accuracy of Light Projection

This is difficult in children who cannot comprehend and follow commands. However if a child looks in the direction of the light when it is shown in a dark room it may be a pointer. One has to repeat this three times to look for consistency of response.

16.4.6.2   Eyelid and Orbit Examination

Assessing for ptosis is not as challenging as proptosis. In *ptosis*, measurement of the interpalpebral fissure (IPF) or marginal reflex distance may not be very accurate. What one needs to pay attention to is whether the eyelid is covering the visual axis. If yes, then is there a compensatory head posture to clear the visual axis? If visual axis is clear in the presence of ptosis, amblyopia (lazy eye) should be ruled out. If the ptosis is covering the visual axis, an effort is made to see how it has affected the developing vision. Intervention then becomes imperative to avoid amblyopia.

Assessment of ptosis towards management follows the same principles given in Chap. 7. Measurement of the ptosis can be difficult. Presence of a lid crease suggest some levator palpebral superioris (LPS) function. If a child cannot straighten out an everted lid even after a blink, it means the LPS muscle function is poor. Getting the mother to fix the head while moving the toy to look for eye movements helps. Move the toy down to see if IPF widens in the ptotic eye. If it does, then the ptosis is more likely due to a fibrotic dysfunctional LPS. A Marcus Gunn jaw winking phenomenon can be assessed by getting the baby to suck at feeding bottle or breast. After all the assessments are over, Bells phenomenon can be assessed by lifting the lids in both eyes simultaneously. While doing this, most children will reflexively close the eye, thus aiding in the evaluation.

16.4.6.3 Examination of Proptosis

If proptosis is painful, child will be in distress and further examination should be carried out under sedation/anaesthesia. If it is painless proptosis, then proptosis measurement with exophthalmometer depends on the cooperation of the child but other observations regarding laterality, direction of proptosis, restricted ocular motility, pulsations, thrill and scleral or corneal exposure can be made without causing any distress to the child.

16.4.6.4 Examination of Nasolacrimal duct block (NLD)

A doctor's hand coming close to the face is a cause of panic to many children. Assessment of NLD block can be done without really touching the child. On torchlight examination one can see matting of the lashes on the side of the block compared to the fellow eye. **Dye disappearance test** is very useful in looking for the effectiveness of the tear drainage system. First get the carer to put a drop of topical anaesthetic (proparacaine) into both the eyes of the child. Touch a wet fluorescein strip at the outer border of the eye as discreetly as possible. After 5 min, with the cobalt blue light of the indirect ophthalmoscope examine the tear lake to look for differential clearing of the dye from the two eyes. Normally there is

no dye held in the eye after 5 min. If the child cries after instilling the topical anaesthetic, apply the fluorescein strip as soon as he stops crying. Incessant crying results in the absence of dye in the eye as it gets washed off by the tears. In such children, with the indirect light on examiner's head, look at the nostrils for the presence of the dye in the nose. The tears due to the crying usually makes the nose wet too! After this, the area over the sac region can be palpated to feel the mucocele and reduce it by pressing on the swelling with the idea of teaching carer the massaging technique to aid in the opening of the nasolacrimal duct block.

16.4.6.5 Examination of Pupils

Pupillary reaction in neonates is very sluggish and they have pinpoint pupils. In very young children it is better to examine pupillary reaction in dim lights rather than in completely dark room. After the lights of the room are turned off, dim torch should be turned on and it is important to wait for a few seconds for the child to settle down before beginning the examination. In older children, ask the child to look up at a 'toy' held up by the parent or to 'look up at the ceiling and count the number of blades of the fan' or 'is the fan stationary or working' while assessing pupillary size, shape and reaction. Swinging flash light test to look for relative afferent pupillary defect can also be done with this position of gaze (Chapter 11). The clinician needs to have two torches, one dim for diffuse illumination and one bright to assess pupillary reaction, especially in dark pigmented iris. It is important to look for pupillary reaction even when the room light are turned on. In children with cone dystrophies when the light is brightened the rods become less effective and the cones which is supposed to be more effective does not work. So the pupils dilate instead of contracting in bright light (**paradoxical pupil**).

16.4.7 Ocular (Eye) Examination

This part of the examination really brings out the 'strategist' side of the examiner. This examination involves the child to be seen on the slit lamp (measuring intraocular pressure), indirect ophthalmoscopy and cycloplegic refraction. It is always necessary to explain to the parents what is being done so that they do not get unduly upset when they see their child upset. In children who are older and can understand what is being done, it is important to take their permission to examine.

16.4.7.1 Slit Lamp Examination

Table-mounted slit lamp examination has many limitations as far as paediatric eye examination is concerned. Adjusting the head and chin rest is not sufficient for the small face of a neonate. The *neonate* thus can be mummified (wrapped in a cloth) and held at the slit lamp by the parents/caregiver or a clinical assistant supporting the head, chin and body of the neonate. The eyelids need to be pried open and in some cases may need to use paediatric speculum to pry open the eyelids. If it is *an infant* (Fig. 16.6), the slit lamp examination would involve the child being held horizontally with his head touching the headband, one hand supports the body of the child while the other holds the face ('flying baby' position). Another person can support the legs of the child if needed. This could be a challenging exercise because some children know how to wriggle and proves to *be stronger* than the person holding him.

Slit lamp examination of an older kid may involve using tactics like, 'come I will take a photo with the machine because you have been such a good kid today' or 'come this machine will show your favourite cartoon character' or 'come let me see if you really drank milk this morning' or 'let me see your eyes on this machine

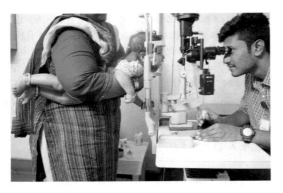

Fig. 16.6 Flying baby position for examining infants on the slit lamp

and I will give you a toy to play with'. For this examination, the child could sit on his parents lap or sit/kneel on an adjustable chair by himself or if tall enough can even stand at the slit lamp. In some anxious children, in order to gain their confidence it is better to show them how slit lamp examination is being done first on their carer. Children who may keep their chin on the slit lamp rest may be inconvenienced by the pointed tip of the applanation plate hitting them and this may have to be removed. When the child is seated on the lap of the carer and the slit lamp is lowered to the height of the child, it can press against the child's thighs and one may need to get the child to spread out his legs to avoid this. Getting the co-operation of the child during the ocular examination depends on the examiner's ingenuity.

Those who cannot sit on slit lamp due to their physical disability or those who have a fear to sit at the 'machine' or parents who do not want their wards upset can be examined with surgical loupes (for magnification) and a bright torch. Portable slit lamp may not be very well suited for an outpatient consultation unless the child is sedated as the examiner has to go quite close to the child to examine and it could be overwhelming for the child.

Getting a measurement of **intraocular pressure (IOP)** in children is the fire test for any paediatric ophthalmologist. This need not be part of the routine ophthalmology examination in children. It should be reserved for children who present with signs and symptoms of congenital glaucoma, juvenile glaucoma, facial haemangiomas or in children undergoing intraocular surgical procedures (cataract surgery, retinal detachment surgery, trauma, glaucoma surgery) and those who are or need to be on long-term systemic steroids (for collagen vascular disorders, bronchial asthma, nephrotic syndrome, etc.) or topical steroids (for allergic conjunctivitis). To measure IOP same strategies are used as with slit lamp examination. The examination technique is described in the Chap. 13 (glaucoma). To calm the child one can fake a measurement in one eye without touching the eye and then go to the fellow eye saying one eye is over and if it is OK to do the fellow eye and then come back to the first eye. In neonates and children who are not cooperative one may have to instil the anaesthetic drops after restraining the child. Portable tonometers like tonopen and Perkin's tonometer are used to check IOP in these children. It may be necessary on occasions to sedate these children to check the IOP. It is important that when the eyelids are pried open, the globe is not pressed upon, as this will give a false high recording of the IOP. While touching the instrument on the ocular surface, care should be taken not to touch the eyelashes as the drops do not anaesthetise the lashes and the chances are that the child may wake up.

16.4.7.2 Dilated Fundus Examination

Dilated fundus examination is usually done to assess the posterior pole up to the equator to look for optic disc pallor, cherry red spots, macular scars, bony spicules of retinitis pigmentosa and retinal hamartomas. The peripheral retinal examination of a child is not of much interest except in case of suspected retinopathy of prematurity, intraocular tumours (retinoblastoma), retinal detachment, and patients with stickler's syndrome or incontinentia pigmenti. This procedure may require some restraining by caregiver or clinical assistant especially in neonates, infants and children with special needs. Examining them on their parent's lap or the pram or their own wheel chair along with satisfying auditory or gustatory inputs is a good way to examine the posterior segment. Children generally calm down when their parents sing to them or talk to them or play their favourite nursery rhyme or give them 'sweet' rewards/soothers when the examination is underway. In older children talking them into showing at the slit lamp usually works especially if they have experienced the slit lamp examination before in the day. If a child needs scleral depression to see the periphery of the fundus, it should be done under anaesthesia (EUA). See Chapter 14 for examination of the retina.

At the end of the consultation when all the queries are answered there is nothing is more gratifying than to see a happy child and equally happy and satisfied parents. A wave, a handshake, a hug, a high-five or a flying kiss is a cherry on the new relationship just established.

16.5 Pupillary Dilation and Refraction

Pupillary dilation is done for static refraction and fundus examination. As the cycloplegic/mydriatic drop sting on instilling in the eye, it is better to precede it with anaesthetising the cornea with topical anaesthetic. Inform the parent and the child that they would experience blurred vision for so many hours (depending on the dilating/cycloplegic drops used), thus avoiding unnecessary anxiety. For cycloplegia and pupil dilatation, one can use cyclopentolate (1% in children more than 1 year and 0.5% in neonates and infants). Combination of tropicamide and phenylephrine is used if only pupillary dilatation is required (0.8% tropicamide with 5% phenylephrine for children older than 1 year and 0.5% tropicamide with 2.5% phenylephrine in younger ones). It is important to instil topical medication especially in neonates with punctual occlusion to avoid systemic absorption of the drugs. For punctual occlusion one should press on the medial canthus of both eyes with the thumb and index finger for about a minute.

Sedating the child for refraction and indirect ophthalmoscopy examination should be avoided if possible as most of the information can be got without it. However, sedation may be useful in children who are violent or those who cannot be restrained. Children with additional neurological disability or are uncooperative for dilated refraction and fundus examination would benefit from examination under anaesthesia (EUA) (discussed later).

In myopes and in patients with astigmatism if the child is able to look steadily at the distant target, an undilated retinoscopy should be done first as the dilating drops can make children unhappy. These children are usually good at subjective refraction too. In hypermetrope and those associated with squint, a cycloplegic refraction is needed. Though in most situations cyclopentolate is enough, atropine may have a role in heavily pigmented eyes to uncover all the hypermetropia especially if there is an element of accommodative esotropia.

After dilatation, some children may be upset because they did not like the experience of the drops instilled in their eye and some may be upset that they cannot see their videogames or too much light is entering their eyes and they cannot see anything. Here is the time for the clinician to showcase his music and story narrating talent. As an upset child enters the examination room, the clinician should either start humming or play a nursery rhyme or start to tell a story. This would calm the child and pay attention to the clinician. Once the clinician knows that he is in control of the situation he should then start doing refraction continuing to entertain the child knowing fully well that he has very limited window of cooperation at hand. Depending on the level of cooperation, the examiner can decide whether to place a trial frame on the child's face or not. **The retinoscopy has to be performed in line with the visual axis to get the true refractive error**, (see Chap. 5) a back-breaking exercise but worth the effort. A dull or blurred retinoscopic reflex suggests high refractive error and so refraction should **not** start with using trial lenses of lower value and then building up, as this is a total waste of time. Some children may want to hold the trial lens; a spare trial lens could be offered to play with as this will help with the ongoing procedure. Throughout this procedure comfortable positioning of the child would ensure fast and accurate refraction.

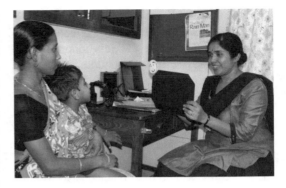

Fig. 16.7 Examining field of a child using black board with puppet faces popping out of the edges

pointing or reaching for the puppet or moving eyes towards the puppet. The distance between the examiner and the child can be varied depending on the response. This test not only allows assessing visual field defects but also areas of inattention and neglect. Modern day automated visual field tests is not useful in children as these are psychophysical tests difficult for many children to perform and moreover the machine lacks normative data on children.

16.6   Visual Field Assessment

A simple, fast, fun-filled, cost-effective and suitable visual field assessment for both normal and developmentally challenged children is the **confrontation test**. It is based on the behavioural responses, reflecting the child's ability to locate target in different areas of the visual field. The examiner is seated about 50 cm in front of the patient. He holds an A4 size board (preferably black in colour) in between him and the child (Fig. 16.7). Puppet faces of different sizes mounted on sticks or sock puppet are then 'popped' into view from behind the board. The child's response is documented as

16.7   Examination in Special Situations

16.7.1   Examination Under Anaesthesia (EUA)

This is done for children in whom clinical examination as outpatient could not be carried out or completed in spite of 'oral pacification or medical sedation', due to poor cooperation or for those requiring scleral depression. Medical sedation depends on the protocols followed by the health system one is working with. When the child is planned for a EUA, the reason for this decision and the procedures planned while the child is under anaesthesia has to be discussed at length with the parent. Many parents think that when their child is taken under anaesthesia, there is something grossly wrong with their ward's eyes. They fear the thought of anaesthesia, coloured by the bad experience of someone else or information got from the Internet. These apprehensions should be addressed. It is a worthwhile exercise if the parents along with the child can have an appointment with the anaesthetist who could clarify the doubts regarding proposed anaesthesia.

Under anaesthesia, the ophthalmologist can do an anterior segment examination using a portable slit lamp, measure intraocular pressure using portable tonometers like tonopen or Perkin's tonometer, do gonioscopy, carry out dilated refraction and scleral depression for fundus examination. Axial length, keratometry, central corneal thickness measurements, corneal diameter measurements, forced duction test, ocular ultrasound and fundus fluorescein angiogram can be done under EUA for diagnostic purposes.

16.7.2 Cerebral Visual Impairment (CVI)

Any child (including neonates) brought into the clinic with a history suggestive of developmental delay, behavioural disorder, intellectual and learning disability is a source of anxiety to the Ophthalmologists. Examination of these children take time as they are either non-responsive or difficult to examine. A lack of understanding of the patho-physiology involved and the preconceived notion of hopelessness in these children demotivates the clinicians further. Unlike most other patients in the clinic these children would not usually have an 'instant' happy ending. Significant progress have been made over the years to understand the patho-physiology in these children and **today it is possible to examine them with an intention to find out the clinical features that will give clues to the underlying defects and plan 'habilitation' dependant on that**. What the medical fraternity needs to understand is that vision is more than the ability to see the 6/6 on the visual acuity chart. One could have 6/6 vision and still be visually impaired. What does this mean? *Interpreting the figure M as M is more complex than one thinks. It could be interpreted as W or E depending on how the brain*

sees M. It means that the way one person understands and relates to the surroundings may be different from another person's way of understanding, both have 6/6 vision on testing but can be functionally very different. Why does this happen? 60% of the brain is involved in processing visual information. Any insult to the brain in the neonatal or early infancy can cause cognitive and perceptual dysfunction. This results in cerebral visual impairment (CVI), which is now the commonest non-ocular cause for visual impairment in children. CVI is a sequel of an insult to the retrogeniculate visual pathway and visual association areas with evidence of retrograde trans-synaptic degeneration of the retinal ganglion cells. In children with periventricular leukomalacia there is associated optic nerve abnormalities.

Any child (including neonates) referred/brought in with a diagnosis of developmental delay or intellectual and learning disability or behavioural disorder should be probed into the birth events and history in early infancy. However subtle the event may seem it may have a devastating impact on the child's personality. Vision is not only for seeing but also understanding and interpreting the surroundings, for communication, for social interaction, giving an emotional value to what is seen and for navigation. In CVI, there can be dorsal (occipito-parietal pathway) stream dysfunction, ventral (occipital-temporal pathway) stream dysfunction and subcortical pathway (connecting middle temporal lobes to dorsal stream) dysfunction. All the pathways are involved in the visual dysfunction and this can be in different permutations and combinations; isolated pathway dysfunction is rare. Since cortical and subcortical structures are involved in CVI, it is preferred to be known as 'cerebral visual impairment' rather than 'cortical visual impairment'.

Features of **dorsal stream dysfunction** include problems with crowd, clutter, splitting attention (simultanagnosia), neglect, impaired visual guidance of upper and lower limbs (optic ataxia) and psychic paralysis of gaze (gaze apraxia not congenital motor apraxia of gaze).

Features of **ventral stream dysfunction** include problems with recognition and orientation.

Features of **subcortical pathway dysfunction**: have problems appreciating movement.

Examination should be geared to unearth the hidden visual impairment so as to corroborate with the imaging results and also plan 'habilitation' strategies based on the examination findings.

After getting the history related to birth and early infancy with respect to events that can cause cerebral injury, attention is turned to the functional capability of the child.

Let us try to understand this by an example:

For an 8-year-old school-going child, with no significant birth or neonatal history and normal milestones, the mother feeds the child, dresses him up, completes his homework, he is a 'bad boy in school'. Is this normal? Yes for parents who think that their child is being 'naughty' or for those who still think that their child is too young to do anything independently. All these reasons are fine. But before accepting the above reasons for the child's dependent nature it is worthwhile quizzing the parents a little more (in fact better still would be to question the child directly if cooperative):

1. How does your child manage in school?
2. What do the teachers' have to say about your child?
3. Does your child like to play with friends or likes to be alone?
4. What kind of games does your child like to play?
5. What does he do when out on walk?
6. What kind of activities does your child engage in when on a holiday?
7. How does your child behave when he goes to a wedding reception or religious gathering?
8. Does he watch television and what are the issues then?
9. Can he manage to go to the friend's house in the neighbourhood on his own?
10. Does he recognise familiar faces in a group photo?

So if the child is a loner, does not like making friends, does not like public gathering, has problems copying from the blackboard and has poor academic records, the clinician knows that the child has features suggestive of dorsal stream dysfunction. If he likes to be in the cheering squad of a football match but does not like to be part of it or often misses the ball in a game of cricket, suggests that he has problems appreciating movement. If he is always holding on to parents clothes or upper arm while walking suggests he may have lower field defect and this can be confirmed by confrontation test as described. One can therefore see that more than any special examination techniques it is the history that gives a clue to the functional capability of the child and the pathology thereby.

If CVI is suspected in any child, for further assessment and training the child should be referred to specialised paediatric ophthalmologists along with neuroimaging.

One must remember that CVI is a diagnosis of exclusion. Delayed visual maturation, uncorrected refractive error, media opacities like cataract can all mimic CVI like symptoms. One should be careful before labelling a child 'CVI'. While discussing CVI with the parents it must be emphasised again and again that the success of CVI habilitation rests with the parents/caregivers. The examination should also be used as an opportunity to demonstrate child's difficulties and explain how the child can be supported, so as to give the child a chance to be independent. Parents need to understand that their child has a different interpretation of the surrounding compared to normal people. Once the parents understand this they partner better in helping the child cope with his differential ability.

16.7.3 Examination for Retinopathy of Prematurity

Looking at the posterior segment of neonates is one of the easier examinations in paediatric ophthalmology. It is not as scary as it would seem. The only precaution that the ophthalmologist needs to take before starting the examination is to inform the parents exactly what he is going to do to their little one. Parents can be given an option of waiting outside while the procedure is on. Before starting the dilated fundus examination, mummify the baby well, put some sugar water drops in the mouth for the child to suck on or the clean little finger of the assistant to suck. After instilling the topical anaesthetic, place an infant speculum to open the eyelids. Scleral depression is easy in these babies because the scleral rigidity is very low. Scleral depression can be done using a depressor or a cotton bud. A +30D lens is better suited for ROP screening as the details are not so important. First the posterior pole should be assessed, especially the calibre and tortuosity of the vessels. Next the extent of the vascularization into the periphery is noted. If the limits of retinal vascularisation is seen with indirect lens without depression, then it is Zone 1 disease. If avascular retina is seen on depression nasally, then it is Zone 2 disease. If only temporal crescent of retina is avascular, it is Zone 3 disease. After ascertaining the extent of vascularization, feature such as neovascularisation and traction is noted. If the pupils are not dilating well, look for neovascularisation of iris with the indirect ophthalmoscope and + 30D lens. After examination and documentation is over, the parents have to be informed about the findings.

16.8 Conclusion

In conclusion, as mentioned earlier in this chapter, examining a child is not easy but it is an art worth mastering. An ophthalmologist will have to come down to the level of the child to befriend them in order to make the whole process of examination a pleasant experience for both the healthcare seeker and healthcare provider. It may not be an essential part of qualifying examinations for ophthalmologist in training. However, it is very important that every ophthalmologist knows how to examine children, who are increasingly becoming healthcare seekers, without having a bias that paediatric ophthalmology is difficult. It just requires the right attitude along with lot of patience. Every child who walks into a clinic is a learning experience for the ophthalmologist, different from the previous patient who walked out and from the next patient who will walk in and a relationship that will last a lifetime.

Systemic Examination and Examination of the Sinuses, Nose and Throat

17

17.1 Introduction

The beauty of being an ophthalmologist is that they are really physicians who operate. Only about 10–20% of patients who come to a general eye outpatient clinic will need any surgery.

The eye is a unique organ in that it is the only place in the body were one can see blood vessels and nerves in vivo. The eye is made of all the embryonic layers except the endoderm. The transparency of these tissues in the eye enables one to see these layers in vivo. Diseases affecting any of these layers may have manifestations in the eye too. If one were to look at the systemic diseases affecting humans, 80% of them have some ophthalmic manifestation during the natural history of the disease. In certain diseases the side effect of the treatment may affect the eye. Therefore, when a patient comes to the ophthalmologist with eye diseases that may have systemic features or referred by colleagues to look for its ocular manifestations or to look for ocular side effects of treatment, the ophthalmologist should not be found wanting, not knowing what to look for or how. Conversely, if the patient presents to the ophthalmologist with the ocular manifestation of a disease, he should be able to look for the systemic manifestation to make a diagnosis and arrange a sensible referral.

Talking about general examination in an ophthalmology setting may make one appear like a dinosaur in this age of sub-specialisation where ophthalmologist do not even want to do a complete eye examination for a patient who comes to them. The joy of clinical ophthalmology is lost when, for whatever reason, the sub-specialist is only interested in their layer of the eye and examine only that (often with a high tech scan) and excludes others. Imagine the plight of a patient whose only complaint is that he cannot see and does not know which of the layers is affected!

History taking has to be targeted; quite often the relevant systemic history is taken based on the findings in the eye. If uveitis is noted, then one has to go back and take history of joint swellings, fever, early morning stiffness of joints, etc.

The general examination skill one requires as an ophthalmologist is primarily inspection. Of course as mentioned before, our mind should know what to look for in order to see it. Neurology examination is dealt with in Chap. 15.

17.2 General Examination

As the patient walks into the room one should observe the patient's build and his walk. An acromegalic face in a patient with pituitary tumour, the stiff and slightly flexed neck of a patient with ankylosing spondylitis, obesity, dysmorphic facial features, etc. should not be missed.

Besides the findings that are obvious; like history, the rest of systemic examination should be

© Springer Nature Singapore Pte Ltd. 2020
T. Kuriakose, *Clinical Insights and Examination Techniques in Ophthalmology*,
https://doi.org/10.1007/978-981-15-2890-3_17

targeted based on the patient's ocular complaints and findings.

In patients who have vasculitis or papilloedema one may have to take the blood pressure (BP) to rule out hypertension. BP may have to be taken in more than one limb in cases of suspected Takayasu's disease. The important thing to keep in mind when taking BP is that the cuff width used should be proportional to the circumference of the limb. The normal adult cuff (about 12 cm wide) cannot be used for small children or to take BP on the thighs.

In patients with thyroid eye disease (TED) or suspected Kearns-Sayre syndrome the pulse rate needs to be checked. Since pulse rates are intimately related to the patient's emotional status, this is best taken as discretely as possible after the patient is relaxed. The endeavour as an ophthalmologist is not to get the exact pulse rate but an idea as to, if the pulse is too fast or too slow. This can be gauged by discretely feeling for the radial pulse.

In some cultures it is difficult to get a history of alcohol intake and even more difficult to get a history of dependence on the same. If a relative is there with the patient, they may have to be questioned alone to get a history. If history is 'suspect' one can try to go close to the patient to see if one can smell alcohol in the breath. Some patients will be agitated and have a mild tremor. In patients with optic neuropathy and ocular surface symptoms suggestive of vitamin deficiency this history and finding may be important.

With growing affluence the world over, nutritional deficiency as a cause of the ocular problem is often overlooked. In the affluent patients it may not be the diet itself but other factors like alcohol abuse, malabsorption syndromes that may be the cause. Besides their dietary history, patients should be asked about history of acid peptic disease, Crohn's disease, intestinal resections, treatment for liver dysfunction, etc. Some patients with cirrhosis will give a history of night blindness. During systemic examination one should look for glossitis (magenta red colour with deep rouge) and angular stomatitis (ulceration with encrustations at the angle of the mouth).

Examination of the lower forniceal conjunctiva may reveal gross anaemia. If Hb is below 5 g/dL, it will look pale. In jaundice the conjunctiva and sclera above the upper limbus which is white normally will appear yellow.

In patients who complain of swelling of the lids especially in the morning one should think of a fluid overload in the body. This suspicion can be further strengthened if the patient has pedal oedema. Pedal oedema can be checked by pressing on a bony prominence in the dependant part of the body. A reliable and easy place to check this is over the medial surface of the tibia just about the angle. The skin here is exposed and inspected first to ensure there is no local pathology causing a swelling here. The examiner's thumb is pressed over the bone for about 15 s and released. If there is a depression on the surface that fills slowly, the patient has pitting oedema suggestive of fluid overload. If oedema is suspected, but there is no pitting oedema, then one should suspect a myxoedema.

Examination of the face give many a clue to the ocular condition one is dealing with. One should stand back and have a look at the face and also go close to see the smaller lesions. A mask-like face may be seen in Parkinson syndrome. The skin over the face may show scaling suggestive of ichthyosis that may be the cause of an ectropion. Nodules on the face or mass on the lids may be seen in neurofibromatosis. In patients with retinal hamartomas fine nodules may be seen on and around the nose. Umbilicated nodules of molluscum contagiosum seen on the face may be the only clue to the red eye the patient has. Red macular lesions on the cheek in rosacea will give clue to the conjunctival congestion the patient has. The ear should be checked for its position. Additional ear lobules may be seen in Axenfeld Rieger syndrome. Absence of eyebrows especially laterally may be suggestive of Hansen's or Myxoedema.

In patients with severe pain on one side of the face, the skin over the forehead, lids and nose should be inspected for blisters suggestive of Herpes zoster. Sometimes there may just be some localised redness without blisters. If the redness is limited to the distribution of a particular branch of the sensory nerve, e.g. ophthalmic division of the fifth CN, then the diagnosis is more likely.

A butterfly-shaped rash on the face may suggest an underlying systemic lupus erythematosus (SLE).

In patients with anterior ischemic optic neuropathy, the possibility of giant cell arteritis (GCA) should be explored. History of fever, malaise and pain in the jaw while chewing are suggestive of GCA. The scalp, face and mouth may have black areas of necrosis. The temporal artery is examined by placing the index, middle and ring finger of both hands of the examiner on the temporal fossa on both sides. The fingers are placed parallel to the eyebrow just inside the hairline. If pulsation is not felt, the fingers are rolled up and down to feel for the chord-like artery.

Leprosy once thought to be an insignificant problem is making a come back. In older chronic patients the eyebrows may be missing. Bilateral facial nerve palsy with poor lid closure is not uncommon. Patients before the advent of triple therapy may have facial deformities like saddle nose (Fig. 17.1). Examination of the skin in other part of the body may show lightly pigmented anaesthetic patches. Palpation of the ulnar nerve at the elbow on the ulnar prominence may reveal a thick chord-like nerve. Patients with leprosy may come with complaints of dry eyes and uveitis in the early stages of the disease.

In patients with subluxation of the lens a Marfan's syndrome has to be excluded. To compare the patient height with his arm span, all one need to do is to ask the patient to stretch out the hand and touch the floor with one hand and keep the other against the wall (Fig. 17.2). The examiner marks the position on the wall and the patient is asked to stand under it to compare the height with the arm span. If the arm span is wider, it is likely the patient has Marfan's. Grasping the fellow wrist with the hand by putting the thumb and the little finger around the wrist, one can check to see if the hand can encircle the wrist. If the hand encircles the wrist easily with some 'little finger' length to spare, it is suggestive of Marfan's syndrome. Auscultating the heart may reveal a murmur due to aortic regurgitation. Just detecting the murmur is enough as an ophthalmologist, the finer details can be figured out by the specialists!

In patients with suspected angioid streaks in the retina one may get a history of the head becoming bigger due to Paget's disease. The skin over the neck should be inspected to see if it has an orange peel like bumpy appearance suggestive of pseudoxanthoma elasticum. Both these conditions can cause angioid streaks.

Examining the neck for a thyroid enlargement is easily done by asking patient to swallow. A prominent thyroid gland can be seen moving with deglutination. To palpate for the thyroid gland one has to stand behind the patient and feel the gland with both hands. The same method is used to palpate for lymph glands on the neck and feel for the carotid artery pulsation. To check for atherosclerosis of the carotid artery, stand behind the patient. Three fingers (index, middle and ring) of both hands is placed in front of the sternocleidomastoid muscle at the angle of the jaw. Normal carotid pulsation can be felt here. The pulsation on both sides should be equal. If pressure is to be applied on the carotid artery, it should be done only one side at a time so as to not compromise the cerebral blood flow. The bell of the stethoscope can be placed over the carotid bifurcation to listen to a bruit that may be present in some cases of carotid vessel narrowing. This examination is useful in patients suspected with ocular ischemic syndrome or who have been found to have suspected emboli in the retinal artery.

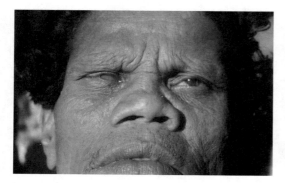

Fig. 17.1 Patient of Hansen's disease with loss of eyebrows, saddle nose and tarsorrhaphy in the right eye for a facial nerve palsy

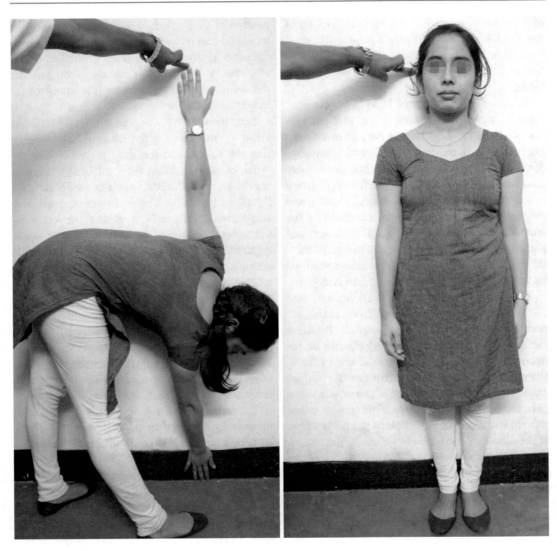

Fig. 17.2 Simple way to estimate a patient's arm span and to compare it with the patient's height

The skin on the trunk of the body should be checked carefully for coffee-coloured (cafe-au-lait) flat lesions with irregular borders. More than six such spots on the trunk is suggestive of an underlying phacomatosis. Nodules on the skin may also be seen in this condition.

Though palpating the abdomen and looking at the genital region are all important and relevant components of general examination that may have eye implications, it may be best left to clinicians who do this on a regular basis for more reliable results. The presence of a chaperone during the general examination cannot be over emphasised.

17.3 Examination of the Sinus, Nose and Mouth

The closest non-nervous system structures to the eye are the ear, nose, sinuses and the mouth/throat (Fig. 17.3). Pathology of any of these

Fig. 17.3 The close relation of sinuses to the orbit

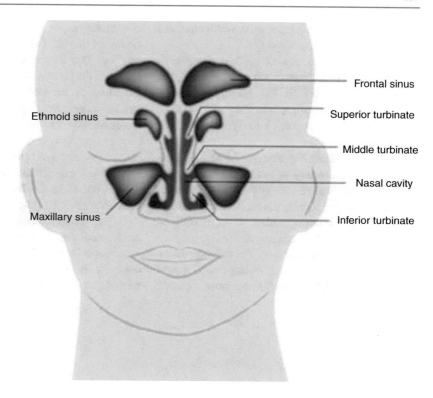

Frontal sinus

Superior turbinate

Ethmoid sinus

Middle turbinate

Nasal cavity

Maxillary sinus

Inferior turbinate

structures may affect the eye. Some patients who present with eye problems have the origins of their symptoms outside the orbit. The ophthalmologist may be the first doctor the patient presents to in the belief that the eye or structures around is at fault. An ophthalmologist must be reasonably familiar with examining the ear, nose, mouth, throat and the sinuses so that he can make a sensible referral to the ENT surgeon. In cases of ocular pain, diplopia and proptosis, examination of the nose, mouth and the sinuses are important. Luckily for the ophthalmologist the indirect headband and light source can act as co-axial light source to look into the throat and nose.

This section will deal with only those examination techniques that can be done by an ophthalmologist in the eye clinic.

Sinusitis can present as eye pain. In severe pansinusitis, due to the inflammation of the periosteum patient may develop proptosis too. One of the simplest way to look for sinusitis is to press over the bone of the sinus. Pressing above the eyebrows medially and over the cheek below the inferior orbital margin examines the frontal and maxillary sinus, respectively. Pressing medially into the upper medial angle of the orbit tests for the ethmoid sinus. On pressing if the patient winces or says there is more pain than what is expected or compared with the other side, a sinusitis should be suspected. Tapping directly on the bones forming the sinuses like one does for percussion can also elicit pain. If a patient comes with a non-axial proptosis, a sinus pathology should be suspected.

A simple way to look to see if the sinus is full is to check its transillumination. Here in a dark room a small rimmed bright torchlight is kept in the mouth and mouth closed. All the sinus area will show transillumination. Lack of transillumination suggest that the sinus is full of tissue/pus and is not hollow. Needless to say these patients need referral for further evaluation.

In the examination of the mouth one should start by looking for angular stomatitis, glossitis, etc. suggestive of vitamin B deficiency. Vitamin B deficiency can cause ocular surface discomfort and dry eye-like symptoms. The cornea may show some stippling. Nutritional amblyopia can be a cause of defective vision.

When mucous membrane graft is planned to be harvested from the mouth and palate, the potential donor sites for the same need to be examined to make sure it is healthy. A high arch palate may suggest an underlying Marfan's syndrome.

While examining the mouth one should look to see if there are any ulcers or necrotic areas, suggestive of giant cell arteritis, or malignancies growing from adjacent structures like the sinus. Loss of upper teeth can also be suggestive of malignancies in the maxillary sinus.

A simple way to check for the patency of the nostrils is to ask the patient to blow onto a steel surface or your fingertip with one nostril closed at a time. Fogging on the steel surface or the sensation of the air blowing gives a clue to its patency. The patient can be told to extend his neck and the tip of the nose turned up to look into the nose. A markedly deviated nasal septum, mass in nose including polyps may be made out. Unfortunately only the anterior part of the nostrils can be seen this way and for seeing more posteriorly one needs a specialist ENT examination. Again one should be familiar with how a normal nostril looks like and not mistake prominent turbinates for polyps.

A general examination and examination of the mouth and sinuses breaks the monotony of eye examination and make one feel a more complete doctor. It also enables one to make the correct referral and gives the satisfaction of having done so.

Putting It All Together for the Patient

There was this patient who went with symptoms of common cold to a doctor who had just opened his first general practice clinic. The doctor heard the patient out and then told him to go and stand under a shower for 5 min and not to dry up after that. The patient found the treatment a bit strange and asked the doctor if he was sure this will rid him of the illness he had. The doctor told him reassuringly that his advice will lead to pneumonia and he knew how to treat that!

Often when a patient comes with a problem, the doctor is looking for a diagnosis to treat rather than trying to address the patient's problems. The scenario where a patient comes with pain in the eye, the doctor cannot figure out straight away why there is pain but finds a pterygium during examination and treats that which was not the cause of his eye pain in the first instance is not uncommon. Focussing on the patients presenting complaint is therefore a must and that needs to be sorted first, not what you know to treat!

What next after clinical examination. If one is not sure of the diagnosis at the end of the clinical examination, one can look at the signs which are more representative of the condition under consideration to increase the probability of the diagnosis. As mentioned, ruling out a differential diagnosis is very effective in narrowing down the differentials and one should work towards that when stuck. Ordering diagnostic tests to make a diagnosis is most effective when the pre-test probability is around 50%. When the pre-test diagnostic probability is above 90%, then diagnostic tests are more useful for quantification of the disease, managing the problem and to prognosticate. Look for one diagnosis that explains all the clinical features if possible.

When a patient presents to the doctor it not only a disease that needs attention. An individual is more complex than the probable disease condition he has. The presenting complaint may just be a mask to hide the real reason for his visit. The real reason behind a complaint of eye strain may just be an eye check-up for a reassurance that all is fine. Often patients come with their own ideas about the condition they may have. These ideas should be respected instead of being ridiculed even if they have no scientific basis. Treatment incorporating these ideas can have powerful placebo effect sometimes. If the patient relates the symptoms to eating a particular fruit, there is no harm asking him to avoid it! It is a good idea sometimes to ask the patient during the history taking if they are particularly concerned about anything that has not come up during the conversation. Concerns if any including possible cost of treatment need to be addressed. Some patients come with unrealistic expectations and if these expectations are not understood and one fails to meet it, the doctor can have a very unhappy patient. This is especially true with refractive surgery and oculoplastic procedures. Finally, for the doctor the patient may be just another case of presbyopia. However, an anxious patient with no

© Springer Nature Singapore Pte Ltd. 2020
T. Kuriakose, *Clinical Insights and Examination Techniques in Ophthalmology*,
https://doi.org/10.1007/978-981-15-2890-3_18

medical background may be stressed, worrying if this is the beginning of the road that will lead him to be blind one day! The empathy of the doctor in such situations is important.

Physical discomfort is often the reason patients go to the doctor. All the discomfort may or may not be caused by the underlying disease. The symptoms of the patient need to be addressed. Sometimes the symptom has to be managed separately along with managing the disease. For example, giving cycloplegics and painkillers along with antibiotics is necessary for patients with infected corneal ulcer. An effort should be made to ease the acute distress of the patient. To assume that by treating the disease the symptoms will resolve is a disservice to the patient as an individual. Treating only the symptoms without making an attempt to find the underlying cause is unethical.

The human psyche plays a role in disease aetiology and response of the individual to diseases. It takes more than good diagnostic skills and up-to-date medical knowledge to be considered a good doctor. Communication and empathy with the patient that is facilitated by a good history taking and physical examination cannot be over emphasised.

Epilogue

In the final analysis, clinical medicine is a humbling experience. When one hears from patients that a particular doctor was arrogant, one wonders where it comes from. Is it from the fact the doctor was smart enough to fend off competition and get into medical school? Is it the trust and respect patients give the doctors that has got into the head? Is it the fact he has the power to manipulate the body functions or is it the social standing and the money they make? There is no other professional that should be more humble than a doctor. Just due to biological variations the diagnosis we make can be wrong. The patient's response to treatment is so variable and what works for one may not work for the other. In the end there is so much we do not know.

A physician is in the unique position where human beings trust their body with you. Entrusting your wealth or reputation with somebody is not that intimate. The physician has the power to kill or heal. All these can only make a person humble and not arrogant.

Does a professional sportsman work or play? When does play become work, or better still when does work become play? In economics, it is said that people get paid for working to compensate for the trouble or lack of enjoyment at work. If one enjoys work can it become play? What better thing can happen in your life if you get paid for something you like to do. Look at every patient as a mystery to solve, relish it. When you decode the mystery of a disease and treat it, a joyful patient at the end of your management is reward in itself. Monetary compensation is a bonus.

The mental stress in treating a patient can be reduced if you see all patients including your parents as human being needing your expertise and care. Bringing in compensation, your reputation and thus the worry about outcomes is what makes such a joyful profession the stressful one it sometimes become.

Doctors often undervalue their worth. In terms of diagnostic worth, history and physical findings contribute more to the diagnosis than a CT scan, yet a scan costs more than the doctor's consultation charge. The diagnostic capability of the doctor comes from years of reading, training, internalising and practice. The diagnostic machine which is the doctor is much more useful and valuable than a CT scan machine. This is something the physician and the lay public should not forget. The comfort in one's self-worth and the humility in the light of this knowledge is what makes a true physician. To be a physician is a calling and not just another avenue to make a comfortable living.

© Springer Nature Singapore Pte Ltd. 2020
T. Kuriakose, *Clinical Insights and Examination Techniques in Ophthalmology*,
https://doi.org/10.1007/978-981-15-2890-3

Printed in the United States
by Baker & Taylor Publisher Services